A PRACTICAL GUIDE TO
BREASTFEEDING

Lisa,

It has been a wonderful experience knowing you and learning so much from you about "*** and girls" since you have 3 of your own. I'm very thankful for our friendship. Thanks again for all your help.

love,
Joy

Lisa,
Many thanks for all your help!

fondly.

Sheila

Lisa,
It was really enjoyable having your thoughts and insights. Thanks for all your help, and advice. Love,

Wendy

A PRACTICAL GUIDE TO
BREASTFEEDING

JAN RIORDAN, R.N., M.N.

College of Health Related Professions, Department of Nursing,
Wichita State University; The University of Kansas,
Division of Health Care Outreach—Wichita, Wichita, Kansas

with 98 illustrations

JONES AND BARTLETT PUBLISHERS
BOSTON

Editorial, Sales, and Customer Service Offices

Jones and Bartlett Publishers
20 Park Plaza
Boston, MA 02116

Printed in the United States of America
10 9 8 7 6 5 4 3 2

ISBN: 0-86720-448-6

Contributors

JIMMIE LYNNE AVERY

Director, Lact-Aid Service & Supplies Center,
Denver, Colorado

EDWARD R. CERUTTI, M.D.

Assitant Clinical Professor of Pediatrics, Case
Western Reserve University, Cleveland, Ohio

BETTY ANN COUNTRYMAN, R.N.,M.N.

Vice-Chairman, Board of Directors, La Leche
League, International; formerly Assistant
Professor, School of Nursing, Indiana
University

KITTIE B. FRANTZ, R.N.,C.P.N.P.

Director, Breastfeeding Infant Clinic; Clinical
Instructor of Pediatrics, University of Southern
California School of Medicine, Los Angeles,
California

RICHARD A. GUTHRIE, M.D.

Professor of Pediatrics and Director of Kansas
Regional Diabetes Center, The University of
Kansas School of Medicine at Wichita,
Wichita, Kansas

PAULA MEIER, R.N.,M.S.N.

Formerly Clinical Nurse Specialist Supervisor,
Special Care Nursery, Michael Reese Hospital
and Medical Center, Chicago, Illinois

Preface

This text provides comprehensive information on breastfeeding for the practicing nurse. Spurred on by the many women who now choose to breastfeed, nurses are increasingly called on to assist families with breastfeeding infants and children. Surely it is no semantic accident that the word *nursing* is used to refer to both breastfeeding and the care-giving profession: both include nurturance and caretaking. However, just being a nurse does not guarantee the ability to give consistent helpful guidance on breastfeeding. Because of the enormous range of required topics in basic nursing education, few nursing curricula are able to give adequate time and emphasis to lactation and breastfeeding. Heretofore nurses have necessarily relied on their own experience and on the many excellent consumer publications that are now available.

Reflecting the shifting role of nursing, this book views the health consumer and the health professional as partners in a common quest. Implicit in the nursing profession and this partnership is a powerful potential for change within the health-care system that is mandatory for an optimal breastfeeding experience.

No pretense is made of presenting here a balanced discussion of breastfeeding vs. bottle-feeding. The buoyant enthusiasm for breastfeeding is obvious. Although not every reader can be expected to appreciate this approach, all readers will find some information that is applicable to their needs and practice.

As I began to write this text, a colleague good-humoredly commented, "You're going to write a whole book *just* on breastfeeding?" This remark was a reminder that for some people the simple act of nourishing an infant at breast is taken for granted. However, the wave of new research on breastmilk, the recognition that breastfeeding facilitates the early love bonds, and the resurgence of breastfeeding validate the need for such a textbook. This book endeavors to add to the nursing literature new, important data from the laboratory, the social sciences, and nursing research. It seeks to integrate those data with practical knowledge that incorporates my 20 years of experience in working with breastfeeding families.

Part One of the text focuses on the "whys" and "hows" of breastfeeding, beginning in Chapter 1 with a historical overview of infant feeding and implications of the trend away from breastfeeding in many areas of the world. Chapter 2 identifies the anatomic structures of the lactating breast, relating the psychophysiologic mechanisms at work while underscoring the differences between the sucking mechanisms of feedings at the breast and with the bottle. Scientific validation of the importance of species-specific milk, one of the great medical advances of the past decade, is detailed in Chapter 3. These chapters are deliberately brief so that more attention can be devoted to the practical aspects of self-care in breastfeeding contained in Chapter 4. In Chapter 5, theory and practice are translated into breastfeeding (and early parenting) education, the cornerstone of nursing practice.

Part Two addresses situations that hamper lactation—the "what-ifs." Although the line that separates infant problems from maternal problems is hazy at best, Chapters 6 and 7 address special circumstances that affect primarily the breastfeeding woman. The remaining chapters in Part Two focus on infant health problems. Jaundice, slow weight gain, and prematurity are discussed by practicing clinicians who are experts in their topics. Ancient methods and new technologies in relactation and induced lactation are explained by another expert in Chapter 13.

The last section, Part Three, discusses the various breastfeeding and early child-rearing concerns among different cultures. The diversity challenges any preconceived, dogmatic framework for "what should be." At the same time the cultural kaleidoscope of child care focuses on a universal theme: any infant has the greatest potential to thrive when optimal nurturance and nutrition are provided by breastfeeding.

To avoid confusion between the word *nursing* meaning the profession and nursing meaning breastfeeding, *nursing* in the text refers in most cases to the profession. The masculine pronoun has been used for the infant or child throughout the text as a matter of convenience to distinguish the child from the breastfeeding woman or mother. Nurses are referred to in the feminine gender—with apologies to my male colleagues.

No individual ever writes a book alone. She stands—however precariously—on the shoulders of others. With deep gratitude I acknowledge the many people who supported and assisted the writing of this text. I wish to thank La Leche League, International, for its steadfast help and for providing much of my education on breastfeeding as a La Leche League leader. Moreover, the collective experiences of my colleagues in the Professional Liaison Department of La Leche League provided a rich and valuable source of practical information.

Patricia Bayles, R.N., M.N.; Betty Bergersen, R.N., Ed.D.; Betty Ann Country-man, R.N., M.N.; Armond Goldman, M.D.; Diana Guthrie, R.N., M.P.H.; Richard Guthrie, M.D.; Donna Hawley, R.N., Ph.D.; Lynn Mason, R.N.; Michael Newton, M.D.; Marianne Neifert, M.D.; G.D. Robinson, M.D.; Gregory White, M.D.; Mary White; and Ethel-Marie Underhill, B.S.N., reviewed sections of the manuscript. Be-tween college semesters my daughter, Teresa Riordan, lent her editorial skills.

Special thanks go to Jean Cotterman, Liz Crofts, Kittie Frantz, Nancy Goodman, Esther Hermann, Lauri Lowen, Chele Marmet, and Karen Moore for sharing their ex-periences and in some cases their homes for a weary traveler on a quest. With good humor and patience, secretarial and computer processing skills were provided by De-lores Serpan, Debbie Livengood, and Elaine Tischauser. Many of the drawings were done by Phyllis Anderson, biomedical illustrator. RoxAnn Dicker, director of The Uni-versity of Kansas, Division of Health Care Outreach—Wichita; the staff of the Instruc-tional Media Department at the University of Kansas School of Medicine at Wichita; and the nursing faculty at Wichita State University provided an indispensable support system. Finally, with love, I dedicate this book to my husband, Hugh.

Jan Riordan

Contents

Appendixes

A PRACTICAL GUIDE TO
BREASTFEEDING

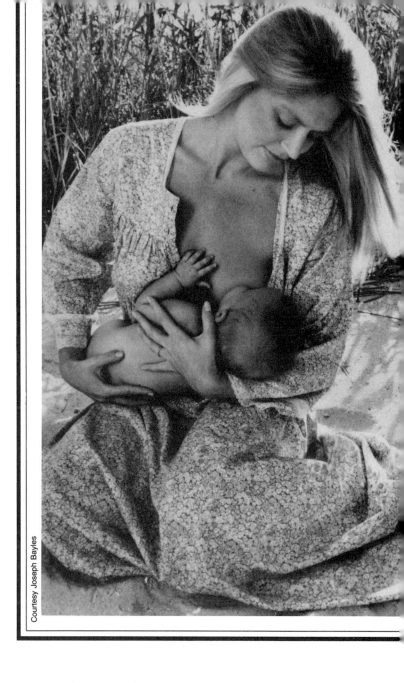

Courtesy Joseph Bayles

PART ONE

BASICS OF BREASTFEEDING
what you need to know first

The photograph of a breastfeeding mother and infant shown here invites the reader to explore the normal process of lactation in this section. Like pieces of a puzzle, these chapters fit together to form a complete picture of breastfeeding, focusing on an ancient process within the context of a scientific age.

Nurses are natural teachers of breastfeeding. Why? We are *there* with the family. Because of the intimate relationship that exists between the nurse and the family, as well as the traditional use of our "therapeutic self," we are able to encourage, guide, and teach and thus achieve our potential in assisting families with breastfeeding.

To do so, it is necessary to assimilate the current broad range of knowledge of lactation and as much as possible base our nursing care on research. The content in the first section therefore lays the groundwork for subsequent sections: the second, which covers specific problems, and the third, which examines cross-cultural perspectives.

1

Infant feeding patterns: past and present

JAN RIORDAN
BETTY ANN COUNTRYMAN

HISTORIC FEEDING PATTERNS
Ancient societies

Imagine if you will a woman as she picks seeds and berries in her trek toward a distant, better land. Where is her infant? Where are all the infants of other women just like her? Swaddled securely, her baby is carried on her body and gently rocked by the mother's movements as she gathers her food at the side of other members of her tribe. At sunset in a suitable place of rest, no longer lulled by the constant motion of his mother's body, the infant becomes more wakeful and hungry. He breastfeeds often, gazes into the mother's eyes, fondles her breast, and responds to the loving cadences of her voice. At nightfall the two lie down to sleep together, and the infant's needs for the breast are constantly met at his mother's side.

Ancient patterns of breastfeeding have important implications for today. The transition of human society from the ways of the tribal hunter-gatherer to agricultural-rural living and ultimately to a predominantly industrial-urban society has been gradual. However, the cumulative impact of these changes on mothers and infants has been profound and sudden—indeed, taking place almost entirely within three generations. Always before, breastfeeding had been the norm in all cultures; intrusion of the bottle followed hard on urbanization. The time involved for evolutionary change is so great that the behavior typical of the breastfed infant today—that is, to feed often, to "bunch" feedings during the late afternoon and evening, and to breastfeed often during the night—may well be a simple behavioral carry-over of ages past.

The rhythmic organization of the infant's sleeping and waking cycle as shown in Fig. 1-1 attests to this tendency for wakefulness in the late afternoon and evening. These wakeful and sometimes fussy periods at the end of the day are often critical ones for the inexperienced breastfeeding mother who is unsure of her ability to breastfeed and unaware that wakefulness and frequent feeding at these times are entirely normal. Nurses can expect that many of the distress calls from mothers during the second and third week after delivery stem from lack of knowledge of this common pattern. Babies, especially those who are breastfed, are frequently fussy and breastfeed almost constantly

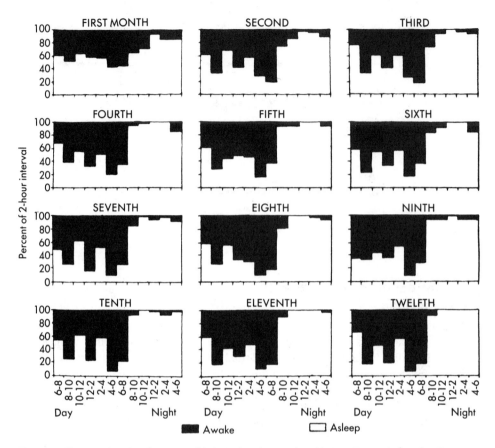

Fig. 1-1. Progressive development of infant sleeping and waking patterns during the first year. (From Emde, R.N., Gaensbauer, T.J., and Harmon, R.J.: Emotional expression in infancy. Psychological Issues, Monograph 37, New York, 1976, International Universities Press, Inc.)

at this time of day. Self-care teaching to these mothers includes reassurance that this daily pattern will change in time and that a lack of milk is rarely the cause.

The practice of breastfeeding is sensitive to cultural and social changes. Although breastfeeding was regarded as the almost universal method of infant feeding until recent times, culturally acceptable alternatives have evolved. In earlier times when a mother died in childbirth, a lactating relative took the baby to breastfeed—the precursor of the hired wet nurse in later societies. Evidence exists that, even some thousands of years ago, artificial feedings were attempted, most often quite unsuccessfully. Feeding vessels have been found in Egyptian graves as long ago as 2500 BC; yet it is known that Egyptian women who enjoyed a relatively high status breastfed their children well into the third year.

The Boulak Papyrus reminds the child with touching wisdom:

> Thou shalt never forget thy mother . . . for she carried thee long beneath her breast as a heavy burden; and after these months were accomplished she bore thee. Three long years she carried thee upon her shoulder, and gave thee her breast to thy mouth. She

nurtured thee, and took no offense from thy uncleanliness. And when thou didst enter school, and wast instructed in the writings, daily she stood by the master with bread and beer from the house.[8]

Other feeding vessels found in Europe appear to have been in use about 500 years later. A pair of spouted feeding cups from the grave of premature twins, circa 600 BC, were discovered in Sudan.[18] Milk from goats, donkeys, and other animals is believed to have been used in the vessels. Direct suckling of animals must have been occasionally resorted to, for reference to this practice is found in Egyptian etchings and Greek myths.

Throughout the centuries, during periods of great wealth and luxury many women turned to artificial feeding or wet-nursing for their babies. Such practices moved Spartan royal lawmakers in 4 BC to dictate that all mothers should breastfeed, and Emperor Caesar Augustus ridiculed mothers who retained wet nurses for their infants.

1600 to 1850

Along with social change, the rapid development of scientific technology during the Industrial Revolution and the spectacular advances in medical science provided a complex matrix that encouraged the trend toward artificial feeding. Mechanized transportation and improved agriculture made urbanization possible. Emigrating from farm to city in Europe and in America, family units became more fragmented and dependent on a cash economy. As a result, women were frequently forced to work soon after giving birth.

Records indicate that pap gruels, the forerunners of modern baby foods, were first used in 1600's. Pap was a liquid, usually milk, combined with bread, rice, or flour. Its use often led to undernutrition, since it had to be diluted to pass through the opening of the container.

Although the life-threatening potential of feeding with other animal milks was well recognized, the eighteenth century marked a major decline of breastfeeding in urban Europe. The literature is replete with references to the high mortality of artificially fed infants from infection, especially diarrhea, during the eighteenth and nineteenth centuries. Diarrhea was persistent and endemic in London, and during the early 1800's seven of eight artificially fed infants perished. Foundling hospitals in the late 1700's had a mortality of 80% or higher.

To avoid the dangers of artificial feeding during this era, affluent mothers employed wet nurses. In the cities wet-nursing became so widespread and profitable that, to obtain easy employment as a wet nurse, girls contrived to have illegitimate babies whom they sent to "baby farms" in the country where they perished more often than survived. Stone[25] describes wet-nursing in this way:

> These nurses were often cruel and neglectful, and they often ran out of milk, as a result of which the baby had to be passed from nipple to nipple, from one unloving mother-substitute to another. If the infant stayed with one wet nurse, then it became deeply attached to her, as a result of which the weaning process at about eighteen months inflicted the trauma of final separation from the loved substitute mother-figure and a return to the alien and frightening world of the natural mother.

Apparently, having the wet nurse stay on as caretaker throughout childhood was enjoyed only by the rich.

In colonial America the mortality of children under the age of 2 was very high—50% by conservative estimate. When the milk of cows and goats had to be used for feedings, mortality rose to 65%. As might be expected, physicians strongly urged women to breastfeed for as long as possible.[6]

As late as 1894 this advice still held, as Jefferis[12] instructed mothers of that era:

> Breast milk is the only proper food for infants until after the second summer. If the supply is small, keep what you have and feed the child in connection with it, for if the babe is ill this breast milk may be all that will save its life.

1850 to 1930

With the great work of people such as Florence Nightingale, Joseph Lister, and Phillip Semmelweiss, reforms in public health and lying-in hospitals began in the second half of the nineteenth century after the end of the Crimean War. For the poor, however, life was wretched, and young children toiled along with their mothers in dark mines and factories. Forced to work, breastfeeding women took their infants with them to the work area, but the child was expected to remain quiet and not interfere with productivity. A popular concoction given to babies who accompanied their mothers to the work site was a liquid called "Godfrey's cordial," a treacle and opium concoction designed to keep the baby quiet during the working day. Not only were these unfortunate children deprived of care, but they also eventually had to endure the agonies of opium withdrawal.[9]

During the postwar years of the 1920's, local authorities began programs to employ midwives and community health nurses to provide free care for childbearing women. In response to the disastrous results of bottle-feeding and following technical advances, artificial feeding improved. Yet gastroenteritis remained a deadly killer, especially during the hot summer months when unrefrigerated cans of sweetened, condensed milk were left open to attract flies until the baby and others in the family finally consumed them. Attacks of gastroenteritis or "summer diarrhea" prompted community efforts for control, such as the innovative "baby camps" of the blistering summer of 1918. These camps or shelters, established by influential women in many communities throughout the country, provided refrigeration for the milk and mosquito netting for the cots of babies cared for while their mothers were working.

Sulfonamides and antibiotics did not come into general use until the 1930's. Sulfaquinadine was the first effective drug developed specifically for combating gastrointestinal infections. Later, discoveries in bacteriology and the emerging science of biochemistry resulted in the boiling, modifying, and canning of cow's milk.

About this time in Britain, the government began providing mothers with a milk substitute called "National Dried Milk" at a nominal fee. This government intervention, instituted instead of an effective national education program for breastfeeding, marked the beginning of the decline of breastfeeding in Western nations and led to the acceptance of bottle-feeding. A further decrease in breastfeeding was facilitated by the development of scientific dairy farming, safe water supplies and sewage systems, public education in sanitation, and the increasing availability of refrigeration. Stabilization for storage of cow's milk through evaporation, canning, and pasteurization contributed further to this decline. The manufacture and promotion of proprietary formula, mass production technology for bottles and nipples, and routine postpartum separation of mother and infant in hospitals significantly increased the problem.

With the widespread use of formulas and cow's milk, other problems, particularly of an allergic nature, have developed in recent decades. Allergies to cow's milk in the form of diarrhea or eczema have become a common problem in infants and are discussed at length elsewhere (see Chapters 3 and 17).

In the attempt to develop a formula "most like mother's milk," vital nutrients were not included, and their absence often led to tragic results. The composition of formulas changed as the lack of essential nutrients became recognized—too late for children who had been permanently damaged. Only in the late 1940's was ascorbic acid added, and in the 1950's formulas were fortified with Vitamin B_6. Vitamin E was a still later addition. Late in the 1970's, one formula was found to have less than half the chloride content recommended by the American Academy of Pediatrics.

In nursing practice we see frequent misuse of formulas. Mothers and others misread instructions or do not read them at all. In the non-English-speaking family, attempts at following container directions are often no more than guesswork. Many Hispanic and Vietnamese babies have been hospitalized after receiving full-strength, concentrated formula because their caretakers were unable to understand the instructions printed in English. Even with the well educated, errors can occur, as happened in the case of father with a Ph.D. who, half asleep, mistakenly offered his baby nondiluted formula at a night feeding. Such a mistake endangers the infant by bringing about an osmotic shift leading to dehydration and possibly a renal crisis, particularly on the immature kidney function of the young infant.

Before 1980 no enforceable law regulating infant formulas existed. Responsive to testimony by physicians, nurses, and others, in 1980 Congress passed the Infant Formula Act (PL 96-359), which sets standards for the content, processing, and marketing of formulas.

The changing role of women from domestic pursuits to jobs outside the home or to professional careers may have contributed to the decline of breastfeeding. Today, however, there is a trend toward breastfeeding by an increasing number of employed mothers who are successfully managing to work and breastfeed their babies. Although some progress is being made, management has yet to establish company nurseries to provide working mothers with easy access to their infants. Such facilities are commonly offered in places of work in several European countries. Another practice in a number of European countries but not in the United States is granting government stipends to mothers for up to 6 months following delivery in compensation for wages lost during maternity leave.

CURRENT PATTERNS
United States

In the United States the pendulum is moving back to breastfeeding once again. Since reports of breastfeeding are not required by law, accurate statistics are not easy to obtain. Currently, formula companies seem to be the best source of breastfeeding data. (Apparently it pays to know the competition!)

Dramatic changes in breastfeeding have occurred in this century.* Over 70% of first-

---

*To avoid confusion, unless stated otherwise the breastfeeding data discussed here refer to initiation of breastfeeding after delivery and not to the number of infants still breastfeeding in later weeks or months.

born infants in the 1930's were breastfed; even in the mid-1940's a national survey showed that approximately two thirds of all infants in the United States were breastfed during the newborn period.[4] The 1950's, however, heralded the beginning of a dramatic decline in breastfeeding. After the late 1960's (Table 1-1) at the nadir of breastfeeding, the decline leveled off at around 18%. It now appears to be rising steadily.[10,11,17] In 1973 25% of babies were breastfed, and by 1975 the number had increased to 35%.

Under close scrutiny a number of discrepancies are apparent in demographic studies of breastfeeding during the last 20 to 30 years. Part of the problem is the exclusion of rural women from sample populations, since most studies have been done in metropolitan areas. Studies in Boston in 1966[23] and 1977,[7] which are frequently cited in the literature, are a case in point. Probably the most valid and comprehensive data come from the 1973 National Survey of Family Growth[27] and the earlier (1965) National Fertility Survey done by the Division of Vital Statistics of the National Center for Health Statistics.[11]

Another discrepancy arises from the fact that these studies are often based on different observational approaches. To say, for example, that 50% of mothers breastfeed their

TABLE 1-1

Percentages of women (ever-married) who breastfed their first child according to the year of birth of the child and selected characteristics

	Breastfed any duration						
	Year of first birth						
	Before 1950	**1951-55**	**1956-60**	**1961-65**	**1966-70**	**1971-73**	**All women**
All women(%)	59.9	49.8	42.9	37.5	27.9	28.7	38.6
Race and ethnic							
White	56.2	48.8	43.0	38.9	29.4	30.2	38.9
Black	72.6	59.1	42.1	23.8	13.7	11.4	35.7
Hispanic origin*	73.2	57.7	55.1	39.1	35.2	19.3	43.1
Geographic region							
Northeast	63.1	41.5	31.3	30.6	26.9	23.1	32.2
North Central	59.4	43.3	42.5	37.4	27.4	26.5	37.0
South	63.9	57.4	43.8	35.1	22.4	21.1	37.6
West	50.5	54.7	54.2	49.5	38.2	53.9	49.1
Education							
Elementary school, 8 yr or less	63.1	62.3	53.0	40.1	32.2	18.1	48.1
High school, 9-11 yr	60.4	49.5	39.8	28.7	17.2	15.7	34.7
High school, 12 yr	54.6	44.7	39.9	32.2	23.3	24.8	33.3
College, 13-15 yr	69.7	57.0	47.6	50.4	35.2	43.5	46.5
College, 16 yr or more	55.6	45.8	50.2	69.2	57.1	52.1	56.0

From Trends in breastfeeding among American mothers, Series 23, No. 3, Washington, D.C., 1979, Division of Vital Statistics, National Center for Health Statistics.
*The Hispanic origin classification was made independently of racial classification and includes women of all racial groups.

infants is not the same as saying that 50% of babies are breastfed. An illustration of such variances is that during nearly the same relative period (1966) in which Salber and Feinlieb[23] found that 22.3% of women in Boston initiated breastfeeding after delivery, the National Fertility Study reported the figure to be 39.5% nationwide. Another example may be seen in the National Fertility Study, which showed that from 1966 to 1970, 14% of black women breastfed their babies after delivery (Table 1-1). However, a few years later in 1970, Rivera[22] sampled black mothers in a low-income section of New York and found that less than 5% initiated breastfeeding. Despite such discrepancies, studies during that period clearly point to one common trend: a rapid decline of breastfeeding among women with 9 to 12 years of formal education.

Regional data during the past few decades show that from East to West in the United States breastfeeding rates increase (Fig. 1-2). In fact, some communities in California informally report that 90% of new mothers in their area are breastfeeding.

As health professionals we should be both challenged and dismayed by these data. Only 7% of babies born between 1971 and 1973 were breastfed for 3 months or more, whereas before 1950 32% were still breastfeeding at 3 months.[27] In 1977 Cole[7] showed that the duration of breastfeeding had increased, with 59% of breastfeeding women in her sample still lactating between 3 and 3½ months after delivery. A recent study[17] indicates that in the decade since 1971 approximately 26% more women have chosen to breastfeed; moreover, the national rate of inhospital breastfeeding was 51% in 1979 (Table 1-2). Undoubtedly the proliferation of support groups such as La Leche League have contributed to the increase.

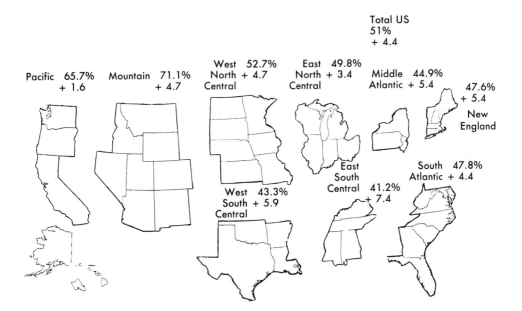

Fig. 1-2. Inhospital breastfeeding in 1979 and 1978 to 1979 percentage point change. (From Martinez, G.A., and Nalezienski, J.P.: Pediatrics **67:**260, 1981. (Copyright American Academy of Pediatrics 1981.)

TABLE 1-2

Percentage of infants breastfeeding in the hospital by selected demographic characteristics

Characteristic	1971	1978	1979	% point change 1978-1979	% point change 1971-1979
Parity					
Primiparous	28.1	51.3	55.6	4.3	27.5
Multiparous	21.9	42.6	47.0	4.4	25.1
Type of medical care					
Pediatricians	26.3	47.3	51.7	4.4	25.4
General practitioners	22.0	44.4	49.5	5.1	27.5
Public clinic	23.8	40.9	46.4	5.5	22.6
Mother's education					
Grade and high school	19.4	40.2	44.5	4.3	25.1
College	42.1	63.4	67.4	4.0	25.3
Home location					
Urban	25.9	47.5	51.9	4.4	26.0
Rural	21.9	43.8	47.8	4.0	25.9
Family income					
Less than $7,000	22.3	34.0	37.3	3.3	15.0
$7,000-14,999	26.7	47.3	49.3	2.0	22.6
$15,000 and above	—*	50.0	55.2	5.2	—
Total all infants	24.7	46.6	51.0	4.4	26.3

From Martinez, G.A., and Nalezienski, J.P.: Pediatrics **67:**260, 1981. Copyright American Academy of Pediatrics 1981.
*Income classification stopped at above $10,000.

Factors influencing breastfeeding. The current trend in breastfeeding may be part of a larger social movement toward the natural, which was led by the youth of the 1960's in revolt against the overmechanization of modern urban living. The convenience, economy, nutritional superiority, and personal satisfaction of breastfeeding certainly express the philosophy of naturalism.

Statistics show that motivation to breastfeed is highest among women with a year or more of college. Certainly breastfeeding has recently become the more common of infant feeding in middle and upper socioeconomic communities. La Leche League groups for breastfeeding education and support rapidly proliferate in suburban communities, while they face a constant struggle for membership in economically disadvantaged areas of a community. Inner-city mothers are therefore less likely to have readily available information on breastfeeding. Additionally, since few of her peers have breastfed their infants, the opportunity of role-model learning for the economically disadvantaged mother is limited. Of those who attempt to breastfeed, not many continue more than a few months. It is ironic that the immunologic and nutritional advantages of breastfeeding are not well used in areas where hygiene may be poor and nutrition substandard.

Also, the adolescent mother, whose nutritional needs are especially great and who may come from an economically disadvantaged community, is less likely to breastfeed. Still struggling to establish her identity, she often finds the constant physical and emotional demand for giving to her infant so difficult that she is psychologically unable to make a commitment of such magnitude to her child.

Since a woman's breasts are an important part of her body image and sexual attractiveness, her feelings about them affect her decision to breastfeed or bottle-feed. To quote one, "I have breasts, therefore, I am!"[3] For example, some women with unusually large breasts, affected by adolescent trauma, choose to bottle-feed because the prospect of their breasts being even larger during lactation is abhorrent. Such deep feelings are not usually expressed to a nurse or physician. Another consideration is society's view of breasts. Especially in our culture, there is a conflict between the erotic and nurturing functions of the breast. Breasts have always been the objects of admiration, but never so much as in our society where "bosomania" constantly influences our visual environment through the public media and in pornography. Conversely, exposure of the breasts in real life is socially taboo, and simple modesty or shame accounts for at least some women's shying away from breastfeeding.[2]

The pregnant woman who undertakes preparation for childbirth and breastfeeding, either through formal classes or individual reading, is more likely to breastfeed and to attend La Leche League meetings in preparation for breastfeeding. A high correlation between participation in self-help groups such as La Leche League and the duration of breastfeeding has been documented.[13] Since breastfeeding is as much a learned skill as an instinctual act in the human mother, both preparation and ongoing peer support are important factors in her initial motivation and continuing performance.

Much has been written about the importance of one-to-one support on the outcome of the breastfeeding experience. Raphael,[20] coining the word "doula," explains the characteristics of such a person as one who is knowledgeable in the breastfeeding process and who "mothers the mother." The doula may be a close relative, a neighbor, a friend, husband, or a nurse who is available to assist the mother in daily tasks, give emotional support, and help guide the mother to a successful solution of her problems. In most non-Western cultures every parturient woman has a relative or some member of her community who has had personal breastfeeding experience and passes her knowledge on to the mother. At the same time she assists the parturient woman with her household work and protects her from the stresses of the outside world. In our mobile and primarily urban society, failure to provide a doula may in large part be responsible for the low rate of long-term successful breastfeeding. In some measure the emergence and proliferation of self-help groups, in which mothers unite and become doulas for one another, fill the gap that society has created.

Implications for practice. According to one study,[15] breastfeeding is more successful when women perceive that their physician is supportive. Of interest is the fact that the pediatricians in this study were reported to be considerably more helpful (76%) than the obstetricians (25%). Since the attitudes of professionals who work with new mothers clearly affects breastfeeding, the question becomes: how important is the nurse's relationship with the mother? The degree of missed potential for assisting breastfeeding mothers in the hospital was shown by Cole,[7] who found that only one third of new mothers reported receiving helpful information from the nurses during their hospital stay. But this same study also demonstrated that most women who were helped were still breastfeeding at 3 months after delivery. The nurse's skills and knowledge about breastfeeding clearly must be brought regularly into use if nurses are to provide optimal nursing care.

A great deal of concern has been manifested over the risk of making the client feel guilty by advocating breastfeeding over bottle-feeding. Although these feelings are of concern to the sensitive nurse, there is little evidence in practice or in the literature that this concern is a plausible arguing point to neglect breastfeeding instruction. In this connection, a study of primiparas showed that bottle-feeding mothers had minimal conflict or guilt about their choice.[5]

Breastfeeding education programs can contribute significantly to a good beginning experience. At present there are only a few hospitals or medical practices that provide mothers with comprehensive patient education on breastfeeding. The development of these programs and some of the problems involved in them are discussed in the last chapter of this section.

Other countries in the Western world

Until recently there has been a steady decline in breastfeeding throughout the Western world. Vahlquist's statistics[28] from Sweden, Poland, and the United Kingdom show a persistent decline until 1977, which is similar among different national social systems (Fig. 1-3).

This trend, however, is reversing in many European countries. In France, from 1972 to 1979 the percentage of French women who were totally breastfeeding increased from 29% to 43%. At the Maternity Clinics in Pithiviers and Grenoble, France, considered

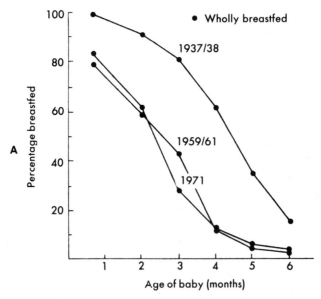

Fig. 1-3. Breastfeeding in, **A,** Poland, 1937 to 1938; **B,** United Kingdom, 1947 to 1968; and **C,** Sweden, 1944 to 1972. (From Vahlquist, B.: J. Trop. Pediatr. Env. Child Health **21:**11, 1975.)

"utopian" for their progressive approaches to childbirth and breastfeeding, 86% to 95% of the infants are breastfed.[26]

At least partially responsible for the increase in breastfeeding rates is the emergence of organized efforts of breastfeeding women helping others to breastfeed. Self-help groups for breastfeeding promotion and education are a common development in Western cultures. The rapid growth of these groups, such as La Leche League International in the

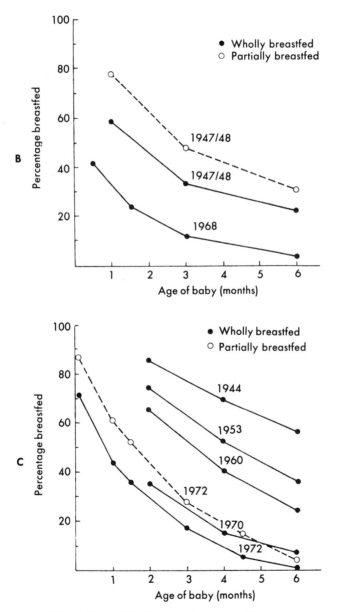

Fig. 1-3, cont'd. For legend see opposite page.

United States and many other countries, Ammehjelpen in Norway, the Nursing Mothers Association of Australia, and Amninghjaelpen of Sweden, demonstrate what can be achieved in filling the knowledge gap. In these countries and many other parts of the world self-help groups perform an invaluable service to breastfeeding mothers.

Developing countries

> *Caracas, Venezuela, July 1977:* In the emergency room of the *Hospital de Ninos,* a large hospital located in the center of the city, lie 52 infants. All are suffering from gastroenteritis, a serious inflammation of the stomach and intestines. Many also suffer from pneumonia. According to the doctor in charge, roughly 5,000 Venezuelan babies die each year from gastroenteritis, and an equal number die from pneumonia. The doctor further explains that these babies, like many who preceded them and those who would follow, have all been bottlefed. He concludes, "A totally breastfed baby just does not get sick like this."[16]

World health leaders view the beginning of a trend away from breastfeeding in developing countries with concern and attribute this phenomenon to the advertising and economic pressures of commercial food companies. Under conditions of extreme poverty, breastfeeding becomes a lifesaving necessity, so the activities of multinational infant food manufacturers must be subject to ever closer scrutiny. Others believe that the problem is not so simple and contend that the nourishment of the breastfeeding mother and of the weanling must be viewed with equal concern.[19]

To support artificial feeding there must be refrigeration, a safe water supply, a reasonable level of literacy, and adequate purchasing power available to the average citizen. By contrast, in Third World countries the average family lives with a contaminated water supply, inadequate facilities for sterilization and storage, insufficient education, and too little money to buy bottles, nipples, and sufficient formula. Safe preparation of infant feeds is therefore almost impossible. Exacerbated by the tropical climate, infectious diseases, especially diarrhea resulting from unhygienic preparation of formulas, pose the greatest threat (Fig. 1-4).

Protein-calorie malnutrition (PCM) is a common and tragic result of many a family's attempt to stretch the costly formula by diluting it, often with contaminated water. To buy a 5-day supply of formula requires the full day's wages of a plantation worker in the Philippines. In the Caribbean, Nestlé's powdered milk, Nido, costs nearly 50% of the family's daily income.[21]

The contraceptive value of lactation is especially important in areas of the world where women have little or no access to alternative methods of child spacing. By inhibiting ovulation, total breastfeeding markedly decreases the incidence of pregnancy during the first 9 postpartal months, and often much longer. In primitive communities like that of the !Kung hunter-gatherers of the Kalahari in Africa who practice no form of fertility control, the average interval between successive births is 44 months. This is thought to be entirely due to the contraceptive effect of breastfeeding. No milk substitute is available in the Kalahari area. There is little doubt that until recently breastfeeding has been the major factor in holding population growth in check. Even today, it probably prevents more pregnancies throughout the world than the cumulative effect of all forms of fertility control[24] except abstinence.

The economic implications of a rapidly expanding population in a resource-poor

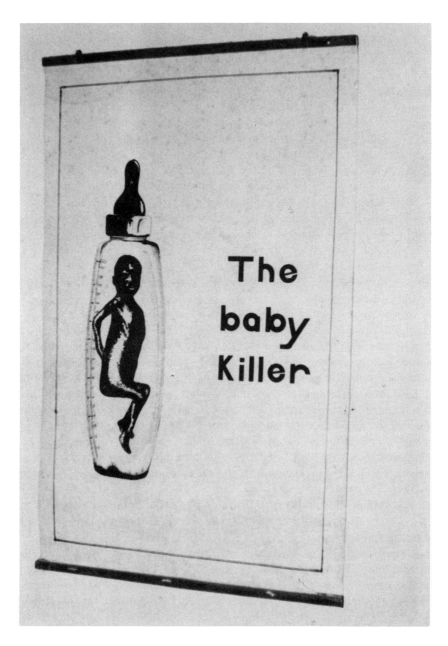

Fig. 1-4. The baby killer. Wall poster in the Under Six Clinic, Baguio General Hospital, Philippines. (Courtesy Michael Riordan.)

nation are far reaching. In the early 1950's pharmaceutical companies began a concentrated campaign to attract Third World consumers. For a quarter of a century now, pictures of smiling healthy white babies have been appearing on formula cans and large billboards in developing countries. The unsuspecting Third World mother is thus lured into believing that breastfeeding is passé and that the bottle is best for her child. In addition, marketing strategies directed toward medical personnel promote the use of formula in underdeveloped countries, often with tragic results.

Reversing the trend. The stormy controversy over bottle-feeding has led to the formation of nonprofit organizations committed to oppose formula sales in the underdeveloped areas of the world. Two such groups are the Infant Formula Action Coalition (INFACT) and the Interfaith Center on Corporate Responsibility (ICCR).

With increasing concern, critics are demanding stronger regulations and codes of ethics for formula advertising in Third World countries. In the fall of 1979 in Geneva, Switzerland, representatives of the baby food industry joined medical experts, members of nongovernmental organizations, and member governments in a meeting sponsored by WHO and UNICEF. Participants agreed that breastfeeding should be "protected and encouraged" everywhere and that promotional advertising of formula to the consumer should be stopped. Participants formulated a draft code of ethics recommending ethical international sales and marketing practices. In May 1981, following several revisions, the code was overwhelmingly passed by the World Health Assembly. The United States cast the only dissenting vote.

To counteract the influence of formulas, governments of some Third World countries and many international agencies are appropriating funds and developing programs for breastfeeding education. A grant awarded to La Leche League International by the Agency for International Development (AID) in 1979 has established a center for the promotion of breastfeeding and the education of professional and lay breastfeeding counselors in El Salvador. The center, called Centro de Apoyo de Lactancia Materna (CALMA), houses a bilingual resource center of references and other documents on breastfeeding and maternal, infant, and family nutrition.

Pointing up international concern with the importance of breastfeeding was the 1974 WHO theme, "Health Begins at Home." In 1978 in Indonesia, a course on breastfeeding education was jointly sponsored by the Department of Child Health and by the Gadjah Mada University in Yogyakarta. In the 1979 International Year of the Child, Health and Welfare of Canada, in collaboration with the Canadian Pediatrics Society and La Leche League, distributed information packets on breastfeeding to health personnel throughout the country (Fig. 1-5).

Also during the 1979 International Year of the Child, the government of Colombia announced the prohibition of all advertising of milk products in hospitals, health posts, and medical centers. A resolution by the Ministry of Health specified measures that aid breastfeeding that were to be used by physicians and nurses in that country.[14] Recently, in Papua, New Guinea, it has been illegal to sell formulas, bottles, and nipples without a prescription.

Larger issues. In addition to the influence of the formula industry, economic hardships and lack of sanitation in Third World countries contribute to infant morbidity and mortality. Poverty correlates with a higher incidence of medical problems in formula-fed infants, and affluence affects child health through general social, economic,

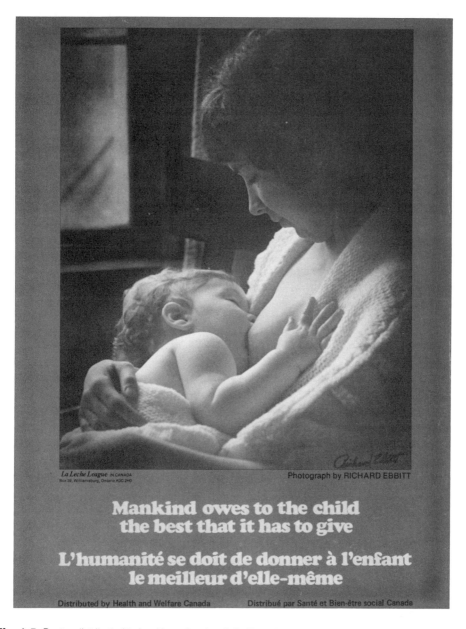

La Leche League IN CANADA
Box 39, Williamsburg, Ontario K0C 2H0

Photograph by RICHARD EBBITT

**Mankind owes to the child
the best that it has to give**

**L'humanité se doit de donner à l'enfant
le meilleur d'elle-même**

Distributed by Health and Welfare Canada   Distribué par Santé et Bien-être social Canada

Fig. 1-5. Poster distributed to health professionals in Canada by Health and Welfare Canada during International Year of the Child, 1979, as part of a national promotion of breastfeeding. (Courtesy La Leche League International.)

and environmental conditions. If the formula industry disappeared tomorrow, there would still be hungry, ill children—but not as many.

Recent observations of mothers and infants in a poor, remote, rural area of the Dominican Republic indicate that infants not being breastfed have significantly more health problems related to malnutrition. Diarrheic illness, usually caused by *Shigella* or *Entamoeba* bacteria, allergies, skin infections, parasites, marasmus, and kwashiorkor are common problems in bottle-fed infants. In more affluent areas of the Dominican Republic, particularly in the larger towns, the situation is somewhat better because of the greater availability of nutritious foods. Bottle-fed urban babies have fewer nutritionally related health problems—except for allergies—than poor rural babies, yet their general health, based on similar medical standards, is not as good as that of breastfed children.

What can nurses do? With the mounting evidence that breastfeeding is superior to other forms of infant feeding, we must now ask ourselves what nurses can do, particularly in the Third World countries. Paramount is the need to influence and educate those individuals who are in a position to lend governmental support to breastfeeding programs. Public health officials, physicians, administrators, and other leaders at local, state, national, and international levels must be persuaded or motivated to provide the needed support. Profound changes can be made, individually or collectively, through national nursing organizations. The resolution[1] sponsored by the Division on Maternal and Child Nursing Practice and adopted by the ANA House of Delegates is a step in the right direction.

INFANT FORMULA MARKETING PRACTICES IN THIRD WORLD COUNTRIES

RESOLVED, that the 1980 ANA House of Delegates go on record as condemning misleading sales promotion techniques in Third World countries

RESOLVED, that the ANA Board of Directors send letters of protest to the corporations involved in promoting the sale of infant formulas in the Third World countries

RESOLVED, that ANA members who are stockholders in any of the corporations be encouraged to voice the association's concern regarding infant formula marketing practices in the Third World countries, and further be it

RESOLVED, that a copy of this resolution be sent to the appropriate federal agencies, legislators, US ambassadors to Third World countries, executive director of the United Nations Children's Fund and all national nurse associations who are members of the International Council of Nurses, and published widely in nursing journals.

Nurses around the world, aware of their significance as primary caretakers in the health-care system, must meet the challenge of promoting breastfeeding and upgrading nutrition of mothers and children the world over.

REFERENCES

1. American Nurses' Association: Resolutions adopted by the House of Delegates, Am. Nurse **12**:12, 1980.
2. Arafat, I., Allen, D.E., and Fox, J.E.: Maternal practice and attitudes toward breastfeeding, J.O.G.N. Nurs. **10**:91, 1981.
3. Ayalah, D., and Weinstock, I.J.: Breasts: women speak about their breasts and their lives, New York, 1979, Summit Books.
4. Bain, K.: The incidence of breastfeeding in hospitals of the United States, Pediatrics **2**:313, 1948.
5. Brown, F., et al: Studies in the choice of infant

feeding by primiparas, Psychosom. Med. **12:**426, 1960.

6. Burns, J.: The principles of midwifery including the diseases of women and children, Philadelphia, 1810, Hopkins & Earle.
7. Cole, J.P.: Breastfeeding in the Boston suburbs in relation to personal-social factors, Clin. Pediatr. **16:**352, 1977.
8. Durant, W.: The story of civilization, vol. 1, Our oriental heritage, New York, 1954, Simon & Schuster, Inc.
9. Gray, A.G.: Breastfeeding: a trilogy. III. The sociologist's tale, Midwife Health Visitor and Community Nurse **11:**391, 1975.
10. Guthrie, H., and Guthrie, G.: The resurgence of natural feeding, Clin. Pediatr. **5:**481, 1966.
11. Hirschman, E., and Sweet, J.A.: Social background and breastfeeding among American mothers, Soc. Biol. **21:**37, 1975.
12. Jefferis, B.G.: Safe counsel, 1894.
13. Knafl, K.: Conflicting perspectives on breastfeeding, Am. J. Nurs. **74:**1848, 1974.
14. La Leche League International, Inc.: La Leche League News **22:**98, 1980.
15. Lawson, B.: Perceptions of degrees of support for the breastfeeding mother, Birth Fam. J. **3:**67, 1976.
16. Margulies, L.: A critical essay of promotion of bottlefeeding, PAG Bull. **7:**62, 1977.
17. Martinez, G.A., and Nalezienski, J.P.: 1980 update: the recent trend in breastfeeding, Pediatrics **67:**260, 1981.
18. Phillips, V.: Infant feeding through the ages, Keeping Abreast J. **1:**1976.
19. Pinckney, C.R.: Third world women and children need more than a boycott! J. Nurse-Midwifery **25:**25, 1980.
20. Raphael, D.: The tender gift: breastfeeding, Englewood Cliffs, N.J., 1973, Prentice-Hall Inc.
21. Riordan, J.: Breastfeeding in the Dominican Republic, LaLeche League News **22:**108, 1980.
22. Rivera, J.: The frequency of use of various kinds of milk during infancy in middle and lower-class families, Am. J. Public Health **61:**277, 1971.
23. Salber, E., and Feinlieb, M.: Breastfeeding in Boston, Pediatrics **37:**299, 1966.
24. Short, R.V.: Lactation: the central control of reproduction. In Ciba Foundation Symposium No. 45: Breastfeeding and the mother, Amsterdam, 1976, Elsevier Scientific Publishing Co.
25. Stone, L.: The family, sex and marriage: in England 1500-1800, New York, 1977, Harper & Row, Publishers, Inc.
26. Thirion, M.: L'allaitement, Paris, 1980, Ramsay.
27. Trends in breastfeeding among American mothers, Series 23, No. 3, Washington, D.C., 1979, Division of Vital Statistics, National Center for Health Statistics.
28. Vahlquist, B.: The evolution of breastfeeding in Europe, J. Trop. Pediatr. Env. Child Health **21:**11, 1975.

ADDITIONAL READINGS

Jelliffe, D.B., and Jelliffe, E.F.P.: Human milk in the modern world, London, 1978, Oxford University Press.

Levin, S.: A philosophy of infant feeding, Springfield, Ill., 1963, Charles C Thomas, Publisher.

The anatomy and psychophysiology of lactation

JAN RIORDAN
BETTY ANN COUNTRYMAN

To be of optimal help to the breastfeeding mother, the nurse needs to know the anatomy of the breast and the physiologic mechanisms of milk production. Cooperation with the natural psychophysiologic mechanisms leads to an uncomplicated breastfeeding experience, while the frustration of these mechanisms results in dysfunction and, ultimately, failure of breastfeeding.

THE BASIC ANATOMY
The mammary glands: structure and function

The mammary glands are modified exocrine glands which undergo numerous anatomical and physiological changes in pregnancy and immediately following birth. The breast is composed of glandular tissue surrounded by adipose tissue, separated from the underlying chest muscles and ribs by connective tissue. The breasts grow during puberty, develop further in pregnancy, secrete minimally in late pregnancy, and achieve major secretory activity after childbirth.

From woman to woman considerable variation exists in the amount of fatty and fibrous tissues in the breast, but these variations seem to have little effect on secretory efficiency. The basic units of glandular tissue are the *alveoli*, which are composed of *secretory cells* in which the ductules terminate (Fig. 2-1). Each cluster of secretory cells of an alveolus is surrounded by a contractile unit of *myoepithelial cells* responsible for ejecting milk into the *ductules*. Each ductule then merges into a larger collecting *lactiferous* or *mammary duct*. Mammary ducts then widen into *ampullae* or *lactiferous sinuses* located behind the nipple and surrounding pigmented area of the breast. There are 15 to 20 subdivided *lobes* in each breast. The breast is highly vascularized and innervated, and the covering skin is modified at the center of each breast to form a *mammary papilla* or nipple into which the lactiferous sinuses open. Surrounding the nipple is the

This chapter is republished from Riordan, J., and Countryman, B.A.: J.O.G.N. Nurs. **9**:210, 1980.

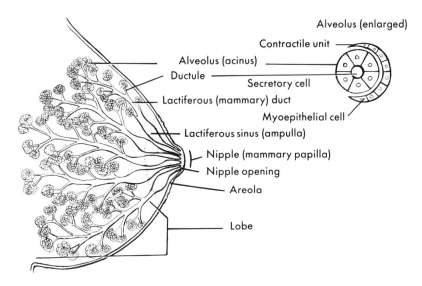

Fig. 2-1. Schematic diagram of breast.

areola within which lie the tubercles of Montgomery, small sebaceous glands which enlarge in pregnancy and provide nipple lubrication and antisepsis.

In pregnancy

During pregnancy the breasts grow larger, the skin appears to be thinner, and veins become more prominent. As the nipples become more erect, pigmentation of the areola is increased and the glands of Montgomery enlarge. Estrogen and progesterone exert their specific effects on the breasts in pregnancy: the ductal system proliferates and differentiates under the influence of estrogen, while progesterone promotes an increase in size of lobes, lobules, and alveoli.[2] Colostrum, the clear yellow-colored early milk, is a secretion of the lining of the alveoli and ductules. Colostrum is present in greater or lesser amounts throughout pregnancy and is the infant's feed for the first day or two after birth.

PSYCHOPHYSIOLOGY
Hormonal influences

Recently, due to technological advances, a great deal of new information on the hormonal function during lactation is becoming known. Radioimmunoassay studies on prolactin show a clear correlation between nipple stimulation during feedings and increased prolactin levels (Fig. 2-2). Previously, it was thought the prolactin level remained low during human pregnancy as it does in animals. Now we know that prolactin levels steadily rise during pregnancy (Fig. 2-3), falling during the 2 to 3 hours prior to birth and peaking around 3 hours after delivery.

As placental and ovarian estrogens decrease following birth, the anterior pituitary gland releases prolactin. Through the mediation of the hypothalamus the alveolar cells respond with the production of milk (Fig. 2-4). The highly vascularized secretory cells extract water, lactose, amino acids, fats, vitamins, minerals, and numerous other sub-

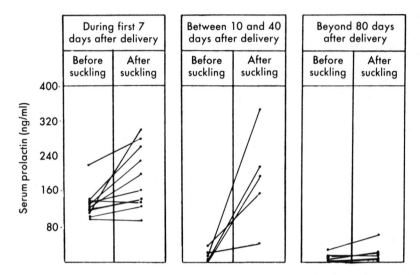

Fig. 2-2. Serum prolactin responses to suckling in normal postpartum women. (From Tyson, J.E., et al.: Am. J. Obstet. Gynecol. **113:**14, 1972.)

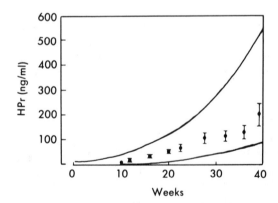

Fig. 2-3. Basal serum prolactin *(HPr)* concentrations during normal gestation. Selected points represent mean and standard error. Zone lines show wide range of values. (From Tyson, J.E., et al.: Am. J. Obstet. Gynecol. **113:**14, 1972.)

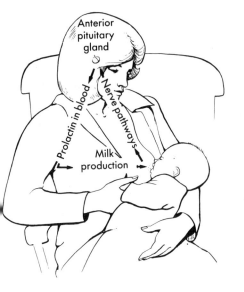

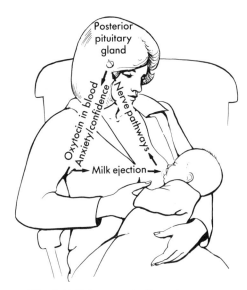

Fig. 2-4. Release and effect of prolactin on milk ejection.

Fig. 2-5. Release and effect of oxytocin.

stances from the mother's blood, converting them to milk for her infant. Responding to suckling, the posterior pituitary hormone, oxytocin, causes contraction of the myoepithelial cells surrounding the alveoli (Fig. 2-5). The secreted milk is then ejected into the ductules and moved along to the lactiferous sinuses where it becomes readily available to the newborn through the nipple opening.

Mechanisms in breastfeeding

To understand milk production and to assist the mother in initiating breastfeeding, one needs a clear understanding of two important mechanisms, the *let-down reflex* and the *supply-demand response*. The let-down reflex is a nerve reflex from the breast to the hypothalamus causing the release of oxytocin by the posterior pituitary gland. Elicited by the infant's suckling, or sometimes even by the mother's thoughts of her baby, this reflex initiates the flow of milk.

Anecdotal reports of spontaneous lactation in mothers who have weaned or who have never breastfed present an intriguing enigma. A case in point is a mother who suddenly began lactating after the death of her 6-week old infant whom she had not breastfed. Along with full breasts and dripping milk, she experienced uterine cramping.[3] In another case, the mother, a pediatrician, spontaneously developed engorgement 4 months after weaning.[1] Trying to relieve herself, she attempted to breastfeed the child, who promptly refused her. The strength of these recalled breastfeeding experiences on the hypothalamus and the pituitary point up the significant psychological mechanisms inherent in lactation.

That the reflex has psychogenic components is also clearly evident in a mother who is insecure, anxious, fatigued, or in pain. A stressed mother may experience considerable difficulty letting down her milk and provide less milk for her baby. Positive reassurance and support as well as efforts toward encouraging her to rest and relax can contribute markedly to an effectively functioning let-down and a feeling of well-being in the new mother.

The baby's sucking controls the amount of milk produced. Conversely, separation of mother and baby, scheduling of infant feedings, substitution of other liquids or solid foods for breastfeeding, and delay of feedings will decrease the production of milk. Despite such separations, schedules, substitutions, or delays, the mother's supply can be increased within a few days if she puts her baby to breast frequently and on demand, offering no other feeds.

Dysfunctions

Among the conditions which may affect breastfeeding are flat or inverted nipples. They should create only temporary difficulties and their care will be addressed later. Another deterrent is improper positioning or "gumming" by the infant at the breast, especially when the woman is a first-time mother. The baby should be carefully positioned to ensure that the nipple *and* much of the surrounding areola are drawn into the infant's mouth so the ampullae will empty as the baby sucks. While the baby feeds, he must be able to breathe freely. The mother can easily manage this by pressing the areola gently inward away from the baby's nostrils with her thumb while cupping her hand under her breast for support.

Milk or lymph stasis resulting from inadequate suckling may also contribute to dysfunction. A mother may become engorged because her baby is not with her to breastfeed *ad lib,* because the infant is sleepy from intrapartal medications, or because bottle feeds are given. At such times her breasts may become full, hard, and painful, and the nipples may no longer project sufficiently for the baby to grasp. Hand removal of the accumulated milk softens the nipple so that the baby can "latch on." Once the baby has begun to breastfeed, the mother should be encouraged to feed her infant at least every 2 to 3 hours.

Instructions for breast massage and manual expression of milk from the breast

A. To prepare the breasts for manual expression, the nurse should first demonstrate a slow and gentle massage of the breast to move milk to the lactiferous sinuses. Then ask the mother to return the demonstration to ensure that she is massaging correctly.

—For the left breast place the left hand at side of chest wall, well back of the breast with fingers pointing down and thumb upward.

—Place right hand flat on chest at midline between breasts (right thumb should also point upward and fingers downward).

—With moderate evenly distributed pressure, slide both hands toward the breast, encompassing it in a circle between the hands. (The circle formed by your hands will become smaller as the hands move more closely together.)

—Continue sliding hands toward each other until you reach the areola. At all times keep pressure *even* and *moderate.* (The mother may feel some discomfort from the pressure, but will find it tolerable.)

—Repeat this procedure several times, being sure to *start well back* on the side chest wall and maintain even pressure throughout.

B. To demonstrate manual removal of milk, use the following procedure and again suggest that the mother follow with a return demonstration.

—To remove milk from the left breast, support the breast with your right hand. Keeping your left hand flat on the breast and encompassing a portion of the breast, place your left thumb above and left fingers below the areola, having thumb and forefinger at areola's edge (Fig. 2-6).

—Push thumb and forefinger gently but firmly toward the chest wall; press forefinger and thumb together well behind nipple and areola and gently roll forward. It is imperative that you keep thumb and forefinger well behind the nipple to encourage emptying of all lactiferous sinuses (Fig. 2-7).

—Repeat this maneuver several times, rotating fingers and thumb around the areola until milk no longer ejects from the nipple and engorgement in the breast is relieved.

C. Repeat both A and B in reverse positions for the right breast until engorgement is relieved.

NOTE: The technique is not easy to do successfully the first few times. Discover this for yourself and encourage the mother to practice until she becomes comfortable with the procedure. If you are in contact with a mother or nurse who is adept with these procedures, you will find it very helpful to observe a demonstration.

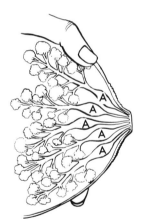

Fig. 2-6. Positioning hands over distended ampulla, A. Left breast, lateral view.

Fig. 2-7. Compressing to force milk out of ducts and ampulla. Thumb and forefinger are behind areola.

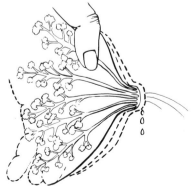

The sucking mechanism of breastfeeding as compared to bottlefeeding

While at the breast, to encourage the ejection of milk, the baby must suck vigorously, using his cheek muscles to draw the nipple well back into his mouth and against the hard palate. Most infants take in very little air because of the tight closure around the areola (Fig. 2-8).

In bottle feeding, complete closure of the baby's mouth around the nipple is seldom effected, allowing for considerable intake of air along with the formula. Also the tongue moves forward or *thrusts* to control the constant drip from the bottle nipple (Fig. 2-9).

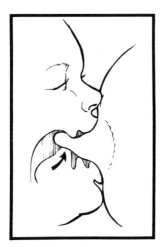 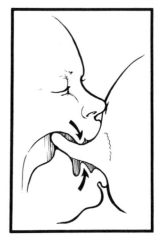

Fig. 2-8. In breastfeeding tongue thrusts up and forward to grasp nipple *(left);* gums compress areola, and tongue moves backward creating negative pressure for suction *(right).* Lips are flattened against areola. Cheek muscles assist.

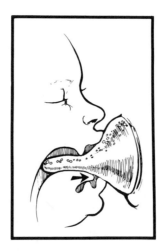

Fig. 2-9. In bottle-feeding *(above)* tongue is forward to control milk overflow from rubber nipple. Gums and lips cannot create compression. Air flows freely. Facial muscles are relaxed.

These two sucking actions are comparable to the separate muscle actions required when, for example, one sucks on a straw as compared to whistling. A few babies can make the required adjustment from one manner of sucking to the others; many, however, are not so adaptable and the stage is set for subsequent lactation failure.

CONCLUSION

In clinical practice the nurse should be aware of the impact which positive attitude, reassurance, and knowledgeable clinical support will have, especially on the first-time breastfeeding mother. Teaching her to position her baby properly, explaining the problems which supplemental bottles cause, and encouraging the mother to nurse her infant frequently, without regard for the clock, are major nursing contributions to a mother's successful start at breastfeeding.

REFERENCES

1. Breastfeeding and Infant Nutrition Conference, Wichita, Kan., 1975.
2. Guyton, A.C.: Textbook of medical physiology, ed. 6, Philadelphia, 1981, W.B. Saunders Co.
3. La Leche League International, Physicians' Seminar, Chicago, 1980.

ADDITIONAL READINGS

Applebaum, R.M.: The modern management of successful breastfeeding, Pediatr. Clin. North Am. **17:**203, 1970.
Bass, C.M., editor: Gray's anatomy of the human body, ed. 29, Philadelphia, 1973, Lea & Febiger.
Brunner, D.L., et al.: Prolactin levels in nursing mothers, Am. J. Obstet. Gynecol. **133:**250, 1978.
Countryman, B.: How the maternity nurse can help the breastfeeding mother, Franklin Park, Ill., 1977, La Leche League International.
Jensen, M.D., Benson, R.C., and Bobak, I.M.: Maternity care: the nurse and the family, ed. 2, St. Louis, 1981, The C.V. Mosby Co.
Marmet, C.: Manual expression of milk: Marmet technique, Franklin Park, Ill., 1981, La Leche League International.
Reeder, S.R., et al.: Maternity nursing, ed. 13, Philadelphia, 1976, J.B. Lippincott Co.

3

The biologic specificity of breastmilk

JAN RIORDAN
BETTY ANN COUNTRYMAN

If breastmilk were to be exactly duplicated and sold on today's market at the price it takes to produce it, we would probably hail it with the enthusiasm the "miracle" antibiotics met in the 1930's. Indeed, formula companies compete for the claim that their product is "most like mother's milk."

Breastmilk has been termed the perfect food for infants because it contains all necessary nutrients in correct proportions and simultaneously provides many antiinfective components. Moreover, through the eons of man's existence, human breastmilk, like the milk of other mammals, has become species-specific, adapting itself to meet the exact nutritional requirements of the human baby. Since the infant's birth weight normally doubles in about 5 months, the nutritional needs of the human baby must be substantially different from those of other mammals, for example, the calf whose birth weight is expected to double in 6 to 7 weeks. Similar contrasts can be found throughout the animal kingdom.

Folklore has often referred to breastmilk as "white blood," considering it similar to the placental blood of intrauterine life. Indeed, human milk is similar to unstructured living tissue like blood and is capable of affecting biochemical systems, enhancing immunity, and even destroying pathogenic bacteria.

Within the past few decades, with the use of sophisticated laboratory techniques, scientific research has substantiated the unique properties of many of the components of human milk. The knowledgeable nurse should know and share this information with mothers who are weighing the pros and cons of breastfeeding.

NUTRITIONAL AND ENERGY VALUES

The diet of the infant must provide sufficient energy in the form of calories to permit normal growth and development. Milk from the well-nourished mother is eminently capable of meeting this demand. During the first month, for example, the breastfeeding mother's normal yield approaches 600 ml/day. In the third month after delivery this becomes 700 to 750 ml/day and reaches 750 to 800 ml/day during the sixth month. Thereafter there is a slow decline in volume as the baby's diet is supplemented by additional foods. Since each 100 ml of human milk yields 75 kcal of energy, the variable volumes produced at different stages of the infant's life correlate appropriately with the needs imposed by age and weight. In addition to these two factors, gender, family (inherited) growth patterns, and the needs of the specific infant tend to affect milk yield to some extent and enable the mother to produce more or less according to her infant's unique requirements. Allowed to breastfeed at will in response to their own needs, infants generally consume milk in appropriate amounts to satisfy energy needs and maintain normal patterns of growth.

Fat

The largest source of calories is fat. The fat content of milk has a diurnal variation, being lowest at 6 AM and gradually increasing to its highest point about 2 PM. At any one feeding the highest concentration of fat is found at the end of the feeding in the "hindmilk."[15] In view of this phenomenon, it is particularly important for the mother not to set rigid time limits for feedings but to allow the infant to suckle until he indicates satiety. Triglycerides, the main constituents of milk fat, are readily broken down to free fatty acids and glycerol by the enzyme lipase, which is found not only in the infant's intestine but also in the breastmilk itself. Thus an initial supply of energy from the free fatty acids is available even before the milk reaches the intestines for ultimate digestion. Of special interest in regard to premature infants is the fact that the energy density of pre-term mother's milk is much greater than that of full-term mother's milk[4] because of a 30% higher fat concentration.

With the discovery of prostaglandins[22] in human milk, it has been proposed that they may play an important role in the infant's intestinal tract. A special group of lipids, prostaglandins are present in most mammalian cells and tissues and affect almost every biologic system. Prostaglandins are formed by numerous body tissues and affect many physiologic functions including local circulation, gastric and mucous secretion, electrolyte balance, zinc absorption, and the release of brush border enzymes. Moreover, they appear to confer what is termed "cytoprotection" of the gastrointestinal tract against many harmful toxins. The full extent of the beneficial effects of prostaglandins in human milk awaits future scientific research. Prostaglandins, incidentally, are not thought to be present in formulas.

The types of fat in the diet of the lactating mother have a significant effect on the types of fatty acids in her milk[13]; dietary counseling of a mother should therefore be an important aspect of teaching care when the milk composition is critical, as with the pre-term infant. Long-term effects of the intake of different types of fats and the resulting cholesterol levels are yet to be determined, but there is some evidence to suggest that reasonable levels of cholesterol may be necessary in the first few weeks of life for the development of later protective enzyme systems. Since cholesterol levels in human milk are generally higher than in formulas using cow's milk or vegetable products, cholesterol levels in adulthood might be expected to be higher in breastfed individuals. The reverse, however, seems to be true. At least one study[20] has shown that coronary artery disease in persons up to 20 years of age is seen less frequently in individuals who were breastfed. This information suggests that the moderate intake of cholesterol present in breastmilk may contribute to a more efficient cholesterol metabolism in adulthood.

Lactose

Lactose is found only in mammalian milk, and it is present in greater quantity in human than in other animal milks. It accounts for most of the carbohydrate in human milk, although small quantities of galactose and fructose are also present. Lactose enhances calcium absorption and metabolizes readily to galactose and glucose, which supply energy to the rapidly growing brain of the infant. Lactose also promotes the growth of lactobacilli, thus increasing intestinal acidity and stemming the growth of pathogenic organisms.

The enzyme lactase is necessary for the conversion of lactose into smple sugars that can be better assimilated by the infant. This enzyme is present in the infant's intestinal mucosa from birth. Congenital or primary lactase deficiency is exceedingly rare, and some authorities even question its existence. Lactose intolerance, however, is common in many mammals as they grow older as a result of diminishing activity of intestinal lactase after the normal time of weaning. In humans it is more prevalent in blacks and Orientals, and affected individuals learn to avoid drinking milk.

Protein

The proteins of milk are casein and whey. Whey proteins predominate in human milk and are acidified in the stomach. As a result soft flocculent curds form and are quickly and easily digested, supplying a continuous flow of nutrients to the baby. By contrast, the primary protein of cow's milk, casein, forms a less digestible, tough, rubbery curd that requires high expenditure of energy for an incomplete digestive process. Although the protein content of human milk is less than half that of cow's milk, the easy digestibility of human milk provides the breastfed baby with an ideal energy-sufficient quantity and quality of protein.

Two amino acids found in breastmilk but almost nonexistent in cow's milk are cystine and taurine. Cystine is essential to somatic growth, and taurine is needed for early brain development and maturation. Both these substances are present in abundance in human milk and are of obvious importance to the newborn, who lacks the enzymes necessary to convert tyrosine to cystine and cystine to taurine.[26,30] Although the blood of breastfed infants contains ample cystine and taurine, that of infants fed breastmilk substitutes contains very little of these essential proteins.

The high quality and quantity of protein in colostrum are especially valuable to the neonate. The percentage of protein in human colostrum is nearly three times greater than in mature breastmilk. This high level is due to the presence of several additional amino acids and antibody-rich proteins, especially secretory IgA and lactoferrin. All ten essential amino acids are present in colostrum and account for approximately 45% of its total nitrogen content.

The importance of available nitrogen cannot be understated. Atkinson et al.[4] have shown that the nitrogen concentration in the milk of women who deliver pre-term infants is 20% greater than in milk of women delivering at full term. They suggest that "the premature infant fed his own mothers' milk rather than mature pooled milk would receive almost twice as much protein during the first two weeks of life if the increased nitrogen was present as available protein." The higher levels of "available protein" and fat in pre-term mother's milk underscore the importance of using the milk of the pre-term infant's own mother rather than pooled milk from mothers in various stages of lactation.

Iron

Normally an infant's hemoglobin level is high (16 to 22 gm/dl) at birth and decreases rapidly as physiologic adjustment is made to extrauterine life. At 4 months normal hemoglobin ranges between 10.2 and 15 gm/dl.

Although iron is present in both human and cow's milk in small quantities (0.5 to 1 mg/L), the healthy breastfeeding infant of a mother who maintained a reasonably adequate diet during pregnancy rarely needs iron supplementation before 6 months of age. The following rationale is given for this phenomenon[19]: (1) the full-term newborn has ample iron stores that do not begin to be depleted until 4 to 6 months after birth; and (2) iron in human milk is used with a superior degree of efficiency (49%) because of the high lactose and vitamin C levels that facilitate absorption. Also, breastfed infants do not risk loss of iron as do cow's milk–fed infants, who can experience microhemorrhages of the bowel as a result of mucosal damage by milk.[31] Table 3-1 compares the metabolism of iron between human milk and cow's milk.

TABLE 3-1

Iron metabolism: comparison between human milk and cow's milk

	Human milk	Cow's milk
Iron content	Low	Low
Iron absorption	49%	4%
Iron facilitators	↑ Lactose	↓ Lactose
	↑ Vitamin C	↓ Vitamin C
Iron loss	None	Sometimes (intestinal microhemorrhages)
Iron deficiency anemia (6-12 mo)	Uncommon	More common

Modified from Jelliffe, D.B., and Jelliffe, E.F.P.: Human milk in the modern world, Oxford, 1978, Oxford University Press.

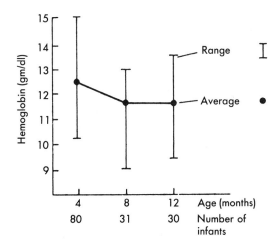

Fig. 3-1. Hemoglobin levels in breastfed infants 4 months to 1 year of age. (From Good, J. In Jelliffe, D.B., and Jelliffe, E.F.P.: Human milk in the modern world, Oxford, 1978, Oxford University Press.)

The results of a study done in Columbus, Ohio (Fig. 3-1), show that hemoglobin levels of breastfeeding infants surveyed remained well within normal limits between 4 and 12 months of age.

Iron supplementation is not usually needed and may in fact be detrimental to the breastfeeding baby during the first half-year after birth. Excess iron tends to saturate lactoferrin and thereby diminish its antiinfective properties.[8]

Vitamins and trace minerals

A significant difference between formula-feeding and breastfeeding is that the direct consumption of breastmilk ensures that all the vitamins present in the milk are transferred to the infant, whereas in formula-feeding vitamins are frequently lost in collecting, processing, reconstituting, and reheating. The levels of vitamins in human milk, especially water-soluble vitamins, are influenced to some extent by a woman's diet. A rule of thumb is that her milk will satisfy the vitamin and trace mineral requirements of a full-term healthy infant if she eats a variety of nourishing foods.

New information relevant to nursing practice indicates a need for brief discussions of vitamins E, D, and K and the trace mineral zinc.

Vitamin D. The amount of vitamin D in human milk, once thought to be 22 IU/L, is currently being reevaluated since the discovery of a water-soluble variant of the vitamin.[17] Although rickets is rarely seen in breastfed children, especially if their mothers are well nourished, some recent scattered reports of rickets have led the American Academy of Pediatrics[2] to recommend vitamin D supplements for children subject to certain conditions. The risk is greatest for dark-skinned children living in inner-city areas, children whose religion advocates clothing habits that deter exposure to the sun, and children of mothers on vegetarian diets that exclude meat, fish, and dairy products. That low birth weight infants need additional vitamin D for a period of time has long been known. However, the child who is adequately exposed to the sun and thus to the radiant precursors of vitamin D and whose mother consumes adequate nutrients does not need routine vitamin D supplementation.[24]

Vitamin K. Required for the synthesis of blood-clotting factors, vitamin K is present in human milk and is absorbed efficiently, but administration of vitamin K to an infant who is to be breastfed may be justified, since the infant usually receives only a small amount of breastmilk during the first 2 days after birth. As far as is known, during the first few weeks of life vitamin K is not manufactured in the infant's gut. Intramuscular administration of vitamin K, however, has recently come under closer scrutiny. An equal dose of vitamin K given orally instead of intramuscularly appears to be absorbed in the intestinal tract in amounts sufficient to prevent hemorrhagic problems.[1,3] Over a 10-year period the Albert Einstein College of Medicine had no known problems after oral administration of vitamin K to newborns.[10] There are in fact several advantages to oral administration of vitamin K: the cost is less; the risk of nerve damage, always present with any intramuscular injection, is avoided; and the infant is spared the pain of an injection.

Vitamin E. A deficiency of vitamin E in infancy can result in hemolytic anemia, especially in the premature infant. The most severely affected infants become edematous. As an antioxidant, vitamin E protects cell membranes in the retina and lungs against oxidant-induced injury. Human colostrum is particularly rich in vitamin E, and

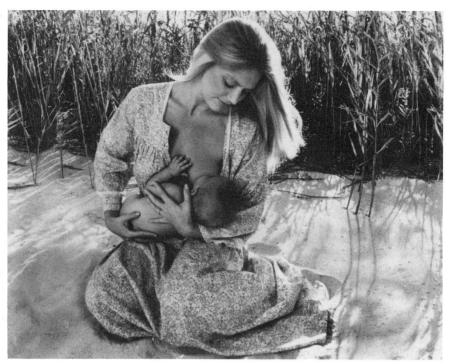

Are you receiving as much vitamin E as the original manufacturer intended?

Fig. 3-2. "Are you receiving as much vitamin E as the original manufacturer intended?"
An abundance of vitamin E is contained in breastmilk. (Advertisement for vitamin E by Hoffman LaRoche, Inc. from Time **118:**86, November 23, 1981.)

mature breastmilk levels, too, are higher than in cow's milk (Fig. 3-2.) Breastfeeding is therefore a preventive measure against hemolytic anemia and other potential problems in infancy. Like vitamin K, vitamin E is absorbed in sufficient amounts when given orally.[6]

Zinc. The trace mineral zinc brings about dramatic improvement in acrodermatitis enteropathica, a serious congenital metabolic disorder that manifests itself in part in severe dermatitis. This disease does not occur in the breastfed infant. Since levels of zinc are high in both human and bovine milk, the question arises as to why human milk has a preventive or curative effect. It is currently thought that the high bioavailability of zinc in human milk is brought about by a zinc-binding ligand that facilitates absorption of the mineral from the intestines.[9]

THYROID HORMONE

Several investigators[25,27] have shown that thyroid hormones are present in human milk in significant quantities, but amounts in commercial formulas and pasteurized cow's milk are negligible. There are, however, conflicting studies[7,18] in the medical literature regarding the degree of protection against congenital hypothyroidism that these breastmilk hormones offer the infant.

Unless routine screening is done, hypothyroidism frequently goes undetected. Even with regular testing, breastfeeding infants may be receiving sufficient thyroxine from their mother's milk to compensate for hypothyroidism, and thus the symptoms may be masked for many months. Since this does not appear to be true for *all* infants, the results of thyroid studies after the first week of life should be interpreted with caution in breastfed infants and should include measurements of both T_4 and thyroid-stimulating hormone (TSH) concentrations.

RENAL SOLUTE LOAD

Another unique aspect of human milk is the effect of the renal solute load on the infant's kidney function and his general state of hydration. Human milk has significantly lower levels of calcium, phosphorus, sodium, and potassium than cow's milk. Because of this and the low protein content of human milk, the solute load on the immature kidney of the breastfed infant is approximately one third that of the infant fed cow's milk.[23] Since excess salts require additional water for excretion, greater obligatory water loss occurs, resulting in increased thirst in the cow's milk–fed infant. All too often this thirst is misinterpreted as hunger, and additional milk is fed. Thus the baby receives a salt overload, and hypernatremic dehydration may result. When ill with diarrhea or vomiting, the infant receiving cow's milk may have a more rapid osmotic shift of free (extracellular) water so that dehydration is more severe than in the breastfed infant. An overconcentrated formula presents a similar hazard. For this reason and for other reasons the risk is generally greater for the nonbreastfed infant when conditions that may result in dehydration are encountered. The breastfed baby, by contrast, does not ingest an overload of salts and needs no additional water under most conditions.

ANTIINFECTIVE PROPERTIES

That breastmilk offers the newborn protection against disease has been recognized for hundreds of years, but only recently have investigators begun to identify the specific antiinfective components of human milk that make it a peerless substance for feeding the human infant. Breastmilk has been looked on from ancient times as a living tissue, and rightly so. This "white blood" contains enzymes, immunoglobulins, and leukocyte cells in abundance. It is these latter components especially that account for most of the unique antiinfective properties of human milk.

Protection against infections afforded by breastmilk is due in part to the direct mode of transmission from mother to baby that eliminates many opportunities for contamination. Yet human milk is not truly sterile. Skin has bacteria, and the mother's areolae are no exception. Cultures of the nipple and areolar skin, however, show a lower bacterial count than other areas of the human body. This is due to the antiseptic secretion from Montgomery's glands in the areola.

Even more important than external factors are those intrinsic to the milk itself. These special components, one frequently enhancing the efficacy of another, prevent infantile diarrhea and numerous other infections during the breastfeeding period and beyond. In some cultures fresh breastmilk is regularly used as eyedrops to treat conjunctivitis; elsewhere it is common practice to rub breastmilk into the skin to heal cracked nipples and prevent mastitis.

Cellular components

Most numerous among the leukocytes of human colostrum and milk are the macrophages and neutrophils. These large, motile, amoeba-like cells literally surround and destroy harmful bacteria by their phagocytic activity. They may also secrete lysozyme and lactoferrin.

Abundant in colostrum and milk are the lymphocytes that produce secretory IgA and interferon, two vitally important antiinfective substances. Individually and together, the living active components of human milk are instrumental in preventing infections in the newborn and the growing baby.

Immunoglobulins

The immunoglobulins IgA, IgG, IgM, and IgD are among the most important protective factors in human milk and supplement the immunoglobulins earlier transferred across the placenta. The most significant of these is secretory IgA, which appears to be both synthesized and stored in the breast itself. Secretory IgA is especially high in colostrum in the first few days after delivery, reaching levels up to 50 mg/ml.[29] It provides the initial bolus of immunoglobulins frequently noted in medical literature to be of immense immunologic value to the neonate. Secretory IgA is present in human milk in many times the concentration found in cow's milk and formulas. This immunoglobulin resists proteolysis by gastrointestinal secretions and functions chiefly within the gastrointestinal tract. Since the infant's own IgA is deficient and only slowly increases during the first several months after birth, secretory IgA received from the mother "paints" the intestinal epithelium and protects the mucosal surfaces against entry of pathogenic bacteria and enteroviruses. Among the organisms against which secretory IgA affords protection are *Escherichia coli, Salmonella, Shigella,* streptococci, staphylococci, pneumococci, poliovirus, and the rotaviruses.

Lysozyme

Lysozyme, a well-known antiinfective enzyme, is present in breastmilk in concentrations up to 5000 times that found in cow's milk. It is specific in its action against certain micrococci as well as against *E. coli* and *Salmonella typhosa.* Lysozyme also may provide protection against several viruses. Lysozyme activity appears to increase during lactation with the highest levels occurring 6 months after delivery.[11]

Lactoferrin

Lactoferrin, a potent bacteriostatic and iron-binding protein, is abundant in human milk but is not present in cow's milk. In combination with secretory IgA, it destroys pathogenic strains of *E. coli.* Because it is an unsaturated iron-binding protein, it readily absorbs enteric iron, thus preventing pathogenic organisms from obtaining the iron they need for survival. Since exogenous iron may well interfere with the protective effects of lactoferrin, the potential disadvantages of giving iron supplements to the healthy breastfed baby must be carefully weighed. The concentration of lactoferrin, lysozyme, and the immunoglobulins during the first 4 weeks after delivery is shown in Table 3-2.

TABLE 3-2 _____

Distribution of immunoglobulins and other soluble substances in the colostrum and milk delivered to the breastfed infant during a 24-hour period

	Concentration in mg/day weeks after delivery			
Soluble product	**<1**	**1-2**	**3-4**	**>4**
Immunoglobulin				
IgG	50	25	25	10
IgA	5000	1000	1000	1000
IgM	70	30	15	10
Lysozyme	50	60	60	100
Lactoferrin	1500	2000	2000	1200

From Ogra, P.L., Fishaut, M., and Theodore, C. In Frier, S., and Eidelman, A.I., editors: Human milk: its biological and social value, Int. Congress Series No. 518, Amsterdam, 1980, Excerpta Medica.

The bifidus factor

The intestinal flora of breastfed babies is dominated by gram-positive lactobacilli, especially *Lactobacillus bifidus*. The bifidus factor in human milk, first recognized by Gyorgy,[14] promotes the growth of these beneficial bacteria and discourages multiplication of pathogens. *L. bifidus* colonizes the intestines of breastfed babies only, whereas formula-fed infants have primarily gram-negative, potentially pathogenic intestinal colonization. The low pH of the breastfed infant's intestinal contents and the large amount of ingested lactose further enhance the action of the bifidus factor and protect against protozoa and enteropathic bacteria.

Other protective factors

Numerous other factors are present in colostrum and breastmilk, some of which have proven protective value, whereas others, as of this writing, remain speculative. Human colostrum has been shown to contain *respiratory syncytial virus* antibodies as well as the enzyme *lactoperoxidase,* a host resistance enzyme system. *Interferon,* produced by the lymphocytes of breastmilk, is believed to protect the infant against various viral infections. An *antistaphylococcal factor* offers known resistance to several staphylococci, notably *Staphylococcus aureus*. Numerous investigators[12,16,29] have reported the presence in breastmilk of antibacterial antibodies to *Shigella, Salmonella, Clostridium tetani, Corynebacterium diphtheriae, Diplococcus pneumoniae, Vibrio cholerae,* and *E. coli.*

Breastmilk is also thought to help prevent acute necrotizing enterocolitis (NEC), a usually fatal disease of the premature baby. Both *Klebsiella* and *Clostridia* are suspected organisms in the intestinal wall infection of NEC, and breastmilk has been found to suppress the growth of both organisms.[5]

Further investigation is needed into the roles played by other known and perhaps some still unknown components of human milk. For example, the reason for the positive reaction to the tuberculin skin test shown by some breastfed infants of tuberculin-positive mothers merits study and explanation. Antibodies to the poliovirus, rotavirus, and to some coxsackie- and echoviruses are known to be present in breastmilk, but the

Table 3-3

Antiinfective properties of human milk

Factor	Function
Secretory IgA and other immunoglobulins	Coat intestinal mucosa and protect from bacteria and viruses; high levels in colostrum, gradually diminishing
Bifidus factor	Creates inhospitable conditions for enteropathic bacteria through presence of *L. bifidus* and resulting acidity
Antistaphylococcal factor	Resists staphylococci, especially *S. aureus*
Lysozymes	Attack bacterial cell wall by cellular lysis; levels increase for 6 months after delivery
Lactoferrin	Inhibits growth of bacteria by chelating iron
Leukocytes	Destroy pathogens by phagocytosis; produce lysozyme, lactoferrin, IgA, and interferon
Interferon	Protects against viral infections
Lactoperoxidase	Kills streptococci
Prostaglandins	Act as cytoprotectors; full effect still unknown

mechanism and degree of protection also need further study. The significance of the presence of nine components of *complement* and of small amounts of *transferrin* awaits further investigation, as do numerous other substances not reported here. Table 3-3 offers a graphic view of the best known protective factors in human milk.

ANTIALLERGIC PROPERTIES

The following discussion deals not with species-specific components present in human milk but rather with the *absence* of certain components, namely food antigens.

Approximately 7% of infants are allergic to cow's milk; if there is a family history of allergies, the probability may be considerably higher. Therefore, in discussions with a mother when there are allergies either in her own family or in that of the infant's father, the nurse should strongly encourage breastfeeding for a minimum of 9 months to minimize potential allergic manifestations. Before 6 to 9 months of age, the infant's intestinal mucosa is permeable to proteins; moreover, his own secretory IgA, which later will "paint" the mucosa and bind sensitizing proteins to itself, is not yet functioning effectively.

Proteins in cow's milk that can act as allergens are lactoglobulin, casein, bovine serum albumin (BSA), and lactalbumin. Modern processing of formula through heat treatment has somewhat reduced without entirely eliminating the allergic potential of these proteins, and the problem is increased by the sizable "dose" of allergens in the formula. At 2 to 4 months of age, for example, a baby consumes his body weight in milk each week—the equivalent for him of nearly 7 quarts a day for an adult—truly a macrodose.

At birth the IgE system is defective in the preallergic infant, and problems arise if this system is activated by allergens. When introduction of foreign proteins is delayed for 6 months or more so that the baby's own IgA system is permitted to become more fully functional, allergic responses may be minimized or occasionally entirely avoided. Breastmilk exerts a protective function by controlling the transport of potentially antigenic molecules into the circulation of the newborn, thereby both facilitating the early maturation of the intestinal barrier and providing an exogenous passive barrier until the baby's own natural barriers develop.[28] The rationale for delay of solids for the first half-year after birth is thus reinforced. Additionally, around 6 months of age the baby becomes increasingly more capable of digesting complex proteins and starches as a result of the maturation of his intestinal enzymes.

When solid foods are ultimately introduced into the infant's diet, the mother should introduce only one food at a time at weekly intervals. In this way the baby can be watched for allergic reactions to individual foods, and those that cause difficulties can be withdrawn from the diet.

SUMMARY

Analysis of the nutritional components of human milk combined with its specially designed immune and antiallergic properties points to its importance as the ideal foundation for good infant health. Practical experience has clearly suggested the benefits of breastfeeding. Now, in recent years, scientific data from all parts of the world and in many areas of maternal, infant, and public health confirm what the practitioner has long known.

Commenting on its unique adaptability, Ratner notes that "human milk has a remarkable fitness in terms of the demands and needs of the infant. . . . The configurations of elements in the milk are like computer information with a reciprocal fitness between the mother and the infant."[21] Moreover, even in special cases such as the accelerated energy needs of the premature infant, this adaptability is seen in the greater availability of energy in the milk of the pre-term mother.

The fundamental importance of human milk needs no further discussion. The next issue is to explore ways in which the nurse can facilitate the transfer of this superior nutrition from the breast to the infant via breastfeeding. This is the subject of the chapter that follows.

REFERENCES

1. Aballi, A.J., and DeLamerens, S.: Coagulation changes in the neonatal period, Pediatr. Clin. North Am. **9:**785, 1962.
2. American Academy of Pediatrics Committee on Nutrition: Vitamin and mineral supplement needs in normal children in the United States, Pediatrics **66:**1015, 1980.
3. American Academy of Pediatrics Committee on Nutrition: Vitamin K compounds and water-soluble analogues, Pediatrics **28:**501, 1961.
4. Atkinson, S.A., Anderson, G., and Bryan, M.H.: Human milk: comparison of the nitrogen composition of milk from mothers of premature infants, Am. J. Clin. Nutr. **33:**811, 1980.
5. Barlow, B., et al.: An experimental study of acute neonatal enterocolitis: the importance of breast milk, J. Pediatr. Surg. **9:**587, 1974.
6. Bell, E.F., et al.: Vitamin E absorption in small premature infants, Pediatrics **63:**830, 1979.
7. Bode, H.H., Vanjonack, W.J., and Crawford,

J.D.: Mitigation of cretinism by breastfeeding, Pediatr. Res. **11:**423, 1977.
8. Bullen, J.J., Rogers, H.J., and Leigh, L.: Iron-binding proteins in milk and resistance to *Escherichia coli* infection in infants, Br. Med. J. **1:**69, 1972.
9. Evans, G.W., and Johnson, P.E.: Characterization and quantitation of a zinc-binding ligand in human milk, Pediatr. Res. **14:**876, 1980.
10. Gartner, L.M.: Personal communication, Sept. 1981.
11. Goldman, A.: Immunologic factors in human milk during the first year of lactation, J. Pediatr. **100:**565, 1982.
12. Goldman, A.S., and Smith, C.W.: Host resistance factors in human milk, J. Pediatr. **82:**1081, 1973.
13. Guthrie, H.A., Picciano, M.F., and Sheehe, D.: Fatty acid patterns of human milk, J. Pediatr. **90:**39, 1977.

14. Gyorgy, P.: A hitherto unrecognized biochemical difference between human milk and cow's milk, Pediatrics **11**:98, 1953.
15. Hall, B.: Uniformity of human milk, Am. J. Clin. Nutr. **32**:304, 1979.
16. Hanson, L.A., and Winberg, J.: Breast milk and defence against infection in the newborn, Arch. Dis. Child. **47**:845, 1972.
17. Lakdawala, D.R., and Widdowson, E.M.: Vitamin D in human milk, Lancet **1**:167, 1977.
18. Letarte, J., et al.: Lack of protective effect of breastfeeding in congenital hypothyroidism, Pediatrics **65**:703, 1980.
19. McMillan, J.A., Landaw, S.A., and Oski, F.A.: Iron sufficiency in breastfed infants and the availability of iron from human milk, Pediatrics **58**:686, 1976.
20. Osborn, F.R.: Relationship of hypotension and infant feeding to the aetiology of coronary disease, Colloques Int. Cont. Natl. Res. Sci. **169**:93, 1968.
21. Ratner, H.: La Leche League International, Ninth Annual Seminar on Breastfeeding for Physicians, Chicago, July 1981.
22. Reid B., Smith, H., and Friedman, Z.: Prostaglandins in human milk, Pediatrics **66**:870, 1960.
23. Reynolds, J.W.: Water: developmental nutrition, No. 10, Columbus, Ohio, 1974, Ross Laboratories.
24. Roberts, C.C., et al.: Adequate bone mineralization in breastfed infants, J. Pediatr. **99**:192, 1981.
25. Strhak, V., et al.: Thyroxine in human and cow milk and in infant formulae, Endocrinol. Exp. **10**:167, 1976.
26. Sturman, J.A., Rassin, D.K., and Gaull, G.E.: Taurine in development: is it essential in the neonate? Pediatr. Res. **10**:415, 1976.
27. Varma, S.K., et al.: Thyroxine, tri-iodothyronine and reverse tri-idothyronine concentrations in human milk, J. Pediatr. **93**:803, 1978.
28. Udall, J.N., et al.: Development of gastrointestinal natural barrier. II. The effect of natural *versus* artificial feeding on intestinal permeability to macromolecules, Pediatr. Res. **15**:245, 1981.
29. Welsh, J.K., and May, J.T.: Anti-infective properties of breast milk, J. Pediatr. **94**:1, 1979.
30. Winters, R.W.: Infant nutrition, Pediatr. Res. **10**:263, 1976.
31. Woodruff, C.W.: The role of fresh cow's milk in iron deficiency, Am. J. Dis. Child **124**:18, 1971.

ADDITIONAL READINGS

Gerrard, J.W.: Breastfeeding: second thoughts, Pediatrics **54**:757, 1974.
Grams, K.: Breastfeeding: A means of imparting immunity? Matern. Child Nurs. J. **3**:340, 1978.
Guthrie, R.M., and Riordan, J.: Infant nutrition: fact and fantasy, J. Kans. Med. Soc. **77**:9, 1976.
Jelliffe, D.B., and Jelliffe, E.F.P.: Human Milk in the modern world, Oxford, 1978, Oxford University Press.
Ogra, S.S., and Ogra, P.L.: Immunologic aspects of human colostrum and milk. I. Distribution characteristics and concentrations of immunoglobulins at different times after the onset of lactation, J. Pediatr. **92**:546, 1978.
Whittlestone, W.G.: The biological specificity of human milk, Leaven **12**:3, 1976.

Self-care

BETTY ANN COUNTRYMAN

Helping new mothers during the lactation process is a rewarding and important experience for the nurse. With a basic knowledge of the anatomy and physiology of the breast and of the nutritional and immunologic properties of breastmilk, she can contribute greatly to a mother's success in breastfeeding; however, she must also be prepared with practical knowledge to help meet the urgent needs of a mother who has little or no breastfeeding experience or who has anxieties or problems. Thus emphasis on self-care by the mother is a major goal of the nursing process.

What the mother learns about breastfeeding and caring for herself and her baby in the medical office or the hospital will affect the breastfeeding relationship for months to come. Recognizing that many who initiate breastfeeding wean by 3 months, we clearly see the necessity for education in self-care skills. Self-care can generally be defined as "the practice of activities that individuals personally initiate and perform on their own behalf in maintaining life, health, and well-being."[32] In the self-care approach to breastfeeding, the nurse assists, encourages, and nurtures the mother and her family toward effective use of their own resources for achieving an optimal breastfeeding experience. This orientation, rather than the familiar patient teaching approach, is more congruent with the current cultural approach to consumer participation. Self-care is especially appropriate for maternal-infant care nursing, where, unlike other areas of nursing function, clients are usually in a state of health. In no other area of nursing is the consumer's involvement in her own care more rewarding for the nurse to observe.

PRENATAL PREPARATION FOR BREASTFEEDING

The mild irritation and nipple discomfort that many mothers experience in the first several days of breastfeeding rarely progress into severe nipple problems for the mother who learns basic self-care skills during pregnancy.

Much has been written about the value of prenatal nipple preparation by manual manipulation. The technique usually involves three modalities: (1) hand expression of colostrum, (2) nipple "rolling," and (3) conditioning the nipple tissue by friction.

A case can be made for the value of hand expression and nipple rolling in familiar-

---

Sections of this chapter are taken from Riordan, J., and Countryman, B.A.: Basics of breastfeeding. IV. Preparation for breastfeeding and early optimal functioning, J.O.G.N. Nurs. **9**:277, 1980. V. Self-care for continued breastfeeding, J.O.G.N. Nurs. **9**:357, 1980.

izing a mother with handling her breasts before lactation begins, but studies regarding their effect on sore nipples and breast engorgement are conflicting. Some[5,39] indicate that these exercises have no effect, but a more recent investigation[1] shows that a prenatal nipple-conditioning regimen significantly reduces the total amount of early postpartal nipple pain. Although a part of its effectiveness may be that the mother is better prepared psychologically for knowing and handling her breasts, many mothers report that nipple friction appears to reduce postnatal nipple soreness. Removing the center portion of a bra cup, thereby exposing the nipples to the friction of clothing, is a simple yet effective method of conditioning nipple skin. Rubbing the nipples gently with a turkish towel is another. An effective and pleasant method sometimes overlooked is oral or manual stimulation of the nipples during lovemaking. One word of caution, however, is appropriate here—women with a known tendency toward premature delivery should not stimulate their breasts, since such action causes uterine contractions. Conversely, some authors promote breast stimulation as a means of preventing postmaturity by inducing labor.

Exposing the breasts to air and sun prenatally to prevent soreness has particular merit when one considers that in regions of the world where women's breasts are normally exposed in daily living, sore nipples are rare. Care to prevent sunburn must be taken, of course.

Probably the most important prenatal preparation involves yet another organ: the brain. As Rubin so effectively demonstrated through nursing research more than a decade ago, the maternal role, far from being intuitive, is learned.[34] For the motivated mother, optimal readiness for breastfeeding is achieved in part through reading a wide selection of available materials, a partial list of which is provided at the end of this chapter.

One final point must be made. Even though a mother may not have prepared her breasts, read about breastfeeding, or attended preparatory classes, she can still have a satisfying breastfeeding experience. She needs reassurance that this is the case. A mother herself often needs mothering and reaffirmation of her own adequacy in nourishing her baby.

EARLY FEEDINGS

Following birth, continuing assessment of the mother's physical condition and psychosocial status is an essential nursing function. The optimal time for initiating breastfeeding depends on these factors as well as on the mother's free choice and will not, of course, be the same for all individuals. However, if the birth process has been relatively uncomplicated, the mother should be encouraged to breastfeed immediately after birth and regularly thereafter. There are several reasons why early and frequent breastfeedings promote an optimal level of functioning for both the infant and the mother:

1. Suckling stimulates uterine contractions, aids in the expulsion of the placenta, and helps control excessive maternal blood loss.
2. The infant's suckling reflex is most intense during the first 20 to 30 minutes after birth. Delaying gratification of the reflex can make it more difficult for the baby to learn the sucking process later on.[11]
3. The infant promptly begins to receive the immunologic advantages of colostrum.
4. The infant's digestive peristalsis is stimulated.

5. Later breast engorgement is minimized or prevented by the early and frequent removal of milk from the ducts and sinuses of the breast.[28]
6. Lactation is accelerated and the milk appears earlier; thus the infant's total weight loss after birth is reduced.
7. Attachment and bonding are enhanced at a time when both the mother and her infant are in a heightened state of readiness.

Promoting attachment

With early and frequent breastfeeding and the mother's full accessibility to her infant, attachment and bonding take place during a time when both mother and infant are most receptive. Klaus and Kennell[21] have demonstrated that a sensitive period for attachment exists shortly after birth. Barring excessive medication of the mother during delivery, a newborn will normally be in an alert state for at least an hour following birth. If the mother has her baby with her during this sensitive period, she will spend a significant amount of time gazing *en face* into her infant's eyes, touching and stroking.

The potential for positive feedback and reciprocal reinforcement between them lies in the infant's remarkable perceptual and sensory abilities at birth: hearing, seeing, smelling, and tasting. Considering the infant's state of readiness for human interaction, hospital routines that promote separation are usually inappropriate, even detrimental to the early mother-infant relationship.

Certain behaviors in the attachment process appear to be species-specific. One is eye-to-eye contact, which has led to our recognition of the infant's ability to see immediately after birth, particularly objects 20 to 25 cm (8 to 10 inches) away—about the distance between the mother's and infant's eyes when he is in her arms[40] (Fig. 4-1). A second is voice pitch, which can be noted when the mother (as well as hospital staff) instinctively speaks to a newborn in a high-frequency range or falsetto voice.[24] A third is the progressive touching phenomenon in which a mother explores her newborn's extremities with her fingertips, then rapidly moves to the baby's arms and legs, and finally caresses the trunk with the palm of her hand.[33]

As attachment becomes established, the newborn is observed to move his arms and legs in rhythm to the cadences of the mother's voice in a synchrony that may be the foundation for later speech.[7] Such interaction is commonly known as entrainment, and its effects carry over into later life.

Several researchers[9,29] have found that children who have minimal separation from their mother after birth have higher levels of parental interaction and personal health in later years. Attachment can certainly take place if a mother does not breastfeed; however, when she breastfeeds, the opportunities for attachment or bonding to take place are enhanced by the frequent touching, holding, and eye-to-eye contact. Although unconfirmed, it is theorized that breastfeeding affects the attachment process because of the higher prolactin levels in the lactating mother. Certainly, the frequency of subjective verbal responses by mothers who state they "feel closer" to their breastfed child merits serious consideration. Rooming-in should be recognized as a valuable adjunct to the beginning breastfeeding relationship because it facilitates "on-demand" feeding and promotes the attachment process.

O'Connor et al.[30] have demonstrated that parental inadequacy, which not infrequently leads to child abuse, is significantly lowered when mother and infant have early,

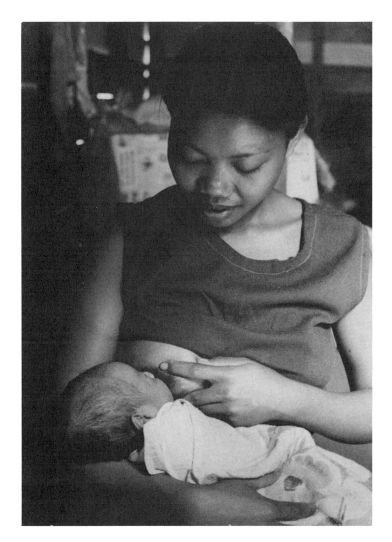

Fig. 4-1. Breastfeeding facilitates direct eye-to-eye contact. (Courtesy WHO, J. Abcede.)

continuous contact. Tables 4-1 and 4-2 show moderate to marked differences in the incidence of accidents and selected illnesses between the rooming-in and control children studies during postpartum follow-up.

Recently the routine instillation of 1% silver nitrate ophthalmic solution in the eyes of the neonate has come under question. Because of its irritating effects, it may interfere with early eye-to-eye contact between the mother and her infant. A delay of up to 30 minutes in instilling the medication does not appear to be harmful and should be routine whenever silver nitrate is to be used. Other less irritating medications are just as effective in the prevention of gonorrheal conjunctivitis and probably should be used instead of silver nitrate. In the Morbidity and Mortality Report of January 18, 1979, the Centers for Disease Control in Atlanta recommended the use of tetracycline or erythromycin

TABLE 4-1

Accidents and selected illnesses

	Rooming-in children	Control children
Total with data	134	143
Infections		
No. of children infected	9	15
Total no. of episodes	10	22
Accidents		
No. of children involved	16	26
Total no. of accidents	20	33
Exanthematous disease	0	5*
Hospitalizations		
No. of children involved	16	23
Total no. of hospitalizations	19	25
No. with gastroenteritis with dehydration	0	3

From O'Connor, S.M., et al.: Pediatrics **66**:176, 1980.
*P < .05.

TABLE 4-2

Comparison of parenting

	Rooming-in children	Control children
Families with parenting inadequacy	2	10*
Substantial	1	9†
Minor	1	1
Children hospitalized with parenting inadequacy	1	8*
Children referred to Protective Services for maltreatment	1	5
Children with nonparent caretakers	0	5*

From O'Connor, S.M., et al.: Pediatrics **66**:176, 1980.
*P < .05.
†P < .02.

ophthalmic ointment. Since some state laws require the use of silver nitrate, changes will ultimately need to be made in the statutes to permit the use of antibiotic prophylaxis.

If there are no intervening complications, the first breastfeeding should take place immediately after delivery. After the airway has been cleared, the infant, wrapped in a blanket, can be placed in his mother's arms to breastfeed. The placenta is normally expelled soon after birth, often before the infant is put to breast for the first time; but if a delay occurs, breastfeeding will usually hasten detachment and expulsion. With the mother propped on her side, a pillow at her back for support, the baby may suckle in the delivery room, and the limitation of a narrow delivery table can be overcome. When the father is present, he can help maintain the positioning of mother and infant and share the enjoyment of these first moments together.

It is not uncommon for newborns to suck minimally at this time; frequently they only lick or nuzzle the nipple. Nevertheless this interaction between mother and infant is advantageous in that it stimulates uterine contractions and may promote colonization of harmless bacteria on the nipple pad and possibly protect the infant from the pathogenic bacteria[21]—a pleasant method of infection control. Explaining this to the mother and telling her not to worry will help to avoid the anxiety she may have if her infant is reticent to take hold of the nipple immediately.

Sometimes the first breastfeeding takes place after the mother and her newborn are transferred to the recovery area or to the mother's room. Wherever it may be, if the mother is awake and oriented, it is best that she, not the nurse, put the baby to breast. As a facilitator of self-care, the nurse is there to guide and assist her. If the mother is breastfeeding for the first time, the nurse can be of significant help to her; on the other hand, if the mother is experienced in breastfeeding, the nurse has an opportunity to observe and learn from her.

There is a demonstrable relationship between success in breastfeeding and early initiation of feeding[20]; for the mother who has not breastfed before, the first several feedings have an imprinting effect. A positive, satisfying experience is important for the development of optimal suckling patterns by the baby and for the mother's own self-esteem. An unhurried and caring approach helps to establish the rapport necessary for the nurse to be an effective health-care partner. Also, it is important to explain to the first-time mother that breastfeeding is not as automatic for the mother as the suckling and rooting reflexes are for her baby. Yet the experience is new to the baby too, and for both the first few times at breast offer an opportunity for each to learn from the other. Following are some suggestions that may optimize the beginning breastfeeding experience:

1. Arrange for privacy. Shut the door or close the curtains around the bed if the mother wishes. Then advise her to cleanse her hands with soap and water or a cleansing wipe.
2. Since first-time mothers often find it easier to breastfeed when sitting, suggest that the mother sit up, either in bed or in a comfortable chair with low arms. At the first feeding, arrange a pillow on her lap or under her arm and shoulder on the side on which the baby is to nurse. The high Fowler's position in bed is recommended following a cesarean birth or if the mother has small breasts. The experienced breastfeeder, however, may prefer to lie on her side, having learned it is possible to relax more completely in this position.
3. Help to position the baby so that his head is snuggled securely in the antecubital fossa of the mother's arm and rotated slightly toward her so that eye contact can be maintained. By cradling the infant's thigh or buttocks with her arm, the mother can control the baby's position and can move him with ease.
4. Suggest that the mother support her breast with her hand: her thumb should be just above the areola, fingers below (Fig. 4-2). In this position the mother is able to guide her nipple in any direction and place more of the areola into the baby's mouth. She can easily maintain the infant's airway by pushing her thumb inward against her breast, as necessary.
5. Explain that her infant should be offered both breasts at each feeding to stimulate

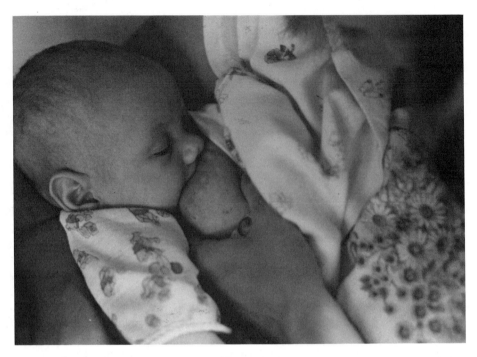

Fig. 4-2. Supporting her breast with her hand, the mother guides it into the infant's mouth.

the supply-demand response. The duration of feedings may be limited if the baby or mother is especially tired or weak; otherwise it should be flexible.

6. Help the mother to break the infant's suction on the nipple by placing her finger in the corner of his mouth. Then she can gently remove him from the breast.

7. Remind the mother to alternate the breast first offered to the infant at successive feedings.

Should feeding times be limited?

In learning self-care skills, breastfeeding mothers sometimes are advised to limit the amount of suckling time in the first few days after birth to prevent sore nipples. Studies have shown, however, that instead of preventing soreness, strict time limitations only delay soreness so that, instead of occurring in the hospital setting, the peak of soreness comes several days after the mother and infant return home.[39] This fact, coupled with the present short hospital stay, has encouraged the erroneous belief that severe restriction of feeding time actually prevents sore nipples.

Strict limitations of the duration of feeding can have definite negative effects. In the early feedings after birth, the let-down reflex may not occur for as long as 3 or more minutes after the feeding begins; following the "learning" period, the let-down usually begins within the first 30 seconds after the baby is put to breast or sometimes even sooner. If feeding time is rigidly limited, let-down may not take place. When this happens, the baby is prevented from receiving the full benefit of the available colostrum in the first few days and later may not receive an adequate supply of milk. Also, the fluid remaining in the ducts and ductules is prone to promote engorgement. Engorgement, which makes the breast hard and nipples inelastic, may render sucking impossible and set in motion the beginning of a cyclic pattern for lactation failure. Rather than limiting the length of feeding, changing the infant's position at breast and increasing the frequency of feeding are more effective measures. Routines that encourage unrestricted frequency and duration of breastfeeding promote optimal lactation and help prevent later problems.

Faulty positioning and suckling patterns

Faulty suckling patterns and improper positioning during breastfeeding should be identified early and corrected as soon as possible. Inadequate suction from faulty sucking or positioning can lead to a variety of problems, especially sore nipples, low weight gain, and frustration for both the mother and her baby. Uncorrected, the problems may ultimately bring about bottle-feeding for the baby and a sense of failure on the mother's part.

It has been hypothesized that faulty suckling patterns can be established if the fetus sucks his thumb in utero; occasionally a tight frenulum is at fault and can easily be corrected surgically. More often, faulty suckling patterns are the result of nipple confusion as an aftermath of bottle-feeding during hospitalization. Nipple confusion may follow the use of even a few supplemental bottles for the normal newborn. The suckling patterns of bottle-feeding and breastfeeding differ significantly, as described in Chapter 2, and some infants simply are unable to make the switch. In bottle-feeding, the milk flows quickly and easily without much active sucking effort, and the baby places his tongue anteriorly against the tip of the nipple to control the flow. The negative pressure exerted by the bottle-feeding infant is far less than that of the breastfeeder; in breastfeeding, a threefold action[13] of suction, chewing, and compression by the posterior part of the tongue and lips forces the milk from the breast.

If the baby is having feeding problems, an assessment for faulty sucking should be made in the following manner:

1. Inspect the baby's cheeks while he nurses. Inadequate suction will cause the cheeks to draw excessively inward. Then determine if the baby is ingesting milk by observing his swallowing.
2. While the infant has the nipple in his mouth, palpate inside the mouth to locate the tongue. (In faulty sucking it will often be curled backwards instead of being placed beneath the nipple.) If placed correctly, the tongue should be visible when the baby's lips are slightly pushed to the side.
3. Listen for a somewhat noisy "drawing" sound of milk being extracted from the breast during sucking. A soft "clicking" sound is indicative of faulty positioning.
4. Test the amount of suction by pulling the breast from the baby's mouth. If suction is inadequate, the breast can easily be pulled away.

Faulty sucking patterns can be corrected by persistently depressing the baby's tongue immediately before the mother's nipple is inserted. Some mothers have successfully retaught babies to suck by judicious, short-term use of an orthodontic rubber nipple, such as the NUK Orthodontic Nipple, between breastfeedings.

The possibility of improper positioning of the baby on the breast should be considered along with faulty sucking, since the two are often related. Sore nipples frequently follow improper positioning and may help in the diagnosis of faulty positioning. Typically, soreness develops in one of the two areas of the breast as described in Fig. 4-3. An antecedent to this problem is positioning the infant's mouth on the nipple rather than on the areola. By tenuously hanging on to the nipple, the baby exerts considerable pressure on the skin at the base of the nipple, causing tissue breakdown and the ensuing sore "stripes." The problem can be relieved by the mother's pulling her baby close to her so that he can more easily grasp the areola as well as the nipple. Also positioning the infant's head slightly backwards will enable the nipple to touch the roof of the baby's mouth and permit his lower jaw and tongue to "milk" the nipple more easily. Once the positional problem is corrected, the mother's nipples should begin to heal within 24 to 48 hours.

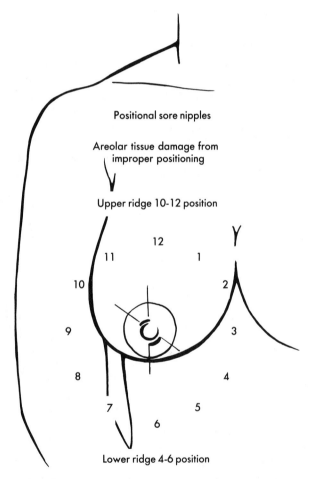

Positional sore nipples

Areolar tissue damage from improper positioning

Upper ridge 10-12 position

Lower ridge 4-6 position

Fig. 4-3. Imagine the face of a clock superimposed on right breast. Soreness usually develops in crescent around perimeter of nipple at 10 to 12 o'clock position and below perimeter of nipple at 4 to 6 o'clock position. With left breast, maximal potential for soreness is, similarly, at 12 to 2 o'clock and 6 to 8 o'clock positions.

EARLY POSTNATAL PERIOD
Engorgement

The most common breastfeeding problem encountered in the hospital is engorgement. As earlier established, engorgement generally occurs on the second or third postpartum day but may be present even sooner, especially in multiparous women.

Engorgement is much less pronounced when an alert and healthy neonate finds that his mother's breast is accessible to him at all times. Therefore the importance of rooming-in cannot be overemphasized. With centralized nurseries and scheduled feedings in hospitals in the United States, we frequently see severely engorged breasts. Nursing interventions, including the application of warm moist heat and the use of mild analgesics and a snug supportive bra, are effective treatment modalities for the breastfeeding mother. A more constructive approach, however, is prevention through early, regular, unscheduled breastfeeding.

Severe engorgement is extremely painful. Sometimes the tissue around the nipple and areola becomes so taut that the baby is totally unable to grasp the nipple. As a result, the newborn draws away from the breast and cries in frustration. The nurse should assist the mother in expressing or pumping out some of her breastmilk to soften the areola before she attempts to put the baby to breast. The milk thus collected is not intended to be saved and given in a bottle; instead, the goal is to enable the infant to suckle directly at his mother's breast. Use of a nipple shield for engorgement should be strongly discouraged, since it generally leads to continuing engorgement and an unsatisfied infant unable to obtain a sufficient quantity of milk through the shield. When expressing milk, immediately before putting the baby to breast it is useful to elicit the letdown reflex so that milk is spurting or dripping from the nipple as the baby begins to feed.

Severe engorgement may occasionally lead to a plugged duct, mastitis, or even a breast abscess. If a plugged duct develops, the mother may obtain relief by taking a hot shower and massaging her breasts from well behind the plugged area toward the nipple while the water continues to flow over her breast. Following this effort, the baby should *immediately* be put to breast. The sucking of the hungry infant will likely dislodge the plug and allow the milk to flow normally from the affected duct.

A higher frequency of plugged ducts has been reported to occur during the winter. The reason for this is currently not clear, although it may be related to the constricting effects of winter clothing. The phenomenon bears investigation.

Some physicians prescribe a low-dose estrogen for severe engorgement. A new nonestrogenic agent, bromocriptine (Parlodel), acts as a dopamine receptor antagonist on the anterior pituitary gland and is sometimes employed to inhibit lactation; it has occasionally been used as a one-time dose for relief of severe engorgement in the breastfeeding mother. As soon as the baby can grasp the nipple, nipple stimulation overcomes the inhibitory effect of the drug.

Although engorgement is generally looked on as a problem of the first week of breastfeeding, it may occasionally occur later as a result of untimely separation of mother and baby. For this reason, instruction in self-care should encourage the mother to avoid separation during the early weeks. Even if the baby or mother should be hospitalized, it is in the best interest of both that they be admitted together, or at least for one to have ready access to the other as soon and often as possible.

Recognizing that severe engorgement is generally preventable, the experienced nurse will encourage the mother to breastfeed regularly and frequently, prevent fatigue and separation from the neonate, and avoid letting the baby suck on rubber nipples of any sort, especially before the breastfeeding relationship is well established.

Breast pain

Among the physical complaints that the lactating woman may occasionally experience are painful breasts. During the first days and even weeks, she may have discomfort or perhaps pain in her breasts during feedings. The nurse may assure her that this is not unusual. It is frequently related to the incomplete let-down that may need some time before functioning with complete efficiency. As the mother learns to relax better and becomes more self-confident, she will generally find that the pain will last only briefly and finally not occur at all. Until then a mild analgesic or a glass of beer or wine may be helpful.

Another less common kind of breast discomfort is a deep, pervasive pain (sometimes described as "shooting" pains) following a feeding. This appears to be the result of a sudden refilling of the breasts and may be expected to disappear when the entire mechanism of lactation has reached equilibrium. Reports of this kind of pain indicate that it may occur intermittently for a period between a week and a month, usually decreasing in frequency as time goes by.

Other possible causes of breast pain are a forceful let-down, adhesions from earlier breast surgery, an untreated breast infection, tension, an uncomfortable or ineffective position for feeding, muscle pain following labor and delivery, and even an ill-fitting bra.

Suggested remedies often include the use of relaxation exercises, supporting the baby or the mother's arm with pillows, an application of warm wet packs to the breasts before nursing, and the use of a heating pad behind the back during feeding. The possibility of an infection, an ill-fitting bra, or an uncomfortable chair or couch should, of course, be considered. Finally, very often the reassurance and support that a knowledgeable and caring nurse can so effectively provide may make the difference between optimism in the midst of bearable discomfort or frustration over a new and frightening sensation, which may be perceived as excruciating pain.

Leaking

A frequent annoyance in the early weeks is the leaking of milk from the breasts. The light, sound, or even the thought of her baby may condition a let-down response in a mother. Some mothers of premature infants who use an electric pump report a let-down when they hear the sound of a motor starting. When a let-down occurs unexpectedly or at an inappropriate time, the nurse may suggest that the mother fold her arms across her breasts and press them gently but firmly against the chest wall. Applying pressure with finger or thumb directly over the nipples also helps to stop the outflow of milk.

SELF-CARE FOR CESAREAN MOTHERS

To the mother who goes into labor prepared for a vaginal birth, a cesarean delivery generally brings major disappointment. For months she has looked forward to the onset of labor as the beginning of a great event in which she, the central figure in the event, will bring about a veritable miracle. Aided and supported by her partner, she will deliver their child, their unique creation.

Already well into labor when the first hint of a cesarean section comes, the mother is nearly unable to cope with this threat to her role, to her plans—in fact, to her very self-hood. Her mind and body cry out against the intrusion of outside forces that seem designed to negate her. After months of hard preparatory work what has happened to her dreams, her anticipation of that beautiful moment when her baby's sounds are first heard, his body first beheld?

The mother who knows early or discovers along the way in her pregnancy that a cesarean section will be her method of delivery has time to come to terms with her situation. When a cesarean section is planned in advance, the office nurse should put the mother in touch with a local support group for cesarean births and with a local breastfeeding group. Through relationships formed in these groups come emotional support and the opportunity to learn to deal with the situation and set a course for the future. Such groups offer films and discussion sessions and provide time for informal sharing of experiences and know-how. Many women welcome hearing from others that this mode of birth will not affect their ability to breastfeed or have a healthy, happy baby.

But it is the mother whose plans are abruptly and so devastatingly changed after labor has begun with whom the hospital nurse must be prepared to cope. It is in this mother that the nurse must recognize the depth of anguish, fear, and loss of sense of self-worth, both before and after the baby's birth. It is for her that the nurse must be ready to exercise her greatest human relations skills.

Almost as soon as a cesarean section is contemplated, and surely when it seems to be a likelihood, the nurse must provide an atmosphere of positive encouragement about the outcome. The mother will undoubtedly be concerned about her own safety, the safety of the baby, and many other aspects of the unknown. If she planned to breastfeed or even entertained the idea that she might, she can be reassured that this, at least, can be one unchanging part of her childbearing experience. She may, indeed, continue with her earlier expectations to breastfeed. The nurse may give her additional encouragement about breastfeeding by sharing with her the knowledge that the breastfeeding woman—delivering vaginally or by cesarean section—frequently recovers more rapidly than if she bottle-feeds.

The nurse should talk with both parents about the expected cesarean section, encouraging the father toward involvement in decision making and support. Often it is necessary to help the couple focus on the importance of the procedure for the infant's health and safety so as to alleviate the personal disappointment that they feel.

It is difficult to be a supportive nurse in such situations. It is far easier to check the monitor and chart, execute routine preoperative procedures, and neglect to relate intimately and compassionately to the client. Easier—yes; but the opportunity to assuage the fears of the anxious mother will not be missed by the caring nurse.

Constructive interventions abound. In most hospitals the father may now stay at his wife's side throughout the delivery, supporting and encouraging her. Many physicians offer a range of choice in anesthetics, and the infant may be delivered while the mother is awake and aware of all that is being done. In some cases, even a modified Leboyer birth is possible. Rooming-in is as much an option for most women who have had a cesarean section (''cesarean mothers'') as for those who have vaginal deliveries. Nursing on the delivery table or at least in the recovery room is also common when both mother and baby are in good condition after the delivery.

Continued explanations, even during surgery if the mother is awake, are a ''must.'' Immediate showing of the baby, even to a groggy mother, is essential to begin the bonding process; and the first breastfeeding should come at the earliest possible safe moment. Before the spinal anesthesia wears off she feels better than she likely will in the next 72 hours. At this point, while she is free of pain and excited about the baby, comes the opportune time to initiate breastfeeding. All the foregoing activities have a significant effect in lowering the mother's (and father's) anxieties and in increasing their beginning attachment to the baby.

''From the waist up, I felt like a success; from the waist down, a failure!'' In these few words one mother summed up the feelings of guilt, frustration, and loss of self-esteem that most cesarean mothers experience to some degree. The concerned nurse recognizes this and makes every attempt possible to encourage a healthy resolution of these nearly universal feelings.

As with a vaginal delivery, the circumstances that surround a cesarean birth can contribute enormously to a good beginning of breastfeeding. If life-threatening problems are not present, the choice of medication is often one that leaves the mother alert and helps her to be a real participant in the birth. As indicated earlier, the father's presence at the birth provides much needed support for the mother, reduces her stress, and better enables her to focus on the baby. When the baby is put to breast on the delivery table or in the recovery room, the father can arrange the pillow to make the mother comfortable or can, himself, be the support that she leans against on the narrow table or bed.

The nurse should not assume that the cesarean mother is too uncomfortable or tired to breastfeed but should individually assess each client's condition. The infant's condition, too, must be evaluated on an individual basis; however, even babies who are receiving nothing by mouth can usually tolerate the small amount of colostrum available during the first few hours after birth.[14]

If circumstances do not allow for immediate breastfeeding, the baby should be taken to the mother as soon as possible after the conditions of both are stabilized. Because of the physical and psychologic advantages to mother and child, no unnecessary delay in putting the baby to breast should occur.

Once the mother returns to her room from the recovery room, it is desirable that the infant be with her as much as possible. If both are in good condition, rooming-in is ideal. It offers the best opportunity for the mother and infant to relate to each other and to initiate breastfeeding. The infant may profitably spend a great deal of time in the mother's bed, and the mother can be helped to learn how to breastfeed and move her infant with minimal discomfort. Once the anesthesia wears off, lateral Sims' position is appropriate for comfortable breastfeeding. The mother can be positioned with her back supported by the guardrail or a firm pillow and with her abdomen supported and protected by a bath blanket. The infant should lie on his side facing the mother, thereby making it easy for her to snug his buttocks in toward her body and position his mouth near her nipple. As she cradles her infant's head in the arm that rests on the bed, her other hand is free to offer the breast. Frantz describes placing the baby to breast as follows:

> The mother now pulls baby toward her breast, using the arm she has around him so that his open mouth bypasses the nipple and manipulates only the areola. (Or she can gently roll her body toward him.) Baby's nose should barely touch her breast. If he gets too close, her thumb is conveniently there to press the breast gently away from his nose.[14]

It is important to establish the mother's independence as soon as possible. The nurse can help her learn to transfer the infant from one breast to the other without assistance, by following Frantz's suggestions:

> The mother's first step is to inch her way from the Sims position to the supine position, holding the baby close to her [Fig. 4-4, A]. With baby held prone one her chest, she then raises her leg for leverage to push herself slowly to the other side of the bed. At this point she can move the pillow that was supporting her back to the other guardrail. Inching her buttocks toward the other side of the bed is easy for the mother. Baby remains quite secure on her chest [Fig. 4-4, B]. Sometimes the baby will even burp while in this position, because of the pressure of the breast against his stomach. Mother lowers baby onto bed at her side once she's moved her buttocks. Then, using the guardrail for leverage, she pushes her upper torso toward the other side of the bed, positioning herself on her side. Once in position, she readjusts her pillows and bath blanket with her free hand (she may need help to reach some of them) [Fig. 4-4, C], then puts the baby to her breast as before.[14]

Some mothers prefer Fowler's position for breastfeeding, and advice about position may depend on the locus of the incision. By the fourth day, however, most mothers can sit upright and prefer the high Fowler's position for breastfeeding. In this position, at least three pillows are needed for comfort (Fig. 4-5): *(A)* one under the arm that holds the infant, *(B)* another over the abdomen to protect her incision and to raise the infant to the height of the breast, and *(C)* a third to support her head and shoulders comfortably. Her legs are flexed slightly and braced by her feet resting on an overturned padded washbasin or other footrest. A small pillow or folded bath blanket can be used to help support her legs, but any direct pressure under her legs should be avoided to prevent thrombophlebitis. An alternative is placing the infant in a "football" hold to lessen pressure on the abdomen. While recognizing the early pain of the cesarean mother, the nurse should remind her that most say the third day is the worst. The pain from the incision noticeably subsides by the fourth day, and all activities, including breastfeeding, will be much easier.

Information and techniques that apply to the breastfeeding woman who has delivered her baby vaginally are equally valid for the cesarean mother. Her baby, too, will feed more frequently than a bottle-fed counterpart because of the quick and easy digestibility of breastmilk. Feeding every 2 hours or so will bring in the milk sooner and make supplements unnecessary. If mother and baby are separated for more than a day, the client should be helped to stimulate milk production either by use of a pump or by manual expression at 3- to 4-hour intervals until the baby can go to breast.

A good diet is as important for the cesarean mother as for other nursing mothers. With many doctors, nothing by mouth (NPO) orders are gradually giving way to early

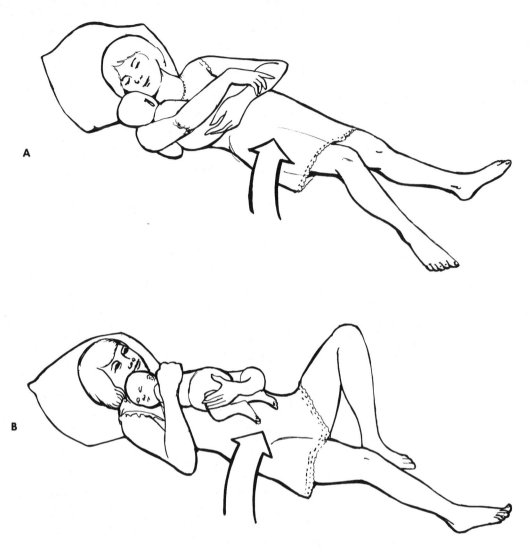

Fig. 4-4. Transferring infant to other breast following a cesarean birth. (Concept from F. Frantz and B.A. Kalmen.)

postoperative encouragement toward a high protein intake. Early feeding and ambulation reduce intestinal gas and cramping. Additionally, protein-rich foods (liquid at first, becoming solid when tolerated) provide the necessary nutrients for rapid tissue healing and plentiful milk.

Parents are often anxious to know about the probability of a cesarean section with future births. The dictum "Once a cesarean, always a cesarean" is no longer valid. Recent studies[27,35] on subsequent vaginal births after a cesarean section indicate that they are being done safely in many areas of the country. Often attempting a vaginal birth is less risky than automatically performing another cesarean section.

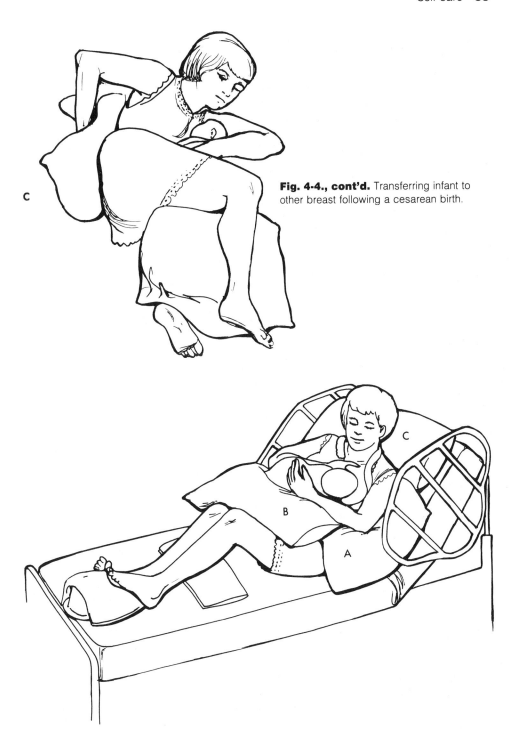

C

Fig. 4-4., cont'd. Transferring infant to other breast following a cesarean birth.

Fig. 4-5. Comfortable position for breastfeeding especially for women who have delivered by cesarean section. (Concept from F. Frantz and B.A. Kalmen.)

Before leaving the subject of the cesarean mother, a few words should be said about medications. Most drugs that the mother is given in normal therapeutic doses will not produce a significant negative effect on the baby. For guidelines consult the drug information in Chapter 6. Also, an excellent drug list is available in *Breastfeeding: A Guide for the Medical Profession* by Lawrence.[26]

Most of all, during the early days after a cesarean delivery, the breastfeeding mother needs an optimistic attitude, emotional and physical support, and many explanations about the value of colostrum, of breastfeeding, and of close physical proximity to her baby. The nurse is in a favorable position to respond to all of these needs.

TWINS

Many nurses who read this text will remember when breastfeeding twins was considered unthinkable, and mothers of twins were discouraged from breastfeeding or were told supplements were absolutely necessary by physicians, nurses, and relatives. Now it is taken for granted that women can breastfeed more than one infant, usually without supplementation. Since women are endowed with two breasts, it is questionable if there ever should have been any doubt about it in the first place.

Although having twins in itself does not create a breastfeeding problem, over half of twin births are premature, and breastfeeding is necessarily delayed if one or both infants must be transferred to the intensive care unit after birth. If well born, both infants should begin feedings shortly after birth and feed frequently on demand thereafter to ensure a rapid buildup of the quantity of milk demanded by two children. In counseling the breastfeeding mother of twins there are special implications for diet, managing feedings, and attachment, although the same principles of lactation such as supply and demand are as applicable to twins as to a single birth.

The simultaneous breastfeeding of twins saves time. When two infants are at breast simultaneously, the milk that would normally be lost in the let-down of the contralateral breast is available to the second twin. When two infants awaken at the same time with cries of hunger, they should both be put to breast, and the mother will initially need assistance (Fig. 4-6).

Sore nipples are a frequent problem for mothers of twins. Alternating between the usual frontal position and the football hold during the first few weeks helps to prevent this by distributing the areas of pressure on the breasts. As the infants grow, it becomes more difficult for the mother to hold both babies on her lap, and she soon learns to experiment with different feeding positions. Some of the time, too, only one infant is hungry, and she feeds each singly. It is best, however, that she feed each infant on both breasts and not favor one breast for one infant. The sucking patterns of infants, even identical twins, vary, and each infant needs the visual stimulation and exercise of both eyes that alternating breasts provides. An excellent publication[16] containing illustrations of feeding positions and a wealth of practical information on the care of twins should be made available to the mother.

When two infants are totally breastfed, the lactating mother of twins is producing over a liter of milk per day in the first few weeks and approximately a liter and one-half in the following months. To keep pace nutritionally, she needs nearly 1000 extra calories daily. Unfortunately, extremely busy and tired mothers of twins tend to grab a

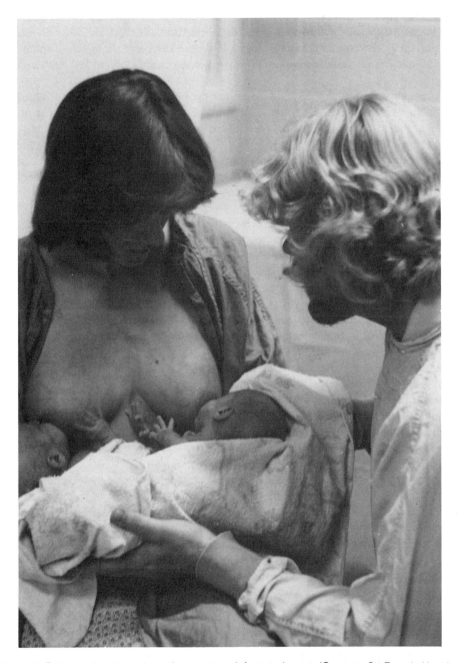

Fig. 4-6. Father assists in putting twin premature infants to breast. (Courtesy St. Francis Hospital, Wichita, Kan.)

bite on the run and are therefore at risk for nutritional depletion, unless they are conscientious about their diet. Exhaustion affects appetite and milk supply, so help with housework for the mothers of twins is almost mandatory. If there are other children to care for, help becomes even more essential. Before discharge from the hospital both parents should know this and make appropriate arrangements for the first few weeks at home.

Although a mother may be unaware of it at the time, it takes longer to attach to two infants than to one infant. Monotropy, the tendency to form a close attachment to only one infant at a time, may account for mothers' interest in dressing their infants alike and choosing rhyming names for the infants. It enables them to perceive their infants as a unit instead of singly.[15] Still, the bonding process is both slower and more complicated with twins.

PUERPERIUM AND BEYOND

Both mother and baby profit when breastfeeding is continued beyond the puerperium. The infant's nutritional needs are best met by breastmilk, and his psychologic needs are most adequately answered by one consistently present and available person. The woman, too, profits physically from the completion of the maternity cycle of pregnancy—birth—breastfeeding. Her uterus returns to its prepregnant state more rapidly when she breastfeeds, and she derives psychologic satisfactions from the certain knowledge that she is uniquely, irreplaceably important to her child. In addition, the bonding that began at birth is further enhanced by the frequent holding, cuddling, and skin-to-skin contact between mother and child.

A survey of the literature reveals a panorama of advantages in continuing breastfeeding beyond the early days after birth. Decreased morbidity is among the most important of these advantages. Breastfed infants are generally healthier than those who are formula-fed, and allergies, gastrointestinal ailments, respiratory problems, contagious diseases, and human errors are all lessened by breastfeeding.

Early days after birth

Increasingly today, more and more parents are electing to have their babies at home or in birthing centers from which they go home within a few hours. This facilitates an early adjustment and provides an excellent milieu for a successful start in breastfeeding. For the breastfeeding couple who were hospitalized after birth and separated during the hospital stay, the early days at home may be attended by numerous, often unnecessary stresses. But even the mother and baby who have been together from the beginning occasionally encounter problems.

Among the most common early concerns of mothers is the frequency with which the baby breastfeeds. The nurse can prepare the breastfeeding mother to deal with this common worry before she leaves the hospital by developing and ultilizing a discharge planning sheet like the one in Chapter 5 for teaching self-care skills. Discharge teaching should explain that the breastfeeding baby needs to feed more frequently in the early weeks, often eight to twelve times a day or even more. As a part of her discharge teaching, the nurse should further explain that since the infant's stomach is small and breastmilk is so readily digestible, he can rarely be expected to go more than a couple of hours between feedings. Most experienced mothers neither know nor care how many times their babies nurse in a 24-hour period, but it is all too often a matter for worry with the new mother.

An inexperienced mother may be unaware that there are days when a baby needs to feed even more frequently than every 2 hours and that this occurs for many different reasons. A common reason for the infant's increased frequency of feeding is simply that he has an increased need for calories. The infant, therefore, may seem to feed almost constantly for a day or two to build up his mother's milk supply and then will revert to fewer feedings. These variances are normal and not an indication she is losing her milk.

Mothers are often very concerned about being tired or tense, and most babies react to maternal tension by fretting and crying. If the mother responds quickly to the baby's cry or to his demand to feed, both relax better. Frequently the infant responds negatively to a mother's overworking or eating improperly; as a consequence, the mother who slows down her activities and begins to eat regular, nutritious meals will see a rapid change in her infant's behavior and her own exhaustion. By reassessing her own life-style and making adjustments that such an evaluation calls for, the mother frequently changes the fretting, apparently colicky baby into a more satisfied and happy little one. Mothers should know that problems of this nature are not unique to the breastfed baby; they may—and, indeed, often do—occur in the bottle-fed infant as well.

When possible, the breastfeeding mother should plan in advance to meet her increased need for rest. Discussions with the mother about putting her own and her baby's needs first and streamlining the care of her house should also be a part of discharge planning for self-care. She should be encouraged to relax, nap when the infant is asleep, and let others take care of house, laundry, and cooking while she devotes herself to her baby. A week or two of making herself and her infant the top priority will yield dividends in the months ahead. Mothers are all too often concerned about the appearance of the house and the welcoming of visitors at a time when they should be cementing their own and close family members' relationships with the new baby.

Sleep

For the new mother loss of sleep often presents a problem, more because she worries about it than because of the lost sleep itself. There are no studies that show that it is essential to have 8 hours of unbroken sleep each night; in fact, though we generally are not aware of it, all sleep has a rhythmic pattern, and most adults normally awaken a number of times during the night in response to their biologic rhythm. Physical rest, even without falling asleep, renews one's energies, and it is partly for this reason that we encourage mothers to lie down to breastfeed and to take the baby to bed with them at night. It may help to suggest, also, that a mother refrain from looking at the clock (which merely serves to awaken her more) each time the baby breastfeeds.

Safety while traveling

A long neglected aspect of infant and child care has recently received much attention from professionals and lay persons alike. Most accidents that lead to the death of children over a year old happen in a car. A mother's arms are the perfect place for a baby—

but not in a moving vehicle. The force of a crash can easily wrest a baby who is not mechanically restrained from the arms of the person holding him. As part of her predischarge guidance counseling the nurse should advise the baby's parents to install a crash-tested carseat in their own vehicle and use it for every trip, including the first one home from the hospital and future short jaunts to the store or in their immediate neighborhood. Such advice has become an integral part of a car safety campaign of the American Academy of Pediatrics.

The breastfeeding mother may wonder if it is possible to feed her baby in a carseat. It is, of course. Far better, however, would be to feed the baby before starting the trip and to stop along the way when baby wants to breastfeed. Feeding breaks, especially on longer trips, may coincide with rest room stops and provide a welcome opportunity to stretch. The recommendation to get out of the car and walk around for a few minutes out of every hour for one's own comfort and health while traveling is all too often ignored; the breastfeeding mother now has an excellent excuse.

Some women find it possible to lean over and feed a baby strapped in an infant safety seat that faces backwards (Fig. 4-7); many find it less than satisfactory but better than having an unhappy baby. In an emergency when for some reason the driver might consider it unwise to stop, the mother may attempt to breastfeed her baby in this manner until a safe stopping place can be found. If the mother is the driver, however, it would be very difficult to justify advising her to breastfeed and drive. The distractions simply are too great to warrant this, and the lives of everyone in the car would be endangered. The mother's thoughtul preplanning should prevent such a crisis from occurring. Both the nurse concerned with discharge planning and the community health nurse who visits in the home can be helpful in instructing the mother in self-care techniques to avoid problems of this sort.

Clothing

On discharge from the hospital or when the community health nurse visits at home the first time, the new mother may need instruction about comfortable and convenient clothing for nursing. Two-piece dresses as well as skirts or slacks with blouses are preferable. Tops can be pulled up from the waist instead of opened from the neck down so that the baby can feed unobtrusively. Bras are often a matter for discussion. Mothers should be encouraged to purchase bras with cups as near to 100% cotton as possible. Bras should never contain plastic liners, straps should not be of elasticized material, and cup closures should be easily managed with one hand. For the mother with average or small breasts, middle-priced nursing bras that close in back and have snap fastners or Velcro on the cups are usually quite adequate. Nursing bras that hook in front between the cups are generally unsatisfactory because they afford too great exposure and too little support. Many stores, including Sears, Love in Bloom Maternity Shops, and large and small department stores that carry the Mary Jane Company's garments, generally have good assortments of high-quality, comfortable nursing bras.

The mother with large breasts frequently has difficulty finding a comfortable bra. When breastfeeding, she needs one with an extra wide back with hooked fasteners to compensate for the weight of heavy breasts. Encourage her to avoid bras with underwires, since the constriction and compression of milk ducts caused by wires may lead to a plugged duct or mastitis.

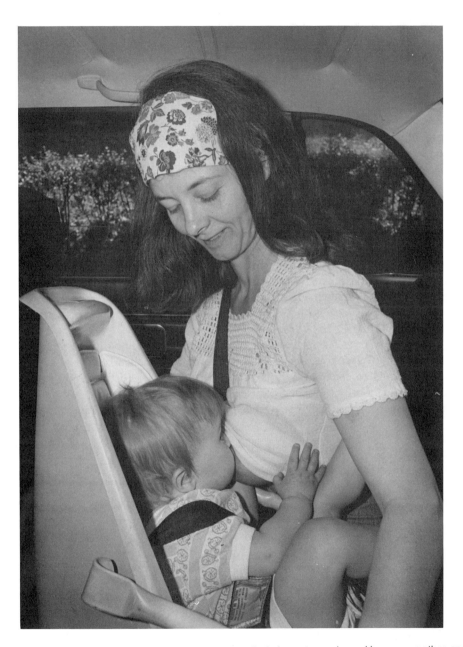

Fig. 4-7. Best place for breastfeeding on a motor trip is in a stopped car. However, mother and child *can* breastfeed as passengers in moving car with mother in shoulder belt and child in secured infant seat. (Courtesy La Leche League International.)

Nutrition

A dietary history and nutritional evaluation are important clinical tools for nursing assessment and teaching self-care to the lactating woman. Her nutritional status when initiating breastfeeding is the result of her lifetime nutrition and is probably at least as important during lactation as in pregnancy. Although lack of an adequate quantity of food is frequently a problem in the less developed countries, in the United States, where food is generally plentiful, quality is frequently a problem. In the adolescent this is all too often the case.

Certain basic information is necessary for the nurse to present in teaching the mother. The goal of nutritional self-care teaching by nurses is to meet the demands of the breast-feeding infant without significantly depleting the mother's own reserves. The lactating woman needs only 500 to 600 extra calories per day. This should include 24 additional grams of protein. Increased fluid intake is essential: a helpful guide is to drink 6 to 8 ounces of fluid (such as water or juices) at each feeding. Increase in the need for thiamin, riboflavin, and niacin, as well as for other vitamins and minerals, occurs during lactation, as shown in Table 4-3, and these needs are generally met by a balanced diet. Although we emphasize the importance of essential nutrients being obtained from the foods that the lactating mother eats, there is no evidence that vitamin supplements in physiologic doses cause harm. They may, in fact, provide a margin of safety against nutritional depletion. Some mothers maintain that they feel better and have more energy when taking dietary supplements. There are, however, conflicting reports about the lactation-inhibiting effect of large doses of pyridoxine (vitamin B_6).[4]

Most women are at least somewhat aware of the various food groups and have a general concept of what a well-balanced diet includes. Each client's level of nutritional knowledge should be determined by the nurse, and, when it is deficient, instruction in this area must be a priority for self-care teaching. The mother who has had poor long-standing nutritional habits may be motivated to improve them for the good of her baby.

TABLE 4-3

Recommended daily nutrient intake for women 19-35 years

Nutrient	Normal activity	Pregnancy	Lactation
Energy (kcal	2100	2400	2600
Protein (gm)	41	61	65
Thiamin (mg)	1.1	1.3	1.5
Niacin (NE)	14	16	21
Riboflavin (mg)	1.3	1.6	1.9
Vitamin C (mg)	30	50	60
Vitamin A (RE)	800	900	1200
Vitamin D (IU)	100	200	200
Calcium (mg)	700	1200	1200
Phosphorous (mg)	700	1200	1200
Iron (mg)	14	15	15

Canada Department of National Health and Welfare, Committee for Revision of the Dietary Standard: Standard for Canada, 1975.

In encouraging good nutrition there are some basic and practical guidelines to give her:
1. Eat a variety of food of different colors, flavors, and textures.
2. Eat foods in as close as possible to their natural state.
3. Avoid processed foods, especially those with refined sugar.

The most common food-related problems in breastfeeding mothers are:
1. Anxiety about being overweight
2. Poor eating habits and reliance on ''junk'' foods
3. Concern over which foods to avoid
4. Anorexia because of fatigue

In dealing with excess weight, self-care teaching should emphasize the probability (and desirability) of maintaining some extra weight—usually 5 to 10 lb in the early months. During pregnancy, well-nourished women add 9 to 10 lb of subcutaneous fat to their normal weight in preparation for the demands of subsequent lactation. This appears to ensure a ready supply of calories for the baby in the early weeks. The mother may be reassured that, by 3 months after delivery, breastfeeding mothers, on the average, lose about 2 pounds more than their bottle-feeding counterparts.[10] The extra weight is gradually lost in the metabolism of milk production. In the rare case of weight gain during the early months of lactation the mother should be encouraged to eliminate desserts and ''empty-calorie'' (highly refined) foods, substituting low-calorie fruits and snacks instead. Many women have lost unwanted weight during lactation. Providing that the necessary nutrients are consumed daily and the woman's motivation is sustained, the period of lactation may well be an opportune time to lose weight.

When a mother's eating habits are poor, there is surprisingly little immediate clinical evidence of deterioration of the nutritional status of her milk, at least in the early months.[19] Even when the extra reserves laid down during pregnancy are gone, breastmilk continues to maintain relatively high levels of nutrition at the expense of the woman. As noted earlier, since poor nutrition may affect the level of water-soluble vitamins, a long-standing poor diet eventually affects both the quantity and quality of the breastmilk. For the mother who needs financial support in upgrading her nutrition, enrollment in the WIC (Women, Infants and Children) programs should be facilitated.

Despite all the available information, some women are unaware that they rarely need to avoid particular foods during lactation because of their spicy or gas-producing qualities. The nurse should dispel old wives' tales about chocolate, beans, and highly spiced foods. Occasionally, however, a mother may discover that a certain food in her diet triggers undesirable symptoms, as discussed earlier, or regularly causes discomfort to her infant. By eliminating the food from her diet, she generally can solve the problem.

A common sequel of fatigue is anorexia, and many mothers complain they are''just too tired to eat.'' With the constant care of their newborn and household responsibilities, the problem then becomes cyclic: lack of certain vitamins, notably thiamin, causes fatigue and irritability and depresses the appetite even more. As well as being mandatory for general well-being, the importance of planning rest periods and minimizing housework cannot be overemphasized from a nutritional standpoint.

Finally, something should be said about the use of tobacco, alcohol, and caffeine during lactation.

It has been demonstrated that smoking negatively affects the nutritional status of the pregnant woman and results in, among other things, a higher incidence of low birth weight babies. Although the effects of smoking during lactation do not appear to be as hazardous as smoking while pregnant, the heavy smoker has been shown to have decreased milk production,[17] with lower levels of vitamin C in her milk, and her infant may be at greater risk for nausea, colic or cramping, and diarrhea.[38] In addition to being subject to the well-publicized hazards to her own health, the mother who smokes in the presence of her infant is also increasing her child's risk of pneumonia, bronchitis,[6] and possibly sudden infant death syndrome.[3] As in nutrition counseling, motivation to do the best for her infant may make the breastfeeding mother receptive to information and advice about the hazards of smoking.

The effects of alcohol on the breastfeeding baby appear to be directly related to the quantity that the mother ingests. Alcohol affects the central nervous system and can inhibit milk ejection[25]; however, when the lactating woman drinks moderately, the amount of alcohol the baby receives has not been shown to be harmful. In case of an upset or colicky infant, the effects of a small amount of alcohol taken by the mother may have a mildly sedative effect on her baby.

Hyperactivity, fussiness, and colic have been reported in babies whose mothers regularly drink sizable quantities of coffee or cola. Each mother needs to determine her own child's susceptibility and level of tolerance. The nursing history of a hyperactive breastfeeding baby should always include information about the mother's intake of caffeine.

Coping with maternal changes

Psychologic and physical changes in the breastfeeding woman are many, and the adjustment to having another person totally dependent on her for all of his needs can be anxiety provoking, particularly for the first-time mother.

A new child brings changes in relationships, sometimes creating complicated problems in the family. The woman's desire to give much time and attention to her baby may bring tensions of no small proportions to her marriage. The mother may be emotionally labile, and her responses to husband, other children, mother and mother-in-law, sisters and sisters-in-law, and even to visitors tend to be magnified and often misinterpreted. The father should be encouraged to run interference for her, since the mother herself may have all she can do to cope with her own and her infant's needs. Although the nurse may not be able to counsel a couple specifically about these problems, it can be helpful to let them know that the mother's coping abilities return to normal as her total biopsychosocial adjustment takes place during the coming weeks.

Sexual relations

Nurses are frequently able to assist the new mother and her husband toward understanding and making marital readjustments after the birth of their infant. Resuming the role of a sexual partner is neither less nor more difficult for nursing mothers than for those who formula-feed, but there are some phenomena that are common in the breastfeeding mother and should be considered here. Dryness of the mucous membranes of the vagina is experienced by some mothers during the first few months after childbirth, and nursing mothers are no exception. Using a lubricant such as K-Y jelly or a vegetable oil to increase comfort during intercourse generally takes care of the matter.

Occasionally in the early days of lactation, as during pregnancy itself, there may be heightened or decreased libido. If the breastfeeding mother and her husband discuss their feelings openly, they generally can arrive at a satisfactory adjustment to this temporary problem. Breastfeeding mothers—and new fathers, too—often are very tired. Such tiredness may contribute to a lack of interest in sexual play and can often be lessened by keeping the baby in or beside the parents' bed at night and by taking turns in infant care and in many household chores during the day.

Some mothers express concern about taking the baby into bed for nighttime feedings, yet many parents do this as a matter of course. The parents' bed is often the focus of fun, comfort, and sleep for the growing family, and there are no validated reports of babies being harmed in any way by breastfeeding and falling asleep in the parents' bed. Ideas and feelings about this should be explored by the mother and father, keeping the baby's needs as well as their own in mind.

Nurses and others frequently hear from both parents, "Will things ever get back to normal?" The answer must certainly be, "No"—at least not to the prepregnant norm. With a new member of the family a *new* norm will eventually be established, and the breastfeeding mother and the father need encouragement and support as they grow into this new way of life. Yet, although it is difficult for the mother—breastfeeding or otherwise—to manage all aspects of her new life, she should be encouraged to remember that her relationships with other significant persons in her life remain, with all their challenges, problems, and joys.

INFANT CARE
Early development and needs

Understanding the infant's development and the changes that normally occur in the early months is valuable for the new mother. Self-care includes awareness that the bright-eyed baby who has six to eight wet diapers a day, whose color and skin tone are good, and who generally feeds every couple of hours is following the expected norms. The mother should know that once or twice a day the baby may occasionally go 4 or 5 hours between feedings, following which he may need to breastfeed immediately and then again in an hour, or even sooner, to make up for the lengthy period without nourishment.

Since it is often necessary to provide a new mother with ongoing reinforcement, the desirability of recommending her to a nursing mothers' group such as La Leche League is evident. If there are no such support groups in her area, a knowledgeable nurse may be willing to talk with her by phone at home. A simple statement like "You must be awfully proud to be doing such a good job of mothering your baby" has an immediately reinforcing effect when used appropriately. Such support, whether given by other breastfeeding mothers or by an experienced and sympathetic professional, may make the difference between the continuation of breastfeeding and early weaning.

If the mother appears to be anxious, listen carefully and ask questions to assess the problem. Often a mother who calls with a problem is primarily in need of a sympathetic ear, someone to whom she can talk without being rushed and who will allow her to work her own problems through without judgment or disapproval. Asking open-ended questions that begin with "how" and "what" will elicit the most insightful responses.

At all times support the unsure new breastfeeding mother with encouragement, reassurance, and your personal conviction about the superiority of breastfeeding.

Crying and colic

Infants cry for many reasons, but it can be said unequivocally that they cry for *some* reason. They are not merely exercising their lungs. Crying is a survival mechanism to express some unmet need, whether it be for food, suckling, cuddling, a change in position, or a dry diaper. A baby's cries should never be ignored; the sooner his needs are attended to, the greater will be the relaxation and enjoyment of both mother and child. In promoting self-care, nurses who have regular ongoing contact with mothers and who wish to contribute to the child's optimal mental and emotional health will place considerable emphasis on the importance of answering the needs of the crying infant.

When crying turns into a high-pitched wail or scream, something is very wrong. It may be colic, but it may also be a more serious digestive problem. Parents should be made aware of the importance of having the baby examined by a physician when such symptoms appear.

Colic is sudden spasmodic abdominal cramping. Often the baby draws up his legs, cries violently, and has a distended abdomen. No other signs or symptoms of illness are usually evident. One of the characteristics of colic is its tendency to recur about the same time every day. Eventually, after about 3 months it disappears.

The cause of colic has not been pinpointed; in fact, it is attributed to many causes, including allergies; overfeeding; underfeeding; too rich or too weak feedings; too much fat, sugar, or protein; too large or too small a hole in a bottle nipple; excessive swallowing of air; the anxious mother; and various other phenomena. Some of the foregoing possibilities clearly show why colic is more prevalent in bottle-fed than in breastfed infants; yet it it not unknown in the baby who receives nothing but his mother's milk.

Although the possible causes of colic are numerous, it is quite likely that the infant is responding as much to emotional phenomena as to physical ones. The human gastrointestinal tract is highly sensitive to tension and stress. Since colic is much more frequently seen in first babies than in others, many authorities believe that parental anxieties and apprehensions may be reflected in the infant, causing colic. Unfortunately, the crying of the colicky infant only increases these anxieties. It has been said that colic is rarely seen in the infant of mature parents. They are sufficiently ready to make the necessary sacrifices that a new baby requires, including responding immediately to his cries, feeding him many more times a day than the once customary 4-hour schedule entails, holding him a great deal of the time, loving him unconditionally, and devoting most of their time during the early weeks and months to him.

Treatment for colic has been varied. Medications combining atropine derivatives and phenobarbital in an alcohol solution are widely marketed to treat colic, yet they have been found to be generally useless and not infrequently harmful.[31] Several years ago a study[18] in Sweden showed that symptoms disappeared promptly in two thirds of colicky babies whose mothers were placed on a diet free of cow's milk protein. On reintroduction of cow's milk into the mother's diet, colic reappeared in all but one of the infants. Efforts to adjust the mother's diet should certainly be made, but perhaps most of all support and reassurance of both parents that colic generally is self-limiting is an effective therapy for a colicky baby.

A practical technique for immediate relief of colic is simple positioning of the infant. In the "colic-carry" position, the infant, with his head slightly higher than his feet, is laid astraddle across the legs of the caretaker and gently rocked.[22]

Growth spurts

Mothers must anticipate that their infants will be subject to growth spurts and that, at such times, the frequency of demand for feeding increases. Growth spurts occur most noticeably around 2 weeks after birth and again about 6 weeks, 2½ to 3 months, and 4½ to 6 months. At these times, an infant is noticeably more active, awake, and sensitive to stimuli. He may fret and cry more easily, and the mother may find that, for a day or two, she seems to be holding and breastfeeding him most of the time. After a day or two, when he has arrived at his new developmental level and his mother's milk has increased to meet his needs, he will once again be contented. At such times, however, a mother should learn to expect a change of the infant's habits with some increase in his quiet alert state and interest in the world around him. Purposeful stimulation of his sensorium with safe objects of varying sizes, shapes, textures, and bright colors enhances his learning and development.

Stools

During the first month or two, the breastfed infant's stools are frequently of concern to the mother. If they are unformed or liquid or if they occur more than once or twice a day, the mother may think the baby has diarrhea. The physician who has dealt primarily with the formula-fed infant may be unaware that the small, soft, or liquid stool that the breastfed baby often passes at each feeding is a wholly usual and normal phenomenon.

Breastfeeding stimulates frequent gastrointestinal peristalsis and stooling in the early weeks; however, if totally breastfeeding, some infants occasionally go without a bowel movement for several days, even as long as a week. Although this can happen any time, it usually occurs in the second or third month. If this entirely normal phenomenon is of concern to the uninformed mother, suggest that she observe her baby for abdominal guarding or signs of pain. If such symptoms are not present and the baby seems content, there is no need to be alarmed or to seek medical intervention. Experienced mothers and others who know and deal with the totally breastfed infant realize that as long as the baby is healthy and alert and the abdomen remains soft, it matters little whether he has half a dozen stools a day or only one or two a week. Whichever it may be, the nurse can reassure the mother that the baby has absorbed the bulk of the valuable contents of breastmilk because it is so readily and quickly digested.

Teaching for self-care should include discussions about the inadvisability of giving supplemental additions of formula, water, and solids to the well infant before they are indicated. Increasingly, it has become clear that most full-term, healthy infants who are breastfeeding regularly need nothing but breastmilk until about the middle of the first year after birth. Many physicians routinely order vitamin supplements. Although breastmilk usually supplies adequate vitamins, the exception is the black infant, particularly in winter in northern climates, where he may have minimal exposure to the sun and absorption of its rays. For these babies vitamin D supplements to prevent rickets is often indicated.

Weaning

Mothers frequently ask, "When shall I wean my baby? How shall I do it? How long will it take?" Such questions on self-care may come even when an infant is only a few weeks old, and the nurse must be prepared to help the mother discover that weaning takes place on its own as the child develops.

Additions of solid foods to the baby's diet around the middle of the first year is the first step in weaning for most babies. Then, as time goes by and the outside world becomes more and more interesting to him, the baby wants to breastfeed less and less. A few babies give up breastfeeding on their own before a year, others around 12 to 15 months of age, and still others seem to need to continue for a little or a much longer period.

Ideally, weaning will occur in response to the child's needs, whatever his age. Some mothers, however, feel a need to wean the child before he is fully ready. At such a time, the mother should be encouraged to wean very gradually. Cutting out one feeding a day for a few days, omitting a second for several more days, and continuing slowly to eliminate additional feedings will enable the baby to adjust with less trauma than in abrupt weaning. Mothers who undertake mother-led weaning should endeavor to give the baby a great deal of additional holding, cuddling, and attention to replace the loss that the baby is experiencing.

If a crisis demands more abrupt weaning, the mother should take as long as possible for the process. She will likely experience engorgement, which can be best relieved by permitting the baby to nurse long enough to make the mother comfortable but not to empty her breasts completely. She may also use a breast pump or manually express her milk if she is not with the baby. Rapid weaning is always physically and psychologically traumatic to both mother and baby and should be avoided whenever possible.

Sometimes a mother believes that it is necessary to wean a baby to take medication prescribed for her by her doctor. Fortunately, there are very few medications that are unsafe in therapeutic doses and for short-term use by the lactating mother, and when an unsafe or uncertain drug is prescribed, it is generally possible to substitute another that is acceptable. Often, too, treatment of the mother may be elective, and consideration should be given to postponing therapy for a few weeks or months until the baby weans more easily on his own. The subject of medications and breastfeeding is discussed further in Chapter 6.

Eagerness for solids, the enjoyment of cup feedings, feeding himself, and going long periods without seeking the breast are all signs that the child is growing and weaning himself. Occasionally weaning may happen very quickly, but generally it is a long, slow process. Sometimes the baby will voluntarily stop for a few days or even more, then want to return to breastfeeding. Weaning patterns differ; the only wholly predictable fact is that, in his own time, each one weans.

Breastfeeding strike

Although it may happen at an even younger age, around 7 to 9 months of age is commonly a time at which some infants suddenly refuse to breastfeed. It is easy for the inexperienced mother to see this as an indication that her infant has weaned himself, yet this is rarely the case. The abruptness of the infant's refusal to breastfeed is usually the mother's best clue to a "breastfeeding strike." Normal weaning seldom happens so rapidly.

Most mothers who have experienced an infant's breastfeeding strike believe the strike is a signal of his distress, dissatisfaction, or confusion associated with feedings. The mother who attempts to get the infant on a schedule that suits her but not the baby or who leaves her infant with a bottle, even of breastmilk, may unwittingly frustrate or confuse him. As a result, in the only way he knows, he refuses to be a partner to the problem that has arisen. Sometimes a physical discomfort like a cold, sore throat, earache, or stuffy nose for several days may bring about a breastfeeding strike. Even the understandable rebuke that the mother may give the teething infant who bites when breastfeeding may confuse and anger the baby, who is not capable of associating biting with hurting mother. One mother reports: "It seems likely to us that he felt rejected by . . . the 'No' from biting and may have decided not to fool around with a situation that seemed unrewarding. . . ."[23]

Once a breastfeeding strike occurs, efforts to resume breastfeeding may require several days. During this time the mother may need to devote herself almost completely to her infant. She should carry him around much of the time and provide a great deal of skin-to-skin contact. It is generally useless to put him to breast while he is awake unless he actively seeks it. Far more effective is to offer the breast to the *sleeping* baby. When he finally accepts it and feeds well several times during his sleep, some mothers have had success in gently awakening their babies during the feeding so that they can see for themselves that it is possible to enjoy breastfeeding again.

The nurse may be truly supportive to the mother whose child has gone on a breastfeeding strike by encouraging her to maintain her milk supply, keep up a good diet, avoid supplementary bottles, and, last but not least, stay with it and have confidence that she can do it. "Relax, cheer up, keep at it, and call me if you need me," tells the mother how much you care.

WORKING MOTHERS

Today more than 50% of employed mothers have children of primary school age or younger, and within 10 years 90% of American women are expected to be in the national work force. Clearly the life-styles of the '80s mandate an in-depth discussion of breastfeeding and working.

The role of the health-care worker in counseling mothers contemplating work outside the home is a new and difficult one. The nurse must walk a fine line. It is important to avoid arousing or reinforcing guilt feelings in the mother who elects to (or must) work, and it is equally essential to ensure that the at-home mother does not feel less adequate, able, or intelligent than her employed counterpart.

Perhaps the nurse must first accept that she will be misunderstood by many of those whom she is trying to help. Even if she presents to the client all aspects of both sides of the coin as dispassionately as possible, her personal experiences, her current choices, and her beliefs will be obvious to some and distorted by others. Despite this, she is in a unique position to offer information and advice, first to mothers who are in the decision-making process and later to those who have elected to work.

Decision-making considerations

More than ever before, today's woman faces difficult decisions in regard to motherhood, childrearing, and self-fulfillment. Soon after the birth of a baby many women return to work for financial reasons; others consider returning to work for personal needs such as to carry on a promising career or because they feel that in staying at home they are wasting their education or talent. Whatever the reason for their dilemma or decision, the nurse must be prepared to help.

Consideration of the infant's needs, as well as the needs of the mother and other family members, is always a part of a caring mother's decision-making process. She and the child's father should generally make the decision together, especially since some of the responsibility for the home and child care is likely to be his if the mother returns to work. Both mother and father, therefore, will generally want all available information when discussing future plans.

Numerous experts strongly encourage the mother's remaining at home as long as possible. In the *New York Times Magazine,* March, 1973, Shaywitz[37] writes:

> We do not know enough about nurturing to be able to tell mothers that if they find a person or an institution that meets such-and-such standards that this will be an adequate mother substitute. We can list people's credentials, pinpoint the standards for a day care center, but just as breastmilk cannot be duplicated, neither can a mother. We cannot put mothering into a formula and come up with a person who has the special feeling for your child that you do. . . . Just as everyone but a mother is excluded from nursing a baby, so they are also excluded from those immense feelings of satisfaction and inner unity with the child. . . .

In *Every Child's Birthright: In Defense of Mothering,* Fraiberg[12] asserts:

> It has been determined that children who do not have the benefit of a single, sustained contact with a loving mother or mother-figure for at least the first three years of their lives, will—depending upon the degree of deprivation—manifest a diminished capacity to love others, impaired intellectual powers, and an inability to control their impulses, particularly in the area of aggression.

To the question, "What's the daily minimum dosage of mothering that an infant or toddler needs for normal, happy development?" Beck[2] in an article in the *Chicago Tribune* answers: "Much of the accepted wisdom about child development in recent decades is conveniently being revised to accommodate the wishful thinking of working parents."

Finally, according to Segal and Yahraes[36] in *A Child's Journey: Forces that Shape the Lives of our Young:*

> The mother's right to an independent life outside the home cannot be denied, but her search for that life without at the same time insuring her baby's security can be costly without measure. Children do outgrow their anxieties about separation, and parents who are sensitive to their little ones will be aware of the time they can tolerate separation without ill effects. Generally authorities believe this time is somewhere between three and five years of age.

On the other side of the ledger, babies are hardy souls, and many a little one has grown well under the loving nurturance of a motherly housekeeper, grandmother, or other person devoted to his physical, emotional, and intellectual development and care. A job with work hours when the father is at home has been satisfactory for many families and enhanced the father-child relationship. Many a mother decides to work while the baby is very young because—for one valid reason or another—she simply *must*. Postponing the final commitment to return to work until after the baby has arrived is often a useful adjunct to the decision-making process.

Many mothers delay their return to outside employment as long as possible. Extended maternity leave is often feasible, as is taking all such leave after the baby's birth rather than dividing it between late pregnancy and the early postpartum period. Job sharing, part-time work, and flexible hours are other possibilities that are becoming increasingly popular with mothers of small babies.

Quality vs. quantity of time spent with a child is often a matter for argument. Certainly, the quality of attention and love that the baby receives affects his future. But quantity matters too. Babies need quantities of quality time—not one or the other, alone.

According to White, founder of the Center for Parent Education, ". . . most children will get off to a better start in life when they spend the majority of their waking hours being cared for by their parents and other family members rather than any form of substitute care." Therefore, when a mother returns to work, supportive counseling will encourage care by father, grandmother, or other close member of the baby's family. There can be no substitute for love in the child's early years.

Many mothers who are gainfully employed find that the home, itself, is an excellent milieu in which to pursue their own interests. Writers, specialty cooks, seamstresses, and women competent in arts, crafts, and gymnastic pursuits can often successfully continue their careers at home. Typists, bookkeepers, and accountants also frequently work in home offices. The presence of a maid, baby-sitter, or other assistant relieves them of the sole responsibility for meeting their child's minor needs, yet they remain available to respond to major ones. Sharing these suggestions is an important aspect of the support that the nurse can offer the working mother.

Perhaps the greatest help the nurse can offer the client who seeks advice about returning to work is to encourage her to come to a clear understanding of her own feelings and conflicts, accept her own decision while making ongoing reevaluations from time to time, and spend most of her nonworking hours with her baby.

In the best interest of the child, counseling the mother who plans to be gainfully employed will include the following points:

- Postponing irrevocable work commitments until after the baby has arrived and the mother is nearly back to normal, emotionally and physically
- Considering all options: home vs. outside employment, full-time vs. part-time work
- Taking as lengthy a leave-of-absence or maternity leave as possible
- Providing the most optimal care possible when leaving the baby by seeking top-quality, consistent, one-to-one or as near as possible one-to-one care, rather than large-group care
- Continuing to breastfeed to avoid potential exposure to allergies and to enhance the mother-child bond

Breastfeeding and working

Even the mother who is gainfully employed outside the home can usually breastfeed her baby for as long as she and the baby wish to continue. Mothers find that breastfeeding helps to maintain the closeness of mother and child and enables the mother more readily to understand her infant's care. It has been suggested that an "auxiliary wife (to provide domestic and child-care services) is important if not essential for optimal career performance" when both parents work outside the home. Such an arrangement is not unlike the norm in many Latin American households, in which the live-in maid is nearly a member of the family and the children often seem to be as responsive to her as to the parents.

For centuries mothers have worked inside and outside the home during their child-rearing years. They have grown crops, tended animals, tanned hides, and performed many other strenuous chores, yet for the most part their infants have been with them. Only in recent decades has it become customary to separate mother and child. One possibility that is long overdue is the installation of crèches or nurseries in the factory or business complex—a not uncommon phenomenon in Eastern Europe. Nurses are in a particularly favorable position to promote such facilities for their own children in the medical complex of which they are a part and to encourage their clients to seek the establishment of similar facilities in or near their work.

The presence of the child in the mother's work area will enable her to provide some portion of the child's care during the day. It also enables the child to see at least one parent involved in her daily tasks. Thus role modeling is begun and continued on a regular basis.

It is good for the nurse to be prepared to provide the mother with practical information and tips to make breastfeeding easier and more satisfying. The most important of these is to have breastfeeding well established before returning to work outside the home.

Once breastfeeding is going well, adjustments are generally quite manageable. These will include feeding just before leaving home, expressing milk at least once (possibly more frequently) during the day while away, and breastfeeding immediately on returning home. The mother should be advised of the importance of full-time nurturing and mothering during the hours when she is not at work. Much holding and cuddling of the baby should be a regular part of the mother's time at home. The suggestion may be made that the baby sleep with the mother at night to provide extra body contact.

It may fall to the nurse to instruct the mother in hand expression or use of a manual breast pump. The Kaneson or Loyd-B pumps described in Chapter 12 are portable and relatively inexpensive. She will also need advice about keeping and transporting her milk. Each day she will need sterilized or clean receptacles into which she can express her milk. Ideally, she will express into each receptacle the approximate amount needed by the baby for a single feeding. For storage during the day, a refrigerator at the work site is very helpful but not essential. The mother can provide her own refrigeration with a thermos or other insulated cold container; for taking the milk home she will definitely need such a container, even in cold weather. On the following day, the milk that she has expressed can be given to the baby by his caretaker. An effective technique for hand expression is found in Chapter 2.

For a week or two before returning to work, the mother should also be encouraged to express and freeze her milk. By so doing she will learn the technique for expressing and building her milk supply, which may diminish somewhat when she begins work. At the same time she will be establishing her own personal milk bank for the baby. Expression can be done following a feeding or between feedings. The milk should be expressed directly into a clean container, and, as earlier stated, each receptacle is most convenient to use if it contains the amount to be given to the baby at a single feeding.

When she returns to work, the mother who is adept at manually expressing her milk will express during coffee breaks and lunch periods, thereby providing breastmilk for the baby's feedings on the following day. If kept under constant refrigeration at 4° C (about 40° F) and refrigerated while in transport, breastmilk will remain safe for about 48 hours without freezing.

Neifert, a Denver neonatologist who breastfed five children while in medical school and as a working mother, offers these additional suggestions:

1. Get outside household help, if at all possible.
2. Breastfeed more often at night and exclusively on weekends.
3. Drink additional fluids at work; the distractions and concentration while at work make this easy to forget. Constipation is a sign of dehydration.
4. Never pump when the infant is available.
5. Keep nutritious snacks in the car for eating going to and from work.
6. Keep a photograph of the baby at the work place.
7. Use assertiveness to get "pump breaks," flex time, and extended maternity leaves at the work place.

A recent letter to the editor of *Pediatrics*,[8] written conjointly by nine professional women who have managed to combine breastfeeding and working, merits attention. The following excerpts should be useful, but the nurse who wishes to provide optimal help to the breastfeeding working mother is referred to the entire text of the letter.

> We have learned that the nursing problems encountered by mothers who work outside the home include all those encountered by mothers who remain at home, and several more. . . . It has been our experience that the earlier the bottle is introduced, the easier is the transition to this form of nourishment. In general late introduction of the bottle is likely to be associated with some resistance on the baby's part, whereas introduction of the bottle after several weeks of exclusive breastfeeding but before 5 weeks of age is not. After it is introduced, the bottle needs to be used regularly (e.g., once daily) to maintain the baby's acceptance of it. Some mothers find that once the bottle is introduced, their infants lose interest in the breast, but this is unusual; it is generally no problem to continue to nurse the baby when the mother is home. . . . Because of the superiority of breast milk, many working mothers choose to express [breast] milk for bottle feeding during their working hours. . . . Unfortunately, many mothers are unable to make this choice freely because they do not receive enough instruction to master the technique of manual expression. Mothers need help in learning to express milk so that lack of skill does not dictate their choice regarding infant feedings. (It is also useful for mothers to be able to express milk at time of engorgement, even if they do not elect to do so regularly for feeding.) . . . Mothers who have expressed milk for their babies—some for as long as several years—have used clean rather than sterile techniques. The mechanical devices mentioned in many books are inefficient at best, and ineffective at worst. . . . It [manual expression] involves compressing the areola in a repetitive fashion, either pressing it back against the rib cage or not, depending on what works better for the individual mother. It usually takes at least 15 to 20 minutes to empty both breasts. . . ." **Travel.** A mother has basically two choices when she travels on business: she can take the baby with her, or she can arrange for bottle (breast milk or formula) feeding in her absence, manually expressing milk [while away]. . . . The most important point is that it is indeed possible to combine breastfeeding and employment outside the home. The unique pleasures of breastfeeding and the resultant bonding with the new baby may be especially precious to mothers who share the infant's care

with others. . . . Mothers who wish to combine breastfeeding and employment should be provided with the information they need and should be encouraged to continue nursing, just as are mothers who stay home.

Every situation is unique and different. Whereas many infants are given a daily bottle well in advance of their mothers' return to work, others manage well without a head start: As one mother said in a letter to La Leche League:

> Don't make elaborate plans for separation from your baby, other than good baby-care arrangements. Don't try to imitate being gone before you go. This includes not avoiding nursings in advance and not substituting bottle feeds until you actually must. The baby will adjust better if all circumstances are generated by reality, rather than pretense.

Some mothers become proficient in the use of one or another of the better breast pumps. Especially if the baby is a frequent feeder when mother and baby are together, a hand pump may be useful. Although the mother cannot rely solely on a pump, many mothers have found that hand pumps are useful for obtaining milk rapidly.

Each working mother needs time and encouragement to develop her own routine and techniques in ways that best suit her and her breastfeeding child. These are the only absolutes.

Although most babies need nothing but their mother's milk until around the middle of the first year after birth, some working mothers find that the baby is better satisfied if solids are introduced a few weeks earlier than this. Whenever other foods are started, the nurse should recommend those that are the most nonallergenic for the baby's first solids and advise the slow introduction of them, one at a time, to minimize allergic responses and to identify more easily those that may not fully agree with the baby. (For recommendations on how and what to feed the baby when starting solids, see Chapter 17.)

Most of the techniques and practical tips that the nurse can provide the employed breastfeeding mother are the same as those that she would offer the mother at home. Yet, as with the baby who receives mother's care full time, the working woman's little one is uniquely his own self, with his own needs, demands, growth, and development. With the help of the observations and reports of the child's other caretaker, the mother is the best person to make judgments or decisions in his interest. The close cooperation of a loving caretaker and the mother optimizes the development of a happy, healthy baby.

Other adjustments

To provide her baby with the greatest possible amount of her time, the mother who works outside the home must make personal adjustments. One of the most frequent laments of working women is that they are so rushed in the morning that they cannot do justice to themselves or their babies. A number of mothers have found that arising half an hour or so earlier than usual provides that much needed extra time to nurse the baby in a relaxed fashion, play with him a little, eat a good breakfast, and leave home with a sense of completion of that phase of the day. Several employed mothers arise 1½ to 2 hours before departing for work so as to have time to devote to the baby and to feel unhurried themselves. Infants also make adjustments and soon learn to breastfeed frequently at night, sleeping longer periods during the day or when the mother is at work.

Occasionally a mother may live close enough to work that she can go home or to the sitter's house at lunchtime. Sometimes it is possible for the baby's caretaker to take him to his mother's place of work at lunch or during a morning or afternoon break. There is, of course, no guarantee that the baby's sleeping or feeding schedule will always coincide with the mother's free time, but often such an arrangement will work very well.

Just as mothers find it desirable to have unrushed time in the morning before leaving for work, so too do they want their return home in the afternoon to be relaxing. If the baby is awake, he will generally want to be held, cuddled, and fed almost immediately. The mother often finds that her breasts are full, and she, too, will want to put the baby to breast on arrival. This should be a complete let-down for them both. The help of the baby's father in setting the table, cooking dinner, and doing certain other domestic chores is a near must, unless the sitter stays on or another helper has been engaged to perform these duties.

Most employed mothers find that they prefer to devote their evenings to the baby. Fathers, of course, are an integral part of this time together. Nor is it necessary to stay home all the time. Snug in a carrier on mother's or father's body, the baby can go walking, hiking, grocery shopping, or visiting in the neighborhood; or safely buckled in the infant carseat, he can take long rides and be a part of almost all of the parents' activities. The security of having the baby nearby makes for the kind of unworried, relaxed evening that would be nearly impossible to experience if the little one were left with someone else.

Bedtime comes early for most working mothers. Yet, each mother should be encouraged to develop her own schedule—one that fits her child's needs and her own and leaves her sufficiently unburdened so that each day is enjoyable for every member of the family.

Finally, a mother needs to recognize that—from month to month, sometimes even weekly—her schedule will need to change somewhat as her baby constantly grows and changes. In responding to the baby's changing needs, she will allow for flexibility in her own life as does the mother who stays at home.

The efforts that the working mother makes to adjust her career and home life often seem prodigious. Yet they *can* be managed and are often very rewarding. The mother's determination to make it work, coupled with her sensitivity to the baby's needs (as well as those of other family members), will often make all the difference—at home and at work, as well.

SUMMARY

With the increased consumer interest in self-care, nursing emphasis has changed from a management approach toward support and education of the client. Guidance given by the knowledgeable nurse not only helps the infant toward a healthy start in life but also provides valuable lifelong health education for the family. The efforts expended may be great but the rewards, both short and long term, are myriad.

76 Basics of breastfeeding

REFERENCES

1. Atkinson, L.: Prenatal nipple conditioning for breastfeeding, Nurs. Res. **28:**267, 1979.
2. Beck, J.: Child care: wishful revisionism, Chicago Tribune, November 20, 1981.
3. Bergman, A.B., and Weiser, L.A.: Relationship of passive cigarette smoking to sudden infant death syndrome, Pediatrics **58:** 665, 1976.
4. Bowes, W.A.: The effect of medications on the lactating mother and her infant, Clin. Obstet. Gynecol. **23:**1073, 1980.
5. Brown, M.S.: Preparation of the breast for breastfeeding, Nurs. Res. **24:**448, 1975.
6. Colley, J.R., et al.: Influence of passive smoking and parental phlegm on pneumonia and bronchitis in early childhood, Lancet **2:**1031, 1974.
7. Condon, W.S., and Sander, L.W.: Neonate movement is synchronized with adult speech: interaction participation and language acquisition, Science **183:**99, 1974.
8. Christoffel, K., et al.: Advice from breastfeeding mothers (letters to the editor), Pediatrics **68:**141, 1981.
9. deChateau, P., and Wiberg, B.: Long term effect on mother-infant behavior of extra contact during the first hour postpartum, Acta Paediatr. Scand. **66:**137, 1977.
10. Dennis, J.K.: Body-weight changes in the puerperium between the 10th and 94th days, Obstet. Gynecol. **22:**14, 1971.
11. Eppink, H.: Experiment to determine a basis for nursing decisions in regard to initiation of breastfeeding, Nurs. Res. **18:**292, 1969.
12. Fraiberg, S.: Every child's birthright: in defense of mothering, New York, 1977, Basic Books, Inc., Publishers.
13. Frantz, K., Fleiss, P., and Lawrence, R.: Management of the slow-gaining breastfed baby, Keeping Abreast J. **3:**298, 1978.
14. Frantz, K.B., and Kalmen, B.A.: Breastfeeding works for cesareans, too, R.N. **42:**39, 1979.
15. Gromada, K.: Maternal-infant attachment: The first step toward individualizing twins, M.C.N. **6:**129, 1981.
16. Gromada, K.: Mothering multiples, Publication No. 52, Franklin Park, Ill., 1981, La Leche League International, Inc.
17. Hervada, A., et al.: Drugs in breastmilk, Perinatal Care **2:**19, 1978.
18. Jakobsson, I., and Lindberg, T.: Cow's milk as a cause of infantile colic in breastfed infants, Lancet **2:**437, 1978.
19. Jelliffe, D.B., and Jelliffe, E.F.P.: Human milk in the modern world, London, 1978, Oxford University Press.
20. Johnson, N.W.: Breastfeeding at one hour of age, M.C.N. **1:**12, 1976.
21. Klaus, M.H., and Kennell, J.H.: Maternal-infant bonding: the impact of early separation or loss on family development, St. Louis, 1976, The C.V. Mosby Co.
22. La Leche League International: A colic aid that worked for us, La Leche International News **20:**110, 1978.
23. La Leche League International: Ever hear of a nursing strike? Information Sheet No. 57, Franklin Park, Ill., The League.
24. Lang, R.: Birth book, Ben Lomond, Calif., 1972, Genesis Press.
25. Larson, B.L., and Smith, V.R., editors: Lactation. Vol. IV. The mammary gland/human lactation/milk synthesis, New York, 1978, Academic Press, Inc.
26. Lawrence, R.: Breastfeeding: a guide for the medical profession, St. Louis, 1980, The C.V. Mosby Co.
27. Merrill, B.S., and Gibbs, C.E.: Planned vaginal delivery following cesarean section, Am. J. Obstet. Gynecol. **135:**555, 1979.
28. Newton, M.: Human lactation. In Kon, S.K., and Cowie, A.T., editors: Milk: the mammary gland and its secretion, vol. I, New York, 1961, Academic Press, Inc.
29. O'Connor, S., et al.: How does rooming-in enhance the mother-infant bond? Soc. Pediatr. Res. **13:**336, 1979.
30. O'Connor, S., et al.: Reduced incidence of parenting inadequacy following rooming-in, Pediatrics **66:**176, 1980.
31. O'Donovan, J.C., and Bradstock, A.S.: Failure of conventional drug therapy in management of infantile colic, Am. J. Dis. Child. **133:**999, 1979.
32. Orem, D.E.: Nursing: concepts of practice, New York, ed. 2, 1980, McGraw-Hill Book Co.
33. Rubin R.: Basic maternal behavior, Nurs. Outlook **9:**683, 1961.
34. Rubin, R.: Attainment of the maternal role. I. Processes. II. Models and referrants, Nurs. Res. **16:**237 and 342, 1967.
35. Saldana, L.R., Schulman, H., and Reuss, L.: Management of pregnancy after cesarean section, Am. J. Obstet. Gynecol. **135:**555, 1979.
36. Segal, J., and Yahraes, H.: A child's journey: forces that shape the lives of our young, New York, 1978, McGraw-Hill Book Co.

37. Shaywitz, S.: Catch-22 for mothers, New York Times Magazine, p. 50, March 4, 1973.
38. Vorherr, H.: Drug excretion in breastmilk, Postgrad. Med. **56**:97, 1974.
39. Whitley, N.: Preparation for breastfeeding: a one-year followup of 34 nursing mothers, J.O.G.N. Nurs. **73**:44, 1978.
40. Wolff, P.: Observation of early development of smiling. In Foss, B.M., editor: Determinants of infant behavior, vol. 11, New York, 1963, John Wiley & Sons, Inc.

ADDITIONAL READINGS

Dery, C.: Lactation. In Fogel, C.I., and Woods, N.F.: Health care of women: a nursing perspective, St. Louis, 1980, The C.V. Mosby Co.
Haire, D., and Haire, J.: The nurse's contribution to successful breastfeeding, in implementing family-centered maternity care with a central nursery, Seattle, Washington, 1971, International Childbirth Education Association.
Hayter, J.: The rhythm of sleep, Am. J. Nurs. **80**:457, 1980.
Murdaugh, A., and Miller, L.E.: Helping the breastfeeding mother, Am. J. Nurs. **72**:1420, 1972.
Newton, M., and Newton, N.: The normal course and management of lactation, Oak Park, Ill., 1972, Child and Family Reprint Series.
Nichols, M.: Effective help for the nursing mother, J.O.G.N. Nurs. **7**:22, 1978.
Salomon, M., Schauf, V., and Seider, A.: Breastfeeding, "natural mothering" and working outside the home. In Stewart, D., editor: 21st Century obstetrics now, vol. 2, Chapel Hill, N.C., 1976, NAPSAC Publications.
Stichler, J.F., and Affonso, D.D.: Cesarean birth, Am. J. Nurs. **80**:466, 1980.
White, G.J., and White, M.K.: Breastfeeding and drugs in human milk, Vet. Hum. Toxicol. **22**(Suppl. 1):1, 1980.
Zambrana, R.E., Hunt, M., and Hite, R.L.: The working mother in contemporary perspective: a review of the literature, Pediatrics **64**:862, 1979. (See also the excellent bibliography at end of article.)

BOOKS FOR PARENTS

Applebaum, R.W.: Abreast of the times, 1979.*
Brewster, D.: You can breastfeed your baby: even in special situations, Emmaus, 1979, Rodale Press, Inc.
Cardoza, A.: Woman at home, New York, 1976, Doubleday & Co., Inc.
Eiger, M., and Olds, S.W.: The complete book of breastfeeding, New York, 1972, Bantam Books, Inc.
Kippley, S.K.: Breastfeeding and natural child spacing, New York, 1974, Penguin Books.
La Leche League International: The womanly art of breastfeeding, Franklin Park, Ill., 1981, The League.*
McDonald, L.: The joy of breastfeeding, Pasadena, Calif., 1979, Oaklawn Press.

*Available from La Leche League International, 9616 Minneapolis Avenue, Franklin Park, Ill. 60131.

5

Breastfeeding education programs

JAN RIORDAN

This chapter discusses current breastfeeding education programs and problems involved in implementing them. The description of these programs is divided into categories based on their setting: community, hospital, clinic, or private practices. In addressing the types of programs I will explore both current breastfeeding education programs and future program possibilities.

As recently as 60 years ago, an inexperienced mother turned to her mother, aunts, or grandmothers to learn the womanly art of breastfeeding. At that time it would have seemed absurd to attend breastfeeding classes or self-care groups such as the ones described in this chapter. During the middle of this century the traditional woman-to-woman conveying of breastfeeding knowledge and skills was lost or at least temporarily misplaced. Into the vacuum came alternative support systems for the few women who still chose to breastfeed their infants. Self-care groups, notably La Leche League, and childbirth education groups began to organize. As the need continued to grow, formal health-care systems began to respond with programs of their own. A listing of worldwide programs and their effectiveness is provided in Table 5-1.

THE CHANGE PROCESS

The programs presented in this chapter reflect the process of change. Instituting new breastfeeding programs in health-care settings requires changing existing practices and policies that may have been ingrained for years. Many change agents are nurses in hospitals and community health settings all over this nation who are expanding their roles and effecting change. Nowhere is this more visible than in maternal-child care, in which childbirth and breastfeeding education programs have instituted successful changes and stress early breastfeeding support and teaching.

For change to happen, several ingredients must be present. Breastfeeding is a controversial subject, and the controversy must be resolved to some extent before initiating a program in an institution. First the power structure must be able to see an advantage, such as an improved public image, increased profit, or a reduction in expenses. These are good motivations for change. Another ingredient is the opportunity to reduce stress,[17] both internally and externally. For example, consumers voicing their preferences create

TABLE 5-1

Summary of selected intervention program effects on incidence and duration of breastfeeding

Source	Place	Type of intervention*	Sample size	Time of measurement	% Breastfeeding or duration of breastfeeding before intervention (or in control group)	% Breastfeeding or duration of breastfeeding after intervention (or in control group)	Net increase in % breastfeeding or duration of breastfeeding
Information and support							
Brimblecombe and Cullen (1977)	Exeter, England	Education of midwives and health visitors on consultant unit (L)	562	Hospital discharge	42.5%	51.0%	8.5%
Burne (1976)	Oxford, England	Continuity of care by stable, familiar health team (L)	73	6 wk postpartum	32.0%	69.0%	37.0%
Coles and Valman (1976)	Harrow, England	Hospital-based education program (L)	±1300	Hospital discharge	54.7%	69.4%	14.7%
Creery (1973)	Cheltenham, England	Education of health professionals (L)	4950	Hospital discharge	45.0%	64.0%	19.0%
De Chateau et al. (1977)	Umea, Sweden	Education of fathers (P)	23	Duration	75 days (fathers not informed)	135 days (fathers informed)	60 days
Halpern et al. (1972)	Dallas, Texas	Positive attitudes of pediatricians (C)	4753	†	14.5% (pediatricians indifferent about breastfeeding)	29.1% (pediatricians not indifferent)	14.6%
Kirk (1978)	Edinburgh, Scotland	Education by doctors and nurses (L)	278	Initiation 1 mo postpartum 4 mo postpartum	43.6% 26.9% 10.3%	68.5% 43.5% 37.0%	24.9% 37.0% 26.7%
Meyer (1968)	U.S. hospitals	Hospital programs to promote breastfeeding (unspecified) [CI]	2951 hospitals	Hospital discharge	18.0% (overall rate)	34.8% (for hospital with breastfeeding program)	16.8%
Rawlins (1978)	Indiana	Obstetric counseling and group support (L)	†	Hospital discharge 5 mo postpartum	33.0% 15.0%	65.0% 52.0%	32.0% 37.0%

From Winikoff, B., and Baer, E.C.: Am. J. Obstet. Gynecol. **138**:105, 1980.
*C, Cross-sectional. L, Longitudinal. P, Prospective controlled.
†Not given.

Continued.

TABLE 5-1—cont'd
Summary of selected intervention program effects on incidence and duration of breastfeeding

Source	Place	Type of intervention	Sample size	Time of measurement	% Breastfeeding or duration of breastfeeding before intervention (or in control group)	% Breastfeeding or duration of breastfeeding after intervention (or in control group)	Net increase in % breastfeeding or duration of breastfeeding
McBryde (1951)	Durham, North Carolina	Rooming-in (L)	2067	Hospital discharge	35.0%	58.5%	23.5%
Salariva et al. (1978)	Dundee, England	Early initiation and increased frequency of breastfeeding (P)	111	Duration	77 days	182 days	105 days
Sosa et al. (1976)	Guatemala City, Guatemala (Roosevelt Hospital)	Immediate suckling after birth (P)	68	Duration	109 days	139 days	50 days
	Guatemala City, Guatemala (Social Security Hospital)	Immediate suckling after birth (P)	40	Duration	104 days	196 days	92 days
Sousa et al. (1974)	Pelotas, Brazil	Immediate suckling and rooming-in (P)	200	2 mo postpartum	27.0%	77.0%	50.0%
Combined programs							
Jepson et al. (1976)	Sheffield, England	Education and changes in hospital routines (L)	11,658	Intention to breast-feed	36.0%	59.0%	23.0%
Svejcar (1977)	Prague, Czechoslovakia	Education of nursing staff and demand feeding and rooming-in (L)	†	1 mo postpartum Hospital discharge	21.8% 67.0%	27.7% 81.0%	5.9% 14.0%
Wong (1975)	Singapore	Support of breastfeeding by hospital staff and no supplementary feeding (P)	†	Initiation	47.0%	72.0%	25.0%

Study	Location	Intervention	N	Endpoint			
(continued)		(L)		2 mo postpartum	22.1%	69.0%	45.9%
				4 mo postpartum	6.0%	39.4%	33.4%
				6 mo postpartum	1.0%	15.4%	14.4%
Sloper et al. (1977)	Oxford, England	Education of midwives and health visitors (L)	256	Hospital discharge	37.0%	52.0%	15.0%
				5 mo postpartum	23.0%	43.0%	20.0%
Sloper et al. (1975)	Oxford, England	Education of midwives (L)	435	Hospital discharge	14.0%	37.0%	23.0%
Smart and Bamford (1976)	Manchester, England	Education of hospital staff (L)	1448	Hospital discharge	37.0%	44.0%	7.0%
Waller (1946)	Woolwich, England	Daily expression of colostrum (P)	200	†	56.0%	83.0%	27.0%
Changes in hospital routines							
Bjerre and Ekelund (1970)	Malmö, Sweden	Rooming-in (P)	3214	Hospital discharge	76.0%	93.0%	17.0%
Clavano (1978)	Baguio, Philippines	Rooming-in, no supplementary food (L)	10,000	†	26.4%	87.3%	60.9%
De Chateau (1976)	Umeå, Sweden	Skin-to-skin contact and immediate suckling after birth (P)	40	3 mo postpartum	26.0%	58.0%	32.0%
De Chateau et al. (1977)	Umeå, Sweden	No routine weighings and no supplementary food (P)	390	Duration	42 days	95 days	53 days
		Skin-to-skin contact and immediate suckling after birth (P)	42	Duration	108 days	175 days	67 days
Jackson et al. (1956)	New Haven, Connecticut	Rooming-in (P)	282	Duration	1.77 mo	3.14 mo	1.37 mo
Johnson (1976)	Seattle, Washington	Immediate suckling after birth (P)	12	2 mo postpartum	16.6%	100.0%	83.4%
Klaus and Kennell (1976)	Guatemala City, Guatemala (Social Security Hospital)	Immediate suckling after birth (P)	40	6 mo postpartum	16.7%	52.9%	
				12 mo postpartum	0.0%	29.4%	

external stress. The advent of birthing rooms and fathers in the delivery room in hospitals typifies the response to this type of consumer stress, as do many of the programs described later in this chapter.

HOSPITAL-BASED PROGRAMS
Ideal vs. reality

A breastfeeding teaching program is usually one of many changes that occur when a hospital institutes Family-Centered Maternity Care (FCMC). FCMC is advocated in our nursing literature and taught as *de rigueur* in nursing education. As a result, the young graduate naively expects to find these practices in full flower. Unless she chooses her place of employment carefully, she will not find Family-Centered Maternity Care, but rather Hospital-Centered Maternity Care. This type of care is characterized by routine mother-infant separation, separate nursing staffs for postpartum mothers and the central nursery, and a regular practice of giving bottles of glucose water and formula (sometimes even surreptitiously if the physician has ordered otherwise). Even in hospitals with all the family-centered trappings, it is possible to find negative, undermining nurses.

The inconsistencies between her educational experiences and these institutional practices lead to disillusionment (internal stress) and eventually burnout. Kramer aptly describes reality shock experienced by new graduates:

> Shock and rejection sets in as the new graduate comes into daily contact with conflicting values and ways of doing things for which appropriate skills, interpersonal cues, and responses are lacking. This is a crucial phase; conflict resolution may well be maladaptive at this point, and progress toward self-discovery and growth arrested.[8]

Where do you start?

Developing a breastfeeding teaching program in an institutional setting takes strong motivation and patience. The change agent, or prime mover, sometimes must persevere against seemingly endless obstacles of committees, protocols, lines of authority, and political infighting. Even so, approval and review are mandatory.

Where you choose to start will depend on the enthusiasm and support you have from individuals in authority within the hospital. A supportive physician is worth his weight in gold. Your approach will also depend on the autonomy of the nursing service in your hospital, since such a program will fall directly under nursing service or staff development. In some hospitals, nursing service has greater autonomy in decision making than others, but the best place to start is with your immediate supervisor. Experience has shown that starting with the apex of political power in the hospital, the top-level administration and medical department heads, may incur unnecessary delay and actually jeopardize the project. Active support by the head nurse, the charge nurse, and the supervisor of the unit, on the other hand, is essential. One nurse-midwife who was the change agent for a breastfeeding teaching program found it a definite hazard to have only lukewarm support from the nursing administration.

> In trying to sell the idea, I spent time with the nursing supervisor. She seemed to like the idea but turned out to be the kind of person not to follow up on it. I realized it

would be going much faster if she had really believed in it. It's the kind of thing where the supervisor has to be dedicated to the idea. The supervisor and the head nurse are the key.

Apparent support for a new project is quite different from real support. Too often, the superficial enthusiasm of apparent support, meant to please, is followed by passive-aggressive behavior that stymies the project. Despite the clarion call for open communication, an honest and forthright approach is still often chastised in nursing.

In starting a new program, be prepared with written proposals that document the need, objectives, and protocol. Back up your proposal with facts. Use nursing studies that validate the effectiveness of a hospital breastfeeding teaching program on breastfeeding success.[6,12,22,24]

Support from consumers in your community helps create the external stress mentioned earlier. In Boulder, Colorado, a group of health consumers conducted a survey on maternity options that resulted in the implementation of FCMC, with an emphasis on breastfeeding education, in a large medical center. Their survey documented what mothers in the area expected in maternity care.[19] When the consumers embarked on a planned effort to change hospital practices and policies, this datum was a persuasive selling point.

Although nursing literature provides very little practical "know how" information on effecting the change to FCMC, there are articles that would be helpful as you plan.[1,20] First, be prepared for a long, slow process. At Chicago Lying-In Hospital, Paukert[13] found that it took over 1½ years of careful planning and steady implementation in small increments to establish an FCMC program that used a single nursing staff for mother-infant care.

In implementing a program, a nurse might expect complaints from the attending physicians who have conflicting views. On the contrary, in surveying many nurses who have been involved in these programs, few reported complaints from physicians. One nurse encountered a physician who stopped by the nursing service to complain about his patients being told not to give routine supplements. After the nurse explained why this was taught, he went off mumbling under his breath but never carried it further. This nurse remarked "I think the *Statement on Breastfeeding* by the Academy of Pediatrics supporting breastfeeding has done more than anything to help back us up."

Breastfeeding education in hospitals can be divided into two programs, one being directed to the staff and the other directed to mothers. Comprehensive programs include both groups. A third area, teaching nursing and medical students, seems to evolve after the program is well established. A case in point is New Haven–Yale University Hospital, where a lactation nurse has been on staff since 1976. Here, in the traditional setting where Jackson did her pioneer work in rooming-in and FCMC, it is not surprising to find that this institution was one of the first to use a lactation nurse. Originally employed for one-to-one lactation counseling on daily rounds and for periodic group sessions for mothers on the unit, the lactation nurse's function has extended to include regular lectures to obstetric residents rotating through the service and to midwifery students at the Yale University Midwifery Department.

Staff education

Regularly scheduled in-services in the maternity unit are an invaluable way for nurses to keep up with new advances and concepts in nursing care, including lactation and breastfeeding. At St. Elizabeth's Hospital in Dayton, Ohio, in-services and orientation in the unit include 4 to 5 hours of extensive content on the lactation process and on breastfeeding problem-solving techniques. Rather than being scheduled, these classes are done ad lib, whenever there is slack time in the unit. Since experience and familiarity with breastfeeding can vary widely from nurse to nurse, an assessment (perhaps a short questionnaire) gives the in-service person an overview of the learning needs of the nurse she is teaching.

Several organizations* regularly offer seminars on lactation and breastfeeding for nursing credit; these seminars are usually well attended and teach valuable information. A number of other seminars have been sponsored by universities, hospitals, and community health departments on a sporadic basis, according to the assessed needs of nurses in their area. In Wichita, Kansas, a seminar on breastfeeding has been held every 2 years for several years. In addition, many La Leche League area conferences all over the country have special sessions with nursing credit. Hospitals have found it economical to send nurses to these conferences and then have them give to the maternity staff in-service presentations based on the new information they have gained.

Mother/client education

Teaching mothers can take place in one of two ways: unit classes and one-to-one teaching. The most effective, but hardest to implement, is one-to-one teaching by the maternity staff (Fig. 5-1). This means that everyone on the staff must have attained an acceptable level of knowledge on the breastfeeding and lactation processes. It also means that there must be some uniformity in the content of what is taught. This is not easy. As women, we have had diverse personal experiences with breastfeeding. Certainly, the lack of personal experience does not preclude a male or female nurse's helping mothers and teaching breastfeeding, but it does mean that we have more to learn, especially since few nursing education programs comprehensively teach breastfeeding information.

A study by Crowder[3] on the level of breastfeeding knowledge of staff maternity and nursery nurses showed that the strongest areas of knowledge were on infant feeding and maternal physiology, whereas the greatest weaknesses in knowledge were on drugs, maternal emotions, and neonatal physiology. Generally the nurses in this study revealed limited knowledge about breastfeeding success factors and concomitant nursing intervention. Surprisingly, few differences existed among the scores of nurses graduating from diploma, associate degree, or baccalaureate programs.

Another problem is the nursing shift system, in which shift rotations mean constantly changing personnel. Sometimes a nurse just gets started helping a mother and discovers it is time to give report. The continuity of the primary nursing concept involving ongoing patient responsibility would go a long way in reducing these frustrations and disruptions in care. Unfortunately, however, primary nursing itself has a long way to go, both in acceptance and in implementation.

A teaching program described by Jarkowsky[7] provides one solution to these problems. In this program the teaching functions are distributed to each member of the nursing staff, who is responsible for making sure her patients have adequate basic information on breastfeeding before being discharged from the hospital. So that the infor-

---

*La Leche League International, Health Education Association, NAACOG.

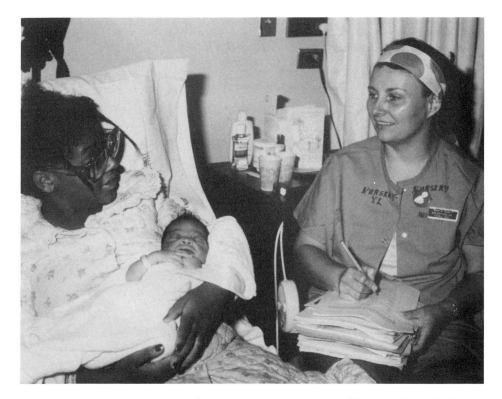

Fig. 5-1. Nurse explaining breastfeeding techniques to new mother. (Courtesy Maricopia County Hospital, Phoenix, Ariz.)

mation giving is consistent, a teaching Kardex with clear and concise information on specific breastfeeding topics, is kept at the nurses' station in the postpartum unit and in the nursery. This Kardex can be carried to the mother's bedside to use as a reference until the staff member is thoroughly familiar with it. Each topic is on a separate index card in the Kardex. The topic number and title correspond to the same topic and number on a checklist. As each topic is covered, a check is made on a checklist sheet similar to the one shown on p. 86. The date and initials of the staff member doing the teaching are included. Comments such as ''Mother is experienced in breastfeeding'' or ''Baby is having difficulty in latching on'' are helpful to the other staff in providing continuity of care. The topics are limited to basic information only; if too much information is called for, the staff is less likely to complete it.

Before this program is implemented, nursing in-services are given to make the staff aware of the new program and to enlist their suggestions. Staff members are less likely to ''forget'' to do the teaching and record it on the checklist if they feel they are part of the planning.

Lactation nurse. Nurses and others who specialize in working with lactating mothers are beginning to call themselves lactation consultants, counselors, or if they are RN's, simply lactation nurses. A general definition of the lactation nurse or counselor is any person professionally engaged in assisting and teaching lactating and breastfeeding women.

SAMPLE CHECKLIST FOR BREASTFEEDING

Hospital breastfeeding teaching checklist to be kept at bedside or on a Kardex for documentation and continuity of teaching.

Name_____ Room number_____

	Date	Comments	Initials
1. Comfortable and proper positioning of infant on breast			
2. Frequency and length of feedings			
3. Care of breast and nipples			
4. Let-down reflex			
5. Prevention of common problems Fear of "losing" milk "Colicky" infant Plugged duct, mastitis			
6. Manual expression			
7. Medications			
8. Home self-care Diet Clothing Child spacing			
9. Special circumstances (prn) Premature or ill infant Inverted nipples Other			

More formal training and breastfeeding education are needed in nursing education programs. In 1977 Whitley was already suggesting that "there is a need for postgraduate training programs in breastfeeding teaching and counseling for maternity nurses."[23] She urged that professional organizations certify nurses who are experts in this area of patient teaching, similar to the certification of a childbirth instructor. To meet the demand for such a specialization within maternity care curriculum, a lactation specialist program could be offered in university nursing education.

Unit classes. The most popular method for teaching any topic in maternity units is regularly scheduled classes in the unit. With this model, mothers are given notice of the time and place classes will be held. The best time of day for the class depends on the routine of the unit and will vary from one hospital to the next. The instructor or leader of the classes can be a staff nurse, a volunteer mother, or sometimes the dietitian. As I stated earlier, it is helpful if she has had personal experience with breastfeeding, but it is not mandatory. Mothers in the unit who are already experienced in breastfeeding should be encouraged to participate, if only to tell the group about their own experiences. Generally speaking, the content structure should be kept open ended and tuned to the needs of the group. A guided discussion will accomplish far more learning than a program so structured that the mother feels that she's back in a high school or college class.

In developing and teaching unit classes for mothers, the nurse should keep in mind that all learning falls into three domains: cognitive (knowledge), affective (attitudes), and psychomotor (skills). Although the content of breastfeeding education falls into all three of these domains, there is a strong affective component, which, used with care, will enhance learning. Using visual aids such as slides, tapes, or charts effectively reinforces the cognitive information in a unit class; however, mothers learn more quickly if they have a role model. Nothing can replace the effectiveness of free interchange and sharing experiences that include personal success, doubts, and fears. Guiding this discussion without bruising the sensitivities of any mother present takes an experienced group leader. Not just anyone with a background in breastfeeding will do. She must have the attributes of wide acceptance, insight, and maturity.

A 50-minute breastfeeding class for mothers could be structured as follows:

Objective: To facilitate a guided small group discussion on lactation and breastfeeding self-care and self-care deficits (problems)

  I. Self-introduction by mothers and a brief description of experience
 II. Assessment of level of knowledge and experience
    A. Prenatal reading or classes
    B. Normal breastfeeding patterns
    C. Proper position and placement
III. Self-care skills
    A. Sore nipples
    B. Engorgement
    C. Maintaining milk supply
    D. Monitoring intake
    E. Normal stool patterns
 IV. Diet at home
  V. Convenient clothing for discreet breastfeeding
 VI. Weaning
VII. Referral persons in the community

Although guided discussion is most effective, visual aids that could be used in unit classes are available from sources listed in Appendix B.

Bedside self-instruction. Closed-circuit television programming for patient education is the newest innovation. It requires sophisticated and expensive equipment, but more and more hospitals are using it effectively. Only a few videotapes of breastfeeding-related topics are available (see Appendix B) at present. Developing your own videotape or slide/tape for your hospital would certainly take time and effort but is a valuable investment considering the potential long-term usage. Many graduate programs award academic credit for such a project. For example, a slide/tape program in constant use in the maternity unit of Wesley Medical Center in Wichita, Kansas, was the graduate project of a charge nurse.

Another alternative is bedside self-instruction with audiotape cassettes, which are inexpensive and easy to use. The tape should be kept short, for even though the mother is in a state of readiness to learn, the lack of visual reinforcements reduces her attention

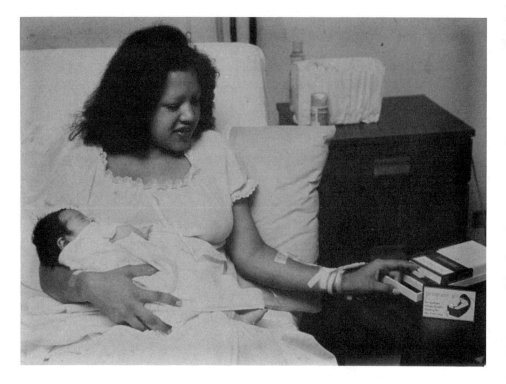

Fig. 5-2. Bedside self-instruction using audio cassette tape. (Courtesy Maricopia County Hospital, Phoenix, Ariz.)

span. At the Maricopia County Hospital in Phoenix, Arizona, a cassette tape is given to each mother who is breastfeeding for the first time (Fig. 5-2). Since many of the mothers speak only Spanish, the tapes are available in either English or Spanish. Dial access programs in which the telephone is used to request a tape on a health topic have been developed as a community service by hospitals, universities, and health agencies. Over the past year, the dial access program at Wichita State University (Tel-Med), which has a tape on breastfeeding, received over 2000 calls per month.

Some hospitals use a sound filmstrip on a Dukane projector that can be placed on a wheeled cart and brought into the mother's room for individual viewing. The advantage is that is can be used any time of the day or night at the mother's convenience. I caution against sole reliance on audiovisual aids for teaching breastfeeding. Ideally there should be the personal one-to-one component of bedside teaching or classes.

Written materials. Written materials are effective teaching tools only when they are presented during learning "readiness" and geared to the mother's educational level and her cultural needs. Women who have done extensive reading on breastfeeding during their pregnancy (an optimal time for learning) are prepared and seem to have fewer difficulties than those who have read little. However, it is important to note that printed teaching materials are *least* valuable during the immediate postpartal period. Rubin[18] described this time as a "taking in" process—a time when the mother turns inward to

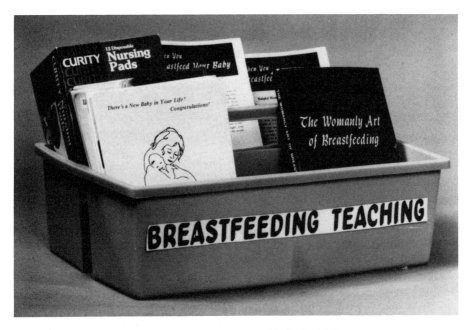

Fig. 5-3. Breastfeeding education basket for bedside teaching.

deal with adjustment of self-concept, self-image, and role. Her energies are spent on physical discomforts, concerns about her new baby, and her new role. Childbirth, in short, is a time of stress, with many new stimuli being absorbed by the mother in a short time. As a result, even oral instructions must frequently be repeated to be remembered.

Another limitation is that many mothers learn better through seeing and doing than through reading. Language barriers must also be dealt with for the mother not proficient in English. If written materials are used, they should be given to the mother to take home. When she has made the necessary psychosocial adjustments, she will be better able to read them with understanding. A basket containing materials on breastfeeding and special aids to lactation (Fig. 5-3) can be kept in the unit and easily carried to the mother's room; this will give her the opportunity to look over a variety of materials and choose the ones she wants and needs.

For evaluating pamphlets on breastfeeding, these guidelines are suggested:

1. Is the information correct? Some pamphlets have rigid rules for frequency, length, and number of feedings. You can discard any of these.
2. Does it read well? It should be written in the active voice and speak to the mother in a conversational style. Long, boring scientific descriptions are completely inappropriate, so avoid pamphlets with detailed explanations of anatomy and physiology. Very few women are interested in how many breast lobes they have or how nutrients are passed through membranes to make milk.
3. Is the educational level suitable for most mothers? A study by Doak[4] showed that at least 20% of adults comprehend only one half of patient education mate-

rials given to them. If it is written anywhere from a sixth to a tenth grade level, it will be readable for most mothers, although many college graduates might find it a little boring. Readability level can be determined by using a standardized formula to determine grade level.[16]

4. Is there a hidden meaning? Most pamphlets printed by formula companies, for example, discreetly drop a phrase such as ". . . and if you decide to stop breast-feeding, our formula provides the right amount of nutrients to support your baby's growth." These implications of inadequacy are particularly destructive to the mother from another culture.

5. Is the information usable over a long time? Some hospitals print their own instructions, which is commendable. But including the names of current staff members and specific hospital policies dates pamphlets very quickly. Too many hospital closets are already filled with outdated literature.

6. What is the cost? Refer back to question 4. Obviously, the least expensive are the pamphlets given free by proprietary companies with a product to sell. Some of them even contain good information. The price of credibility, however, is high, and some mothers are critical of the obvious irony. A few hospitals solve the cost problem of purchasing pamphlets by having reading materials available in the unit for mothers to check out and return. Even with occasional disappearances, the low cost of materials available from the following organizations makes them worthwhile.

La Leche League International
9616 Minneapolis Avenue
Franklin Park, Ill. 60131

Health Education Associates, Inc.
520 School House Lane
Willow Grove, Pa. 19090

International Childbirth Education Association
ICEA Book Center
P.O. Box 20048
Minneapolis, Minn. 55420

Prenatal classes. Hospital-based programs that teach breastfeeding prenatally, which are being offered more and more frequently, usually function as a special section of parenting classes. Since these classes are usually self-sustained, through parent fees, limited hospital budgets are not a problem. Also, hospitals are mindful of the positive public image they create.

These classes may be organized by and under the responsibility of either the clinical nursing supervisors or the staff development department. Nurses often do the teaching. But since many nurses are overworked, experienced mothers in the community often help with these popular classes. A teacher of one of these classes praised the nurse organizer as "extremely open to nonnurses as a part of the prenatal program. Her skill in getting and creating opportunities for breastfeeding education of parents coming to the hospital makes her contribution very special."

At the Washington Hospital Center in Washington, D.C., two antepartum classes in breastfeeding are taught by a nurse each month. Before a couple complete the class they are assigned to a support person, usually a La Leche League leader, to whom they can turn during the postpartum period. About half of the fathers attend these classes. The lactation nurse also gives in-service classes to the nursing personnel using a curriculum that includes background reading, hospital rounds, assistant teaching in the parents'

TABLE 5-2

Effect of breastfeeding education on breastfeeding outcome among three groups of mothers

Group	Duration of breastfeeding (days)	Days increase over Group A (days)
Group A		
No treatment	62	
Group B		
Breastfeeding counseling only	82	20
Group C		
Breastfeeding counseling, staff in-services, audio cassette project, hospital policy changes	96	34

From Operation Collaboration, Maricopia County General Hospital, Phoenix, 1979.

TABLE 5-3

Actual project costs of Maricopia County Breastfeeding Program in 1979

Services	Amount ($)
In-hospital counseling	6760
In-services	265
Toll calls	95
Literature, mothers	420
Literature, staff	500
Postage, supplies	75
Facilities	0
Equipment purchases	
ACCP (4-year depreciation)	145
Prorated costs	
Medical supervision, counsel	1000
Secretaries, clerical	150
TOTAL COSTS	9410

From Operation Collaboration, Maricopia County General Hospital, Phoenix, 1979.

class, a lecture on anatomy and physiology, case studies, and role playing of counseling techniques.[21]

Model program

Some programs begin seemingly spontaneously. At the Maricopia County Hospital in Phoenix, a 525-bed hospital serving the indigent population of that area, the begin-

TABLE 5-4

Breakdown of problems called into the Lactation Clinic Hot Line at the University of California, San Diego Medical Center, during a 12-month period

Problems	Number
Maternal	
Pumping and storage	82
Drug and contaminant questions	73
Nipple problem	69
Milk production problem, too little	63
Engorgement	51
Maternal illness	38
Other	36
Breast infection, mastitis	35
Maternal diet and supplements	24
Clogged, obstructed duct	19
Milk production problem, too much	17
Nursing adopted baby	6
Prenatal nipple preparation	2
Let-down problem, inhibition	2
Let-down problem, excessive	1
TOTAL	518
Infant	
Weight, too little	
Weaning, how to	47
Miscellaneous health	46
Special babies, premature	42
Refusal to breastfeed, cause unclear	26
Refusal to breastfeed, nipple confu-	25
sion	20
Latching on problems	16
Feeding frequency, too often	14
Feeding frequency, infrequent	13
"Vomiting," spitting up	11
Special babies, twins	11
Supplements, milk	10
"Colic"	8
Supplements, solids	7
Thrush	7
Weaning, when	4
Special babies, handicapped	3
Special babies, allergies	2
Supplements, vitamins	2
Supplements, water	2
Special babies, triplets	1
Special babies, heart problem	1
Weight, too much	0
TOTAL	318

From University Hospital, University of California, San Diego Medical Center.

ning was a casual conversation between the Director of the Nurse-Midwifery Services and a bilingual La Leche League leader. Shortly thereafter, the leader was invited to come into the maternity unit two mornings a week to visit breastfeeding mothers and give them basic information in both English and Spanish.

Since that time this service, called the Breastfeeding Education Program, has grown. Four breastfeeding counselors are now employed, and in-service sessions on breastfeeding are given regularly to the maternity staff, including physicians. In addition, an audio cassette has been developed for bedside teaching, and an informal milk bank has been established to provide breastmilk for high-risk infants in the intensive care unit. Gradually, following implementation, the hospital's written policies had to be modified. Since the beginning of the program, over 4000 mothers delivering at this hospital have been served by this program.

Administrators who are wary over the costs of such a program should be aware of this fact: a cost-benefit analysis of the Maricopia program showed that it is paying its own way in the county system. A survey of this program's impact on the long-term outcomes of breastfeeding showed a significant increase in the mean duration of breastfeeding between those who received breastfeeding education services and those who did not (Table 5-2). Overall costs of the program are given in Table 5-3.

LACTATION CLINICS

Specialized lactation clinics have a great potential for helping mothers. Two of these clinics are located in southern California at The University of California in San Diego and The University of Southern California in Los Angeles. Their function is futuristic in concept, and within 20 years there will probably be clinics like these all over the world. According to Naylor, the Director of the Lactation Clinic at the University of California University Hospital in San Diego,* "successful breastfeeding requires more than words of encouragement. It requires a continuum of skilled services designed to enhance the synchronous breastfeeding duet learned by the mother-infant couple." In this clinic and in the one in Los Angeles† women clients and their babies are seen by nurse practitioners, interns, and resident physicians.

These clinics provide an invaluable service during the first few weeks after delivery, when the risk of breastfeeding problems is greatest. They offer intermediate care if the mother is having breastfeeding problems before consultation with her physician at the traditional 6-week well baby visit. Many, but not all, of the mothers attend the clinic as part of a prepaid medical maternity package that includes this visit as an added service. This gives the clinic a sound economic base. Because these programs are comprehensive and successful, I describe them here as possible models, worthy of study by nursing and medical personnel interested in developing similar programs.

San Diego clinic

The San Diego Lactation Clinic is part of a larger lactation program that involves multidisciplinary contributions from several departments of medical, nursing, social,

---

*Breastfeeding Infant Clinic, Pediatric Pavilion CDI, Los Angeles County, University of Southern California Medical Center, 90033.
†Lactation Clinic, University of California Medical Center, San Diego, University Hospital, 92103.

and dietary services. Through this combined effort, a four-part breastfeeding program has been developed that includes (1) prenatal guidance in which parents attend a series of childbearing classes, (2) skilled immediate postpartum assistance with rounds by the nurse practitioner or midwife, (3) postpartum evaluation of mother-infant progress and problem solving in the clinic, and (4) a 24-hour telephone consultation service. Nearly all new mothers room-in in this medical center, which has a policy of early and on-demand feedings. No breastfeeding mother is sent home with a discharge pack of for-mula, because this implies potential failure to the mother. The pediatric nurse practi-tioner, who coordinates and oversees the nursing services, works closely with the hos-pital midwives in prenatal teaching of breastfeeding. She makes daily hospital rounds, as well as seeing the women and babies in the clinic. When the clinic is closed, a "hot line" (sometimes known as the "warm milk line") is answered by the midwives who rotate on call at the hospital. An analysis of the problem calls is shown in Table 5-4.

In the San Diego Lactation Clinic, each client completes a Data Base Sheet (Appen-dix A; note the emphasis on her diet) before she is seen by the staff. This information is then transferred along with other pertinent information to a Chart Review Sheet. Before the interview begins, the attending staff (physician, midwife, nurse, dietitian, and social worker) briefly review her case, pooling their knowledge and insights to make recommendations for teaching and intervention. The clinic visit itself includes (1) a breast and nipple assessment, (2) a well baby physical assessment, and (3) observation of the feeding. It is a cardinal rule that the baby be with the mother during the clinic visit and that the observation assessment of the feeding be made whenever the infant is hungry. During the feeding the nurse or physician has an opportunity to correct any positioning or sucking pattern problems. During the physical assessment of the baby, the nurse explains and points out normal infant characteristics to the mother and looks for any physical problems that might hve been missed in the hospital. Each visit lasts approximately 1 hour; this gives plenty of time for self-care health teaching and oppor-tunities for the mother to express her concerns and ask questions. The whole process is quite relaxed and unhurried. Much of the visit time is focused on areas in which the mother lacks confidence. Demonstrating and explaining as needed, the staff make cer-tain that each mother is complimented for what she is doing well. In fact, "stroking"

TABLE 5-5

Use of postdischarge services and duration of breastfeeding*†

Age at time of weaning	Program services utilized			
	Yes		No	
	N	%	N	%
Less than 3 mo	21	22.6	28	32.2
3-5 mo	17	18.3	20	23.0
6 mo or more	55	59.1	39	44.8
TOTAL	93	100.0	87	100.0

From Naylor, A.J., Johnson, D.D., and Wester, R.A.: Teaching health professionals how to promote lactation: ex-ample of a successful program, Symposium on Human Milk Banking, Hradec Kralove, Czechoslovakia, 1981.
*p = <.205.
†Services include lactation clinic and telephone consultation.

for reinforcement is a priority. Before she leaves the clinic, the mother might be referred to the dietitian or social worker if it is warranted.

Over 80% of the women leave the hospital breastfeeding. The effectiveness of this program on the duration of breastfeeding is documented in Table 5-5. In the first 2½ years of the program, 1039 families were served by the clinic. Since it began in 1977, over 350 health professionals have visited and observed this clinic as a learning opportunity.

Los Angeles clinic

At The University of Southern California Medical Center in Los Angeles, where approximately 16,000 babies are born annually, a breastfeeding clinic serves many Hispanic mothers who have recently come to this country, legally or otherwise, to find work and a better life. They receive packaged maternity services, which include prenatal care, delivery, visits after delivery, and visits to the Lactation Clinic. By coming to the clinic approximately 2 weeks after delivery, these mothers break a traditional Hispanic postpartum confinement of 40 days.

The clinic, directed by the pediatric nurse practitioner, also serves as a teaching/learning experience for health professionals and students. Before the clinic begins, nurses, medical students, and residents are briefed with basic information on the lactation process and interventions, with particular emphasis on the cultural influences. For instance, in the history and assessment sheet, a question that asks how many wet diapers the baby has in a day is singled out as a question that has special implications for families with limited resources. The pediatric nurse practitioner explains that most of these mothers prefer disposable paper diapers to cloth diapers and probably pay a high price for them in local stores, since getting transportation to large discount stores is often difficult. Therefore such a mother tends to keep a diaper on her baby longer and changes it only when it becomes supersaturated—an important point to consider in evaluating the infant's hydration and intake of breastmilk and in teaching prevention of diaper rash.

This clinic visit closely parallels the one in the San Diego clinic, except that medical students and medical house staff do the assessments here. Once they complete their assessment, they report their evaluation to the nurse practitioner for review before making recommendations or doing self-care teaching.

COMMUNITY SELF-CARE GROUPS

The emergence of many self-care groups and organizations within the last decade is a phenomenon worthy of investigation. Before describing those related to breastfeeding education, we need to know more about the origin and function of self-care groups per se.

People who help people

The essence of people coming together for mutual support stems from (1) the failure of other support systems and (2) the need for significant others to help individuals use their resources and share tasks, skills, and cognitive guidance. Self-care groups operate by collecting and storing information on one subject that relates to a role or a problem. They offer guidance and direction to the individual and can be a refuge or sanctuary from a stressful environment.

Self-care groups are usually outside established systems, although they may interface with them in dialogue and sometimes even in organizational structure. Interestingly, these groups are usually more aware of the established, or, in this case, the professional health system than the reverse. Once aware, the professional health system tends to view self-care groups with a condescending eye. In doing this, the professionals negate to their own satisfaction the importance and vitality of self-care groups. It seems that our culture has a high value for services that demand remuneration and a lesser value for those that do not. To undervalue the important role of self-care groups in health care is a serious omission. Health services have traditionally been designed to cure; self-care groups are designed to care.

With a mobile society and the absence of the extended family, self-care help plays a surrogate, complementary role to the traditional family support system. In addition to caring, self-care groups educate through these educational processes[2]:

1. The general goal of self-care education is to *increase an individual's effective capacity to self-manage.*
2. The psychosociopolitical perspective reveals self-care as a process that encourages a *shift in the locus of control in health decision making from the health professional to the lay person.* A key attribute of this process is the demystification of health, disease, and medical intervention.
3. Self-care educated persons, by reason of their expanded base of knowledge, skills, and confidence in personal health management, are more able participants in actions to *achieve social programs responsive to individual and community health interests.*
4. The content of self-care education should reflect the preferences of the clients and be *offered in the context of the life-styles of the users.*

Individuals in self-care groups learn through interactions with one another: group learning. Coping with situational or developmental crises, such as impending parenthood, is enhanced through talking with others who are in a similar situation. People learn best what is of immediate concern to them when they are creatively involved in learning through active listening and free response. Since the topics of self-care groups are emotional as much as intellectual, the group leader's empathy with and acceptance of each member's experience is essential.

La Leche League

Without question, the largest and most effective self-care group for breastfeeding help is La Leche League International (LLLI).* Founded in 1956, the organizational base is small neighborhood groups, in which approximately 6 to 20 women attend monthly meetings in the homes of members and volunteer leaders. Members learn of the organization through friends, nurses, physicians, or the news media. Structured topics of these meetings are (1) the advantages of breastfeeding to the mother and the baby, (2) the art of breastfeeding and overcoming difficulties, (3) the arrival of the baby (childbirth), the family and the breastfed baby, and (4) nutrition and weaning. Essentially these talks focus on helpful information about breastfeeding, childbearing, and child rearing.

---

*La Leche League International, Inc., 9616 Minneapolis Avenue, Franklin Park, Ill., 60131.

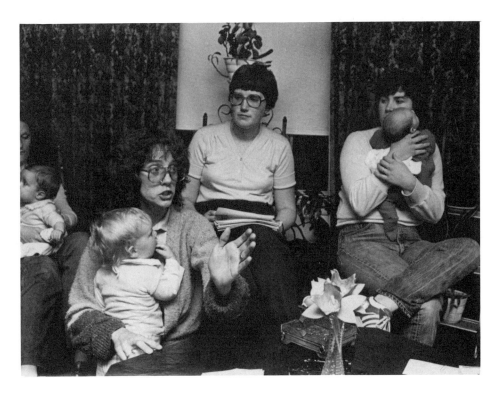

Fig. 5-4. Principles of adult learning in action: a La Leche League meeting. (Courtesy La Leche League International.)

Between meetings, the leaders make themselves available to mothers for guidance, support, and problem solving. Each group maintains a lending library of pertinent books and information sheets, and members receive a bimonthly newsletter. Although they may no longer be in their childbearing years, some experienced women continue to lead or simply attend League meetings to give assistance to first-time mothers who are learning to breastfeed and to parent. Following the scheduled topic, an informal discussion provides friendly, relaxed interchanges between women with a common role and interest in breastfeeding (Fig. 5-4).

La Leche League leaders are regarded as local authorities on breastfeeding and have various socioeconomic backgrounds, although most are white, middle-class women with some college preparation. These women are chosen carefully and become certified leaders after completing a period of training that involves reading, having discussions with experienced leaders, and attending workshops. The last two decades of rapid growth are evidence of this self-help organization's spectacular success in filling the vacuum of breastfeeding education needs that have not been met by health-care professionals. As of this writing there are almost 5000 active groups reaching 100,000 mothers monthly. Although most of these are in the United States, La Leche League groups are found in 49 other countries.

Adult learning principles. In trying to analyze the growth and success of La

---

ADULT LEARNING PRINCIPLES—
ANALYSIS AND APPLICATION IN LA LECHE
LEAGUE GROUP MEETINGS

Principles	Rationale
A. *Readiness to learn* Voluntary attendance after seeking out information about meeting. Participation in discussion. Checking out reading materials.	Importance of new learning for social roles; developing mental maturity.
B. *Problem-centered learning* Hints on ways to improve family nutrition: free discussion. Frequency of breastfeedings and how long? Weaning—how long? Methods of weaning. Modesty during nursing—wearing the right clothing. Mother's diet—what foods can affect the milk? Breast cancer—will breastfeeding protect? Introducing solid foods—what, when, and how?	Immediate application in daily coping; directly related to real problems.
C. *Climate for learning: informality, comfort, and friendliness* Home setting; comfortable chairs, pillows on floor. Babies and small children present—"relaxed" atmosphere facilitating socialization.	Creating a psychologic climate conducive to adult learning.
D. *Involvement of learners in planning and goal setting* Group decides when and where future meetings will occur. Individual problems and needs are discussed following the scheduled topic.	Validating self-concept; adults see themselves as self-directing and needing respect.

Leche League, I looked at what makes the organization "tick": the group meetings. I discovered that the elements of these meetings are closely aligned to adult education principles. By their informal yet goal-oriented format, the small group meeting has captured the ingredients of how adults learn best. These principles and their relationship to the dynamics of the meeting are organized in the box above and were developed from a meeting on family nutrition. They would be relevant and useful to the community nurse who is developing a parenting or breastfeeding education program.

Making a difference. The effectiveness of any program can only be verified by outcome data. In the mid-70's, Meara[11] conducted a research study on the perspectives

TABLE 5-6

Percentage of respondents who follow LLL perspectives and whose breastfeeding experience was only before or only following affiliation with LLL.

Perspective	LLL affiliation	No LLL affiliation
Timing of feeding		
Breastfeeding infant on demand	96%	93%
	(446)	(84)
Weaning		
Introducing first solids at 4-6 mo	87%	31%
	(379)	(13)
Gradual and cooperative	87%	37%
weaning	(347)	(13)
Nursing longer than 9 mo	80%	50%
	(296)	(36)
Hospital routines		
Breastfeeding infant on demand	60%	29%
in hospital	(262)	(34)
Rooming-in at hospital	43%	23%
	(173)	(28)
Breastfeeding soon after	54%	20%
delivery	(233)	(24)

From Meara, H.: J. Nurse-Midwifery **21**:20, 1976.

and behavioral differences of women before and after affiliation with La Leche League (Table 5-6). The results demonstrated significant changes in attitudes and in infant care patterns. Criticism of LLL advocacy of breastfeeding for inducing guilt feelings is an issue appraised by Meara as "rarely tempered by acknowledgement of the many occasions where helpful support does not exceed reasonable bounds. One can readily imagine, however, that there are far more casualties in the unaided battle of healthy and willing infants and mothers to breastfeed against a resistant culture."

Other groups

Nursing Mothers' Counsel. Primarily based in northern California, the dedicated members of this organization give personal counseling (hence the name) to breastfeeding mothers. Much of this counseling is by telephone, since there are no meetings for mothers. Information is conveyed by members who visit mothers during their hospital stay and at home during the postpartum period. The organization gives in-services to hospital personnel and publishes a professional bulletin with the latest information on breastfeeding. It also maintains a lending library and publishes a number of excellent booklets on breastfeeding topics.*

Nursing Mothers' Group (Philadelphia CEA). In the metropolitan Philadelphia area, a growing organization called the Nursing Mothers' Group is sponsored by the Childbirth Education Association.† Here, small monthly group discussions on breast-

*Nursing Mothers' Counsel, Inc., P.O. Box 50063, Palo Alto, Calif.
†CEA of Greater Phildelphia, Nursing Mothers, 129 Fayette St., Conshohochen, Pa. 19428.

feeding topics are offered in private homes, much like La Leche League, In this organization, one mother helps another within a loosely structured setting.

Most women hear of this program when they are contacted by the group during their
hospital stay. Attendance is generally free, and like La Leche League, the women in
charge volunteer their time. Periodic fund-raising events and sales of infant care products, such as baby carriers, help pay some of the program expenses. Depots for breast
pump rentals are located in strategic areas in and around Philadephia and are accessible
to mothers of sick infants or those returning to work. Like other self-care groups, the
Nursing Mothers' Groups are available for telephone counseling and provide speakers
for meetings.

Childbirth preparation classes

Since the advent of the childbirth education movement in the 1950's, there has been
a dramatic proliferation of childbirth education groups under the umbrella organizations
of the American Society for Psychoprophylaxis in Obstetrics (ASPO),* the International
Childbirth Education Association (ICEA),† and the National Association of Parents and
Professionals for Safe Alternatives in Childbirth (NAPSAC).‡ The content and structure
of these childbirth preparation classes vary according to the method espoused by the
teacher. Most, however, contain some breastfeeding information. Unlike La Leche League
meetings, the father or some significant other attends with the mother to serve as her
coach. For many of these parents, this is the only structured information on breastfeeding they receive before delivery. Childbirth instructors make liberal use of audiovisual
materials in teaching basic aspects of anatomy, physiology, and breastfeeding. Because
childbirth, not breastfeeding, is the main focus of the classes, the breastfeeding information is usually not extensive. Potential problems are covered only if they are brought
up by the parents. Often, the teachers of these classes are under the sponsorship of local
CEA affiliates and are paid through parent fees. The classes use hospital facilities or
other places in the community where rooms are available. There is, however, a current
trend toward hospital-sponsored classes that employ teachers. Many of the instructors
are nurses who have had additional training and certification through ASPO. Some are
also certified as La Leche League leaders.

A group method of learning, in which the parents themselves help set the goals and
provide the answers, is used with great success in this setting. At the beginning of
childbirth education classes taught by Perinelli,[14] couples complete a registration card
that includes a question about the planned feeding method. Then during one class couples are asked to discuss their feeding choices. This allows probing parents to share
what they feel are benefits in breastfeeding. Some of the reasons given for choosing
bottle-feeding were the need to return to work, anxiety about birth control, and modesty.
Each reason provides an opportunity to deal specifically with possible solutions if the
couple does want to breastfeed. In another group taught by Crofts in Connecticut, a
breastfeeding mother, baby, and father who are "graduates" of a former class attend to
tell the group about their experiences. This uses a role model in transferring knowledge

*ASPO, Suite 410, 1523 L. Street NW, Washington, D.C., 20005.
†International Childbirth Education Association, P.O. Box 20048, Minneapolis, Minn. 55420.
‡National Association of Parents and Professionals for Safe Alternatives in Childbirth, P.O. Box 1307, Chapel
Hill, N.C. 27504.

and skills and is a teaching method nurses need to use as often as possible.

Fathers. The presence of fathers at class adds a rich dimension (including male humor) to the discussion. Breastfeeding, after all, is a family experience and is not limited to the mother and baby. Fathers are quick to point out the bonuses when their mate breastfeeds their baby:

> So who wants to get up at night to feed the kid?
> Besides just the milk, I can see our baby getting the nurturance.

They are full of practical suggestions:

> Don't play with your baby during the night feeding or he will want to boogie all night.

And a philosophy of parenting:

> What is spoiling? It's a way of describing a kid you don't like. Your kid is spoiled; my kid is nurtured.

While promoting esprit de corps:

> My wife walked into the women's room at Bloomingdale's last week to breastfeed the baby and found 12 other women doing the same thing!

Fathers help each other realize they are not alone in having ambivalent feelings about the closeness between their breastfeeding wives and babies:

> If I'd been more prepared that they would be this complete unit unto themselves, it would have been easier. For a while I felt left out, like I was around only to bring home the money and wasn't a part of it. I felt bad and then guilty about feeling bad. Before the baby came, my wife really spoiled me, you know, really adored and lavished attention on me. Then, whammo, she was pregnant 3 months after we were married and I wasn't getting that kind of treatment anymore. I resented it.

And offer a resolution:

> Things really broke loose and we had a showdown. I finally had to open up and let her know how I really felt. After that, when it was all in the open, things got better. With the next one, I don't think I'll go through those feelings again.

Special classes. A few CEA groups offer more extensive breastfeeding information. In Dayton, Ohio, an "In-depth Preparation for Breastfeeding" is offered as an optional class at the end of the prenatal childbirth preparation series. These 2½ hour classes were started by Cotterman in 1974 and have increased in number because of the popular demand for them. In addition to giving the mothers practical information on lactation, a private assessment is done in which the mother learns self-care skills that include assessing her nipple function, correct positioning of the baby on the breast, breast massage, and hand expression. In cases of nipple dysfunction, the mother is taught interventions such as exercises and nipple rolling and is given plastic breast shields, if needed. According to the instructors, 80% of the mothers who attend these classes are still breastfeeding at 1 year.

Home birth self-care groups

Parents planning home births almost invariably intend to breastfeed. As a result, organizations whose purpose is assisting parents in having childbirth at home have breastfeeding education materials as a part of their service. A national organization for Home Oriented Maternity Experience (HOME), organized by Hermann, offers parents helpful information on breastfeeding in their manual and through newsletters. The same services are available from the Association for Childbirth at Home, International (ACHI).

PRIVATE PRACTICE

When word gets around that the new medical practitioner in town is supportive and knowledgeable about breastfeeding and lactation, the practice builds very quickly. If parenting and breastfeeding groups are offered as well, the practitioner is soon overwhelmed with clients.

Nurse-midwives

Realizing the need for parenting and breastfeeding classes, an encouraging number of practitioners offer them as a vital service in total maternity care. These classes are taught by nurses or women with special educational preparation and experience. One such parenting teching program is provided by a nurse-midwifery obstetric practice* in the Washington, D.C. area. A parent educator leads a series of four classes. The first, an antepartum class, includes breastfeeding and is required for parents. They are called classes for lack of a better term—they are really informal, lively, discussion groups that encourage free parent-to-parent interaction, expression of feeling, and problem solving. "What do you do with a fussy baby?" asks one pregnant mother. "Put him in a warm tub with you" answers an experienced father. In postpartum sessions, these group discussions deal with changing relationships of the couple and adjustments of fitting the parents' life-style to the baby, among many other topics. Many of the deliveries are at home, and parents are asked to call in within the first 48 hours after delivery to relate the progress of breastfeeding and to allow intervention before any problems arise. The data of this program are impressive: 98% are still breastfeeding at 1 month and 75% at 1 year. These figures are in vivid contrast to the national statistics cited in Chapter 1.

Medical practice

A sensitive, knowledgeable nurse is an invaluable asset to a physician in private practice. After receiving more phone calls than he could possibly handle from distressed breastfeeding women, Gustafson,[9] in Royal Oak, Michigan, hired such a nurse to help him.

The nurse soon found phone conversations too limiting and initiated home visits, much to the relief of the women clients who were spared a trip into the office. During home visits, she found a further need: prenatal instruction to help mothers prevent some of the breastfeeding problems they were encountering. "By the time I made my home call, I found the ball game [breastfeeding] was over."

When another staff member was needed, a La Leche League leader who was not a nurse was hired to help teach the prenatal breastfeeding classes. Currently five lactation consultants are employed and evening pre- and postnatal classes are held in a separate

---

*Maternity Center Associates, Bethesda, Md.

education building, which was purchased for that purpose. Each lactation consultant carries a caseload of approximately 55 mothers and does much of her work by telephone from home. This practice also has a number of electric and hand pumps for their clients' use.

Everyone benefits in this type of practice—mothers, babies, fathers, nurses, staff, and physicians alike. As other medical practitioners realize the advantages of this approach, they will incorporate extended teaching services into their practices.

BIRTH CENTERS

The number of freestanding birth centers increases every year in this country to meet the needs of people generally committed to a natural life-style that encompasses childbirth and breastfeeding. Virtually all these centers have prenatal and postnatal classes that offer breastfeeding information for their clients. In canvassing various centers, I found that the teaching took place on two levels: (1) a formal method of required, structured prenatal classes that use abundant audiovisual aids and (2) ongoing voluntary postnatal parent groups. The parent groups are often led by graduate parents who have experience and superior communication skills and who serve as role models and doulas to the less experienced parents.

An example of this model is the Childbearing Center, a part of Maternity Center Associates in Manhattan. Maternal nutrition is a high priority in their antenatal care, and a nutritionist on staff works closely with the nurse-midwife in monitoring the mother and in teaching the family.

Birthing centers use community resources freely in referring their clients for follow-up support and care. The bulletin boards at these centers almost invariably carry a listing of breastfeeding support groups and other community health services.

PRIVATE LACTATION SERVICES

A unique private breastfeeding consultation for lactating women is located in southern California. The Lactation Institute,* a staff of women experienced in tackling breastfeeding problems, offer their services for a fee. They maintain an ample supply of breast pumps, breastfeeding aids, and written materials for mothers who contact them. Some of these women need only a breast pump to use at work, but others have more complicated problems like inverted nipples. Marmet, the head of the Institute, is an expert on nipple inversion, having overcome this problem herself. In fact, it was because of her difficulties in breastfeeding that she became interested in providing services as a lactation consultant. Successful self-care, in this case, motivated her to build a private service in which breast assessment, teaching of basic skills, and problem solving takes place outside the traditional health-care system. Like the in-depth breastfeeding classes described earlier, these women offer an alternative to mothers who are not receiving this care in physicians' offices, hospital, or elsewhere.

PROGRAMS FOR WOMEN WITH LIMITED RESOURCES

Over the past decade a number of community-based programs have been developed for mothers who have limited financial resources. They are usually referred to as inner-

---

*Lactation Institute, 3441 Clairton Place, Encino, Calif. 91436.

city programs if they are located within the city core area. Sponsored by La Leche League or by community health departments, these programs have met with only limited success. Although breastfeeding rates among black women are on the rise, as a group they are still the least likely to breastfeed. Undoubtedly, one of the problems with programs of this type is the cultural gap between the instructors and the women or parents who attend. Later in this book I discuss cultural differences on a more global scale. Here we see that cultural differences among various socioeconomic groups can be just as challenging and frustrating to overcome. According to an instructor of an inner-city clinic breastfeeding education program:

> One of our biggest problems is that of communication. Most of the mothers we see are very quiet, shy, reserved, and insecure. They do not ask questions and barely open up to us. Most of them don't have phones and change apartments often. Some only visit the clinic a few times, maybe only once. It is very difficult for us to build a relationship seeing them maybe just at one clinic session. For some, using the birth control pill is a deterrent to breastfeeding. Many of the mothers wish to resume this type of contraception a week or so after delivery. Others return to work in 4 to 6 weeks. Life is very trying for many of these mothers, and they lack confidence in their ability to breastfeed and can't face any more disappointments. The ones who did seem interested in breast-feeding were more self-confident, better informed, and more out-going women.

In addition to the health, nutritional, and bonding advantages of breastfeeding, saving the expense of formula is especially important for mothers with limited financial resources. Also, having a positive experience with breastfeeding gives them confidence, as this statement from a midwife working at a county hospital attests:

> These mothers have rarely been in control of their lives, and life has treated them badly. That's why they are at County Hospital instead of a private institution. If I can help these women to give birth, rather than be delivered, and to actively participate in the feeding of their infants by producing milk, rather than passively receiving another dole, a supply of formula from the County, then I have helped them realize that they can control their bodies—and their lives. They find that they are worthwhile human beings, vitally important to the well-being of their babies, and they are competent to nourish and care for them. I think that successful nursing is so important to the deprived mother, perhaps even more important than to a mother who has had things going her way since she can remember.[15]

The challenge

Working with disadvantaged breastfeeding mothers poses other special challenges. They move frequently, making it difficult to keep in touch. By the time the nurse finally finds their new address, a crisis may have already happened and the baby is being bottle-fed. Few have telephones, and home visits, which are time consuming, are the only method of contact. This mother may look on the nurse, particularly if she is of another race, as an imposing stranger. Special communication skills must be used and trust established before any help is effective.

These mothers are intelligent, but they are less interested in the written word than are mothers with more education, so reading materials must be simple and short. Two good pamphlets for this purpose are available from La Leche League and ICEA.[5,9]

Several years ago as a school nurse in an inner-city area, I worked with young mothers, most of whom chose not to breastfeed. As I knew them better, I discovered their reasons were mainly related to going back to work, not realizing they could work and breastfeed. Others said, ''My friends are all bottle-feeding'' or ''it's too much trouble.'' A few stated that their physicians had advised against breastfeeding.

An experimental group

While gathering data for a graduate nursing research project, I became aware that less than half of the mothers in an outlying low socioeconomic area breastfed their babies. If they did start breastfeeding, most of the babies were weaned prematurely, often within the first 2 weeks. Thinking that this probably was a direct result of the lack of the support system for breastfeeding, I looked for an opportunity to organize a La Leche League group in one of these areas.

The opportunity arrived one evening when I received a call from a mother to help her sell her own extra breastmilk, since she urgently needed money. Failing to help her contact a ''buyer,'' I tried to help in other ways, such as sharing food and clothing. From this beginning, we held our first La Leche League meeting. It was a disorganized last minute affair that was held in another home because this first mother abruptly moved out of her home following a family fight.

Our small groups continued to meet every month on a tentative basis. The ground rule was that the need for meeting and maintaining the group must come from the mothers themselves. Each meeting followed a series format with assigned topics discussed first, followed by an open discussion. Our ''audiovisual'' equipment consisted of other nursing mothers and babies. The cohesiveness of this group, like all other La Leche League meetings, was the one-to-one sharing and friendships that ''happened'' without specific effort or planning.

The area, Planeview, was built during World War II as ''temporary'' housing during the years of frantic manufacture of Boeing bombers at the nearby plant. The structures were poorly built quadplexes that provided inexpensive housing for Boeing workers. It was in this area that our first meetings were held at the home of Jolene.

Jolene had breastfed her first baby for 7 weeks before regular formula supplements and solid foods had gradually diminished her milk to a point of complete weaning. Now her second baby was due in a few months and she was enthusiastic about learning more about breastfeeding. She and her husband, who worked nights at the Boeing plant, were part of an extended family for whom this area of Planeview was a place to call ''home,'' allowing them to raise their children within a few blocks of their relatives' homes.

It was crowded in the tiny living room, but somehow we all managed to squeeze in. Several toddlers played in the center of the rug, running back to their mothers from time to time for a reassuring pat. We went around the room and introduced ourselves. Except for myself and one other mother, none of the women there had ever breastfed for more than 2 weeks. One mother explained that she had breastfed that long ''so that my breasts wouldn't be so hard.'' During the discussion that evening, someone mentioned that Princess Grace, Susan St. James, and Natalie Wood breastfed their babies. The room was silent for just a moment before the quiet redhead in the corner ventured,

"You mean all of them?" This bit of information seemed important, presenting an admired role model for emulation.

The group continued to meet during the summer, long after my class had ended. During one of the meetings, I recorded the discussion and analyzed the interactions for positive communications. The topic of this meeting happened to be nutrition.

Positive communication	Example
1. Accepting	"I can understand the way you feel. . . ."
2. Giving recognition	"You really tried, didn't you?"
3. Offering self (most frequent)	Introductions by each woman and telling about personal experience.
4. Giving broad openings	"Is there something we haven't mentioned that you'd like to discuss?"
5. Making observations	"She sure seems to be healthy despite her problems. . . ."
6. Encouraging descriptions and perceptions	"Didn't you have some of the same experiences she had?"
7. Encouraging comparison	"Was this something like. . . ."
8. Reflecting feelings	"It bothers you then, to nurse when your relatives are around?"
9. Focusing and relating	"You seem to be tuned into this already. . . ."
10. Giving information (second most frequent)	Numerous nutritional tips and information given.
11. Seeking clarification	"Do you mean you like using the blender better than the grinder?"
12. Summarizing and encouraging evaluation	"When I feed my family better, they don't seem to have as many colds. . . . Does anyone else feel this way?"

After Jolene gave birth, she excitedly called me from the hospital. "What a difference! We're breastfeeding up a storm and so far no problems." The affiliation with this support group appeared to make a difference in Jolene's ability to breastfeed. This time she did not give supplements: she was confident and knew what to expect. Although she had planned to wean at 6 months, somehow she never got around to it until her baby was 16 months old.

SUMMARY

Implementing changes in breastfeeding policies and providing more education and support go hand-in-hand with larger policy changes in which the nurse can play a vital role. Garnering political and administrative support is absolutely essential, as are data that support its need and effectiveness. Without a doubt, the proliferation of educational programs and resources on breastfeeding of the past few years will continue, as health agencies recognize the need. Likewise, the growth of community-based self-care groups related to childbearing and child rearing show no signs of slowing down.

More and more, nurses find themselves moving out of the institutional walls and into ambulatory settings, where young families who choose to breastfeed are often the focus of nursing care. Perhaps we are late in getting started in breastfeeding education, but we are not too late. In presenting an overview of breastfeeding programs in this chapter, I hope the suggestions and insights can be useful to nurses involved in planning, implementating, and evaluating breastfeeding education.

REFERENCES

1. Bird, I.S.: Breastfeeding classes on the postpartum unit, Am. J. Nurs. **75**:456, 1975.
2. Bureau of Health Education: Self-care: public health service, Washington, D.C., 1978, Department of Health, Education, and Welfare.
3. Crowder, D.S.: Maternity nurses' knowledge of factors promoting successful breastfeeding: a survey at two hospitals, J.O.G.N. Nurs. **10**:28, 1981.
4. Doak, L.G., and Doak, C.C.: Patient comprehension profiles: recent findings and strategies, Pat. Couns. Health Educ. **2**:101, 1980.
5. Haire, D.B.: Simple instructions for nursing your baby, Minneapolis, 1967, International Childbirth Education Association.
6. Hall, J.M.: Influencing breastfeeding success, J.O.G.N. Nurs. **7**:28, 1978.
7. Jarkowsky, M.S.: How to prevent breastfeeding problems, Superv. Nurse **11**:43, 1980.
8. Kramer, M.: Reality shock: why nurses leave nursing, St. Louis, 1974, The C.V. Mosby Co.
9. La Leche League International, Inc.: When you breastfeed your baby, Publication No. 124, Franklin Park, Ill., 1966, The League.
10. La Leche League International, Inc.: Physician's Seminar, Rosemont, Ill., July 1980.
11. Meara, H.: A key to successful breastfeeding in a nonsupportive culture, J. Nurse-Midwifery **21**:20, 1976.
12. Ouellette, M., et al.: The impact of an educational and support program upon modern breastfeeding patterns, unpublished study, Ann Arbor, Mich, 1980.
13. Paukert, S.E.: One hospital's experience with implementing family-centered maternity care, J.O.G.N. Nurs. **8**:351, 1979.
14. Perinelli, M.: Preparation for breastfeeding: a component of childbirth education classes, Keeping Abreast J. **2**:30, 1977.
15. Rapp, E.T.: Female sexuality and lactation, Unpublished paper, Phoenix, Ariz., 1976.
16. Redman, B.K.: The process of patient teaching in nursing, ed. 4, St. Louis, 1980, The C.V. Mosby Co.
17. Rodgers, J.A.: Theoretical considerations involved in the process of change. In Berger, M.S., et al. editors: Management for nurses: a multidisciplinary approach, ed. 2, St. Louis, 1980, The C.V. Mosby Co.
18. Rubin, R.: Attainment of the maternal role. I. Processes. Nurs. Res. **16**:240, 1967.
19. Scaer, R., and Korte, D.: A survey of maternity options, Boulder, Colo., 1977.
20. Selby, M.: Fostering breastfeeding: a pediatric program, Keeping Abreast J. **2**:180, 1977.
21. Taylor, V.: Personal communication, Oct. 1980.
22. Verronen, J.K., et al.: Promotion of breastfeeding: effects of a campaign. In Frier, S., and Eidelman, A.I., editors: Human milk: its biological and social value, Amsterdam, 1980, Excerpta Medica.
23. Whitley, N.: Barriers to effective breastfeeding counseling, Hosp. Top. **55**:40, 1977.
24. Whitley, N.: Preparation for breastfeeding: a one year follow-up of 34 nursing mothers, J.O.G.N. Nurs. **7**:44, 1978.

ADDITIONAL READINGS

Auerbach, A.: Parents learn through discussion, New York, 1968, John Wiley & Sons, Inc.
Marram, G.D.: The group approach in nursing practice, ed. 2, St. Louis, 1978, The C.V. Mosby Co.
Nunnally, D.M.: A new approach to help mothers breastfeed, J.O.G.N. Nurs. **3**:34, 1974.
Stranik, M.K., and Hogberg, B.L.: Transition into parenthood. Am. J. Nurs. **79**:90, 1979.

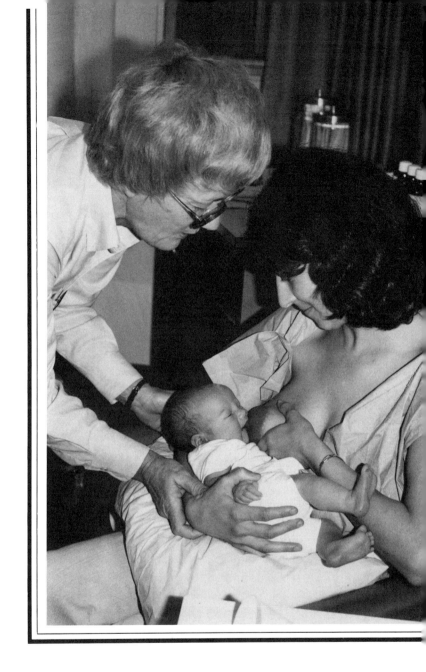

PART TWO

BREASTFEEDING PROBLEMS AND NURSING SOLUTIONS

In nursing practice, as elsewhere, an ounce of prevention is worth a pound of intervention. Many difficulties women encounter while breastfeeding can be prevented by the self-care measures and breastfeeding education discussed in the preceding chapters. When a woman fully understands how to breastfeed, she is at less risk for frustration and failure when she encounters a barrier to breastfeeding. I turn now to problems or self-care deficits that can occur, identifying how nurses can help and giving a clinical foundation to work from.

Special situations in breastfeeding arise much more frequently today than in the past. With the technologic advances in the care of premature infants, concerns over infant jaundice, and the common use of over-the-counter and prescription drugs, nurses are increasingly called on for information and guidance. More often than not, the breastfeeding mother will at some point require extra help and information from nurses and other health professionals.

Self-care deficits of the breastfeeding mother

JAN RIORDAN

As a complement to the self-care approach described in Chapter 4, concern now focuses on deficits in the ability for self-care in breastfeeding, when a problem prevents or hinders normal breastfeeding and professional assistance is needed. The term *self-care deficit* is used here to mean an inability of a mother to maintain optimal breast-feeding for a health-related reason that requires specialized help and guidance.

What effect do maternal self-care deficits have on the outcome of breastfeeding? Not surprisingly, Evans et al.[9] established that women with early deficits were significantly less successful at breastfeeding. In helping these women, surely nurses, since they have the opportunity for direct, continuous care, are key figures for support, guidance, and teaching. There is a tendency to consider self-care deficits as being the responsibility of the hospital-based nurse. But as the length of the hospital stay shortens, more families choose alternative birthing options, and women breastfeed longer, nurses in community health practice and in the medical office are often the ones working with lactating women.

Those who have helped breastfeeding women agree that the most common deficits are breast and nipple problems and medications. Therefore this chapter begins with a discussion of the former and ends with the latter, along with a drug chart for easy referral. The potential effect of specific medications on the breastfeeding infant is also discussed under specific health problems.

First, attention must be given to a situation that rarely receives any notice. Occasionally when an illness or a breastfeeding problem occurs, health professionals are put in the difficult position of giving permission to wean to a woman who no longer really wants to continue but needs official sanction to stop. Even if there is no reason to wean, a relatively minor difficulty can occasionally present a mother with a socially acceptable ''out'' from a situation that she finds emotionally uncomfortable or inconvenient for her life-style. For the nurse or physician who is enthusiastic about breastfeeding, personal feelings and the knowledge of the benefits of breastfeeding conflict with the subtle response from the client that suggests she would rather wean. Granted, this situation is the exception, rather than the rule; yet the comment that the physician or nurse ''told me to wean'' because of a problem might be partially due to the mother's own wishes.

Sections of this chapter are taken from Riordan, J., and Countryman, B.A.: Basics of breastfeeding. V. Self-care for continued breastfeeding, J.O.G.N. Nurs **9**:357, 1980.

Forcing her to continue breastfeeding under these circumstances is neither appropriate nor desirable.

PROBLEMS RELATED TO THE BREAST AND NIPPLES
Prevention of problems through prenatal assessment

Usually little attention is given to prenatal assessment of the breast and nipple, probably because of cultural inhibitions about the breast and a lack of recognition of its importance by health professionals. As a consequence, mothers may unnecessarily encounter immediate feeding difficulties after delivery that could otherwise have been prevented. Nurses practicing as primary caretakers are the ideal persons to do a prenatal assessment, particularly since physicians (especially male ones) are reluctant to do so.

Ideal for teaching as well as for data gathering, a physical assessment of the breasts and nipples is done by inspection and palpation. In inspecting the breasts the following observations and questions are relevant to the future course of lactation.

Inspection. Although varying considerably from woman to woman and from one breast to the other, the size, symmetry, and shape of the breasts proper have minimal effect on lactation. The assessment provides the opportunity to reassure the woman with small breasts that she will be able to breastfeed and have a sufficient supply of milk. It also should be pointed out that having one breast larger or smaller than the other is normal. For the woman with large breasts, discussing the importance of a support bra and where it may be obtained is helpful. Holding and feeding her infant will not be the same for her as for mothers with average-sized breasts. Because of the larger breasts, instead of simply holding the breast the mother should expect to hold or push part of the breast back for her infant to grasp the nipple and have an adequate airway, particularly if the infant is below the average birth weight. During this discussion, she may talk about some of her deeper feelings about having large breasts and her decision to breastfeed.

Now is the time to ask "have your breasts grown during pregnancy?" and "have you had any tenderness or soreness?" An increase in breast size, swelling, and tenderness indicates adequately functioning breast tissue responsive to hormonal changes.

The skin of the breast should be inspected for any deviations. Skin turgor and elasticity can be assessed by gently pinching the skin, although the effect of elasticity on lactation is questionable: whereas multiparous women have more elastic skin, since it has been stretched from a previous pregnancy, primiparas have firmer tissue. If there is a scar, then the type of surgery or injury should be investigated. A simple incision for removal of a benign tumor, for instance, may have little effect on the mother's ability to lactate, whereas any extensive excision of tissue is significant; however, a scar from a lateral incision in the vicinity of the cutaneous branch of the fourth intercostal nerve (left breast, 4 o'clock position; right breast, 8 o'clock position) may mean a severed innervation of the nipple and areola.[10] Note should also be taken of any skin thickening or dimpling of the breast or nipple. Although rare in a woman of childbearing age, it is conceivable that such a change could be an early sign of a tumor.

Next the nipple should be carefully inspected. (For the purpose of this discussion "nipple" includes the areola as well as the nipple proper.) If the nipples appear small, explain that the size of a woman's nipples is of secondary importance to their functional ability. Likewise, any nipple structural abnormality such as inversion should be assessed only in terms of function.

TABLE 6-1

Assessment form for indicating nipple function

Nipple function	Right	Left	Intervention teaching
Protraction	___	___	
Retraction			
Minimal	___	___	
Moderate to severe	___	___	
Inversion			
Simple	___	___	
Complete	___	___	

Palpation. After thorough hand washing, assess the nipple by compressing or palpating the areola between the forefinger and the thumb just behind the base of the nipple (the "pinch test"). This action simulates the compression that occurs when the infant is at breast. Because of possible nipple adhesions within the underlying connective tissue, a nipple that initially appears normal can retract inward on stimulation so that the infant has difficulties as he attempts to grasp the breast. Conversely, a nipple that appears flattened or inverted can, on palpation, protrude normally; therefore a differentiation must be made between structure and function in assessing the nipples.

In the absence of a standard terminology to describe nipple function and dysfunction, the following classification is suggested with an assessment form to record nipple function (Table 6-1). Before this classification is introduced, it must be stressed that although many primigravidas[37] have nipples that tend to retract, it is unusual for the retraction to interfere with breastfeeding.[31]

Classification of nipple function. When the nipple is compressed using the "pinch test," it responds according to one of the following categories indicating function:

Protraction	Nipple moves forward; considered a normal functional response. No special interventions are needed (Fig. 6-1, *A*).
Retraction	Instead of protracting, the nipple moves inward.
Minimal	An infant with a strong suck exerts sufficient pressure to pull the nipple forward. A weak or premature infant may have difficulties at first.
Moderate to severe	Retracts to a level even with or behind the surrounding areola. Interventions are helpful to stretch the nipple outward and improve protractility (Fig. 6-1, *B*).
Inversion	On visual inspection all or part of the nipple is drawn inward within the folds of the areola (Figs. 6-1, *C*, and 6-2, *A*).
Simple	The nipple moves outward to protraction with manual pressure or when cold (pseudoinversion) (Fig. 6-1, *C*). A variation of simple inversion is the "dimpled" nipple in which only a part of the nipple is inverted. Breast cups and nipple exercises are indicated in both cases.
Complete	The nipple does not respond to manual pressure (Figs. 6-1, *D*, and 6-2, *B*) because of adhesions binding the nipple inward or, very rarely, congenital absence of the nipple. Hoffman's exercises, exercising, and breast cups should be used prenatally.

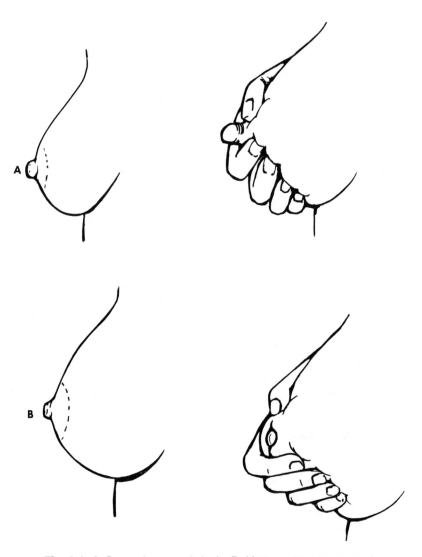

Fig. 6-1. A, Protracting normal nipple. **B,** Moderate to severe retraction.

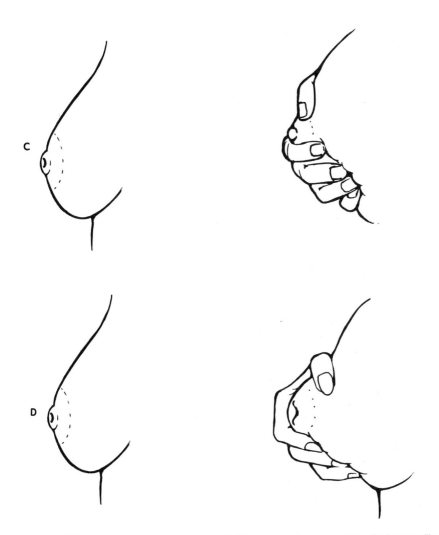

Fig. 6-1, cont'd. C, Inverted-appearing nipple *(left)* when compressed using pinch test will either invert farther inward *(middle)* or protract forward *(right)*. **D,** True inversion.

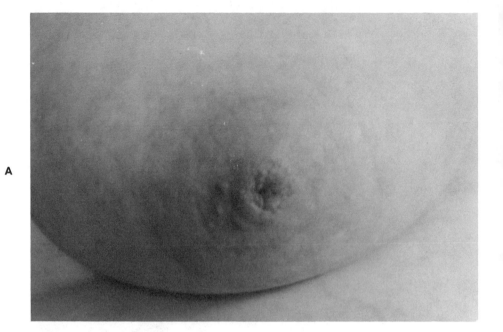

A

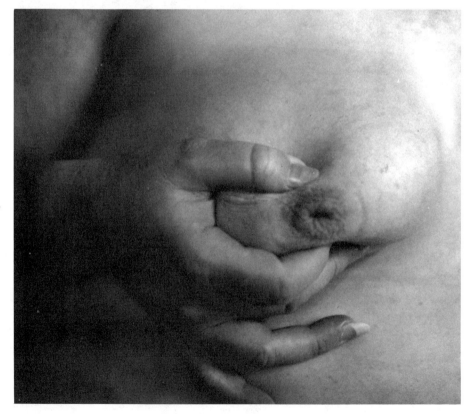

B

Fig. 6-2. A, Frontal view of nipple with apparent inversion on inspection. **B,** Same nipple shows true inversion with compression.

Dysfunction can be present in one nipple while the other is perfectly normal, or it can be present in both nipples. Retraction or inversion can prevent the infant from milking the lactiferous sinuses that lie beneath the areola. The mother with a unilateral problem discovers quickly that her infant prefers feeding from the normal nipple, crying or even refusing the other side. Cases of infants feeding at only one breast are not at all unusual and do not present any particular hazard to the infant, if feedings are frequent; however, unilateral feedings are uncomfortable for the mother until the other breast involutes to a prelacteal state.

If retraction or simple inversion is identified in early pregnancy, time is on the mother's side. As her pregnancy progresses, hormonal changes increase the size and protractility of the nipples. She also has time to use the following interventions that help prevent subsequent feeding problems.

Interventions

Breast cups. Special plastic doughnut-shaped cups are available for correcting inversions or retractions (Fig. 6-3). By a continuous, gentle pressure exerted around the areola, the nipple is pushed through a central opening in the inner shield. These cups should be worn during the last 2 trimesters of pregnancy, starting with an hour or two each day and gradually increasing the length of wearing time. Various trade names of these cups are Woolwich, Netsy, La Leche League Cups, Nurse-Dri, Free and Dry, and Hobbit Shields. They can also be worn after childbirth, but the mother should be cautioned against using milk that collects in the cup. Since body warmth can foster rapid bacterial growth and contamination, this milk should be discarded and not fed to the infant. The use of breast cups, even if there is no nipple problem, is becoming more popular. Some hospitals routinely give them to breastfeeding mothers, a practice that should be *strongly discouraged* for the following reasons: the constant pressure of the cups against the breasts constricts the ducts and may lead to plugged ducts; it is an unnecessary expense; and some mothers may unknowingly use the collected milk for feedings.

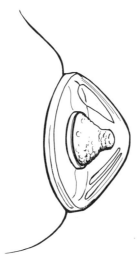

Fig. 6-3. Breast cup for inverted or retracted nipple.

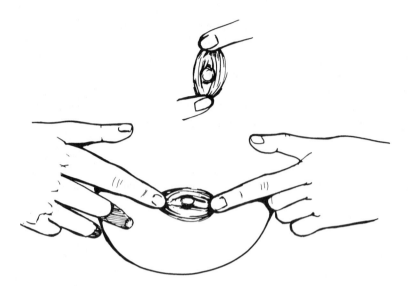

Fig. 6-4. Hoffman's exercises. Mother places her thumbs opposite each other on either side of nipple, then gently draws thumbs distally or away from nipple. Repeat with thumbs above and below nipple.

Nipple exercise and stretching. As originally suggested by Hoffman[16] and explained in Fig. 6-4, nipple exercises are especially effective for separating adhesions that cause retraction or inversion. Several times a day stretching the nipple forward and holding it outward also is generally effective. Since the nipple has tiny muscles that are highly elastic, the infant will also stretch the nipples during feedings. Mothers who have had this deficit find that with the second child the nipple stretches more easily and a previous retraction or inversion diminishes or is even nonexistent. In lovemaking during breast foreplay, oral suction of the nipples helps too—a built-in nipple preparation during the love act.

Suction device. Another method of correcting inversion is suction. A device (Fig. 6-5) designed by Cotterman[7] creates an effective suction for drawing out the nipple. As pictured, the mother will need to have available (1) a glass and rubber shield, (2) an all rubber shield, and (3) a hand breast pump (an inexpensive bicycle-horn pump is sufficient). For the first week or two of using this device, the mother should hold a clean, very warm washcloth over the areola for a minute or two before following this procedure:

1. Place glass shield with rubber gasket directly over areola with nipple centered in opening.
2. Squeeze pump bulb before carefully placing bell of pump over gasket.
3. Maintain constant gentle pressure *backward toward ribs with bell of pump*.
4. Gradually release, then compress bulb to give alternate suction and to rest the nipple tissue, permitting good circulatory exchange.
5. Guide the strength and length of the suction phase by sensation and an occasional look at the color of nipple tissue.
6. Alternate breasts every few minutes to allow nipple unrestricted circulation period.

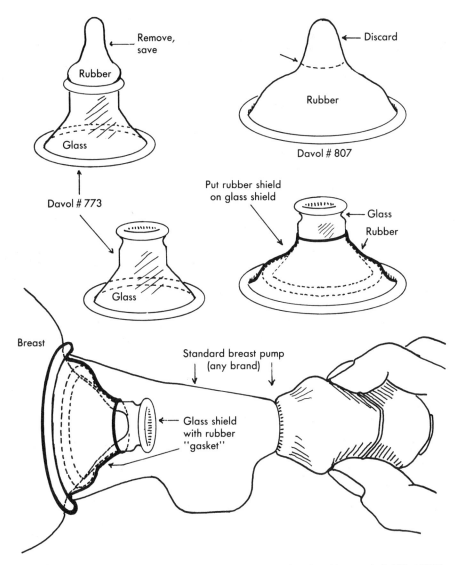

Fig. 6-5. Cotterman's device. (Courtesy Cotterman, J.: Keeping Abreast J. **1:**330, 1976.)

7. Total time: 10 minutes each breast, three times daily, 8 to 10 days. Increase to 15 minutes each breast, four times daily thereafter until nipples appear to function normally and continue to do so. Test this by observing the nipple while compressing areola with fingers backward against chest wall.

Severe inversion will respond after about 2 to 3 months of this schedule. Less retracted nipples will show improvement in 2 to 4 weeks or less.

Using this suction device or the nipple exercises can, of course, stimulate uterine contractions; therefore these procedures are contraindicated for someone with a history of premature labor or delivery. On the other hand, they decrease the likelihood of a postmature labor and delivery.

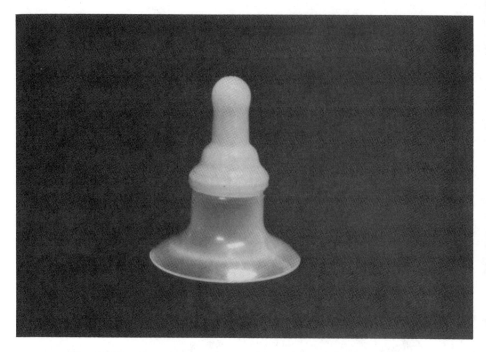

Fig. 6-6. Nipple shield with standard nipple. (Courtesy Charles Cooley.)

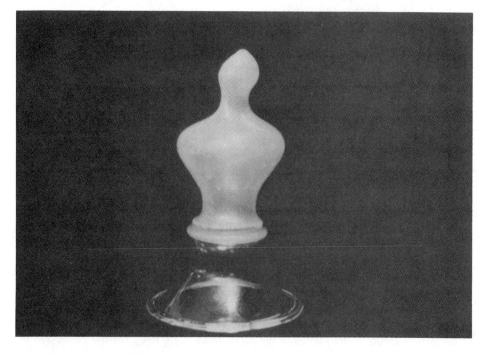

Fig. 6-7. Nipple shield with NUK nipple. (Courtesy Charles Cooley.)

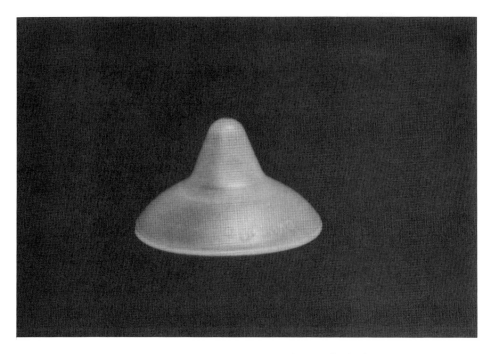

Fig. 6-8. Breast shield. (Courtesy Charles Cooley.)

Breast and nipple shields. Using a breast or a nipple shield is sometimes useful if done judiciously. Although their functions are similar, the breast shield is slightly different from a nipple shield. The nipple shield is made of both plastic and rubber (Figs. 6-6 and 6-7), which can be separated. The breast shield is made entirely of rubber and has a convex shape that molds to the shape of the breast (Fig. 6-8).

Some women with nipple inversions have found that using a nipple shield helps to bring the nipple forward with the plastic part serving as a gasket with the suction from the infant. Light moisture on the inside of the shield acts as a lubricant. Once the infant begins to suck vigorously, however, the nipple shield should be immediately removed so the infant can feed directly from the breast. The breast shield should be used only during the temporary period of engorgement until the breasts become softer and the infant is able to grasp the nipple. There are other situations when its use is warranted: in one case is which the infant had Down's syndrome, the nipple shield was effective until the child developed an adequate suck.[3]

Conservatism is the key point in the use of these shields, but unfortunately they are overused as a fast catchall remedy in many hospitals. A nurse, wanting to assist the frustrated mother and infant through an initial difficulty in latching onto the breast, will often bring a breast or nipple shield to the mother as a first instead of a last resort. Shields should never be used for sore nipples—instead of alleviating the problems, they aggravate them. Rather the nurse should try to correct the underlying cause of the soreness, particularly noting whether the infant is poorly positioned on the breast, tenuously hanging onto only the nipple and not drawing in a part of the areola.

Prolonged use of a shield usually creates more problems than it solves. The infant's

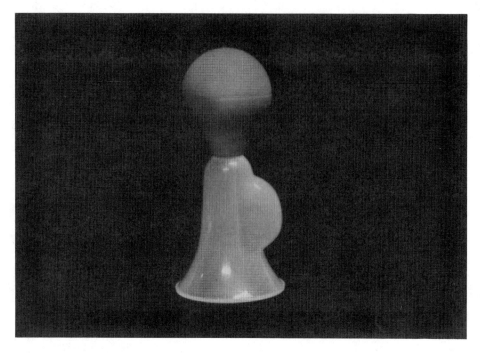

Fig. 6-9. "Bicycle-horn" pump. (Courtesy Charles Cooley.)

sucking pattern becomes imprinted on the shield as much as it does on a rubber nipple from a bottle. In addition the shield makes it impossible for the infant to grasp far enough onto the areola to compress the underlying lactiferous sinuses. Thus sensitive nerve endings on the nipple and areola are not stimulated to release a full flow of milk. Often the mother is never able to establish an adequate milk supply, and as she gives supplements to compensate, she heads toward lactation failure.

Other interventions can be just as effective without the risks of using the shield, although they may take more time. If an electric pump or a bicycle-horn hand pump (Fig. 6-9) is available in the unit, it can be used for either pulling inverted nipples forward or relieving the pressure from engorgement so the infant can get hold of the nipple. A firm but gentle shaping of the nipple, attained by pulling it forward manually and flattening it, is sometimes all that is needed. Once the infant has successfully grasped the nipple and receives the milk, he has cognitively "learned" and will probably do it again the next time with less difficulty.

If an infant is already "hooked" on the shield, refusing to feed without it, some mothers find this technique effective: Trim off 0.6 cm (¼ inch) at a time from the nipple portion of the shield after each feeding. If this is done, the infant gradually becomes conditioned to the breast without the shield. When only a small portion remains, the infant usually decides it isn't worth the trouble and breastfeeds without it.

Sore nipples

Nipple soreness is a common deficit, especially in the first few weeks of breastfeeding. In fact, most women experience a temporary soreness of the nipples after the infant

TABLE 6-2

Commonly used agents for nipple soreness

Name	Description	Main ingredients	Comments
Bag Balm (Dairy Assoc. Inc.)	Jar—yellow stiff ointment	8-Hydroxyquinoline sulfate, 0.3% in a petroleum lanolin base	Claims to be antiseptic. Intended for veterinary use. Must be removed before feeding.
Balm Barr (Mennen Co.)	White cream, spreads easily, tube or jar	Water, emulsifying wax, cocoa butter, mineral oil	Avoid if mother is allergic to chocolate.
USP Lanolin (Merck "Lanum")	Tubes or bulk form: bulk very sticky	Hydrous lanolin	Effective, does not need to be wiped off before feeding. Avoid if mother is allergic to wool.
Mammol Ointment (Abbott Lab.)	Tube—white cream	Bismuth subnitrate, castor oil, anhydrous lanolin, ceresin wax	Instructions advise washing and drying nipple before applying cream, which is not necessary.
Masse Cream (Ortho Pharmaceutical Co.	Tube—white cream	Water, glycerol monostearate, glycerin, cetyl alcohol, lanolin	Must be cleaned off before feeding. Avoid if allergic to wool. Keep out of reach of children.
Rotersept	Antiseptic spray	Chlorhexidine gluconate, propellant gas, water, alcohol, acetone	Manufacturers claim it reduces risk of cracked nipples and mastitis. Research does not support this claim. Distributed mainly in European countries and the United Kingdom.
Vitamin A & D (Schering Corp. and other brands)	Tube—colorless cream	Anhydrous lanolin, petrolatum	No added vitamins A and D are listed on tube.
Vitamin E (Hudson Co. and numerous other brands)	Cream, oil gelatin, vitamin capsules	Vitamin E in suspension; capsules—400 IU each	No known adverse effects (but potential overdose of vitamin E) in infant. If used, must be wiped completely before feeding.

begins frequent feedings. Putting a time limit on the length of the feeding only delays the soreness. Moreover, imposing an arbitrary time schedule for the length of feeding has no advantages and should be left to individual infant demand. In the usual postpartum course, the most severe soreness occurs at the end of the first week, the beginning of the second week after birth, or earlier if the infant and mother are never separated. Then it rapidly subsides. Nipple cream appears to help soothe and heal the nipples, but research on the effectiveness of various creams or ointments is abominably lacking. A listing of agents used for nipples during breastfeeding is given in Table 6-2.

If sore nipples persist, a further assessment should be made to uncover the cause. The answer to the question "Does the pain or soreness last throughout the feeding?" will reveal important information. Discomfort for only the first minute or so of the feeding indicates that the nipple tissue will probably continue to "toughen" to the sucking and eventually disappear. Some infants' sucking (the "barracuda") is so strong that it simply takes longer for nipples to heal. Discomfort throughout the feeding, however, can be a symptom of a deeper problem. *Monilia* is one possibility. Discomfort can also indicate improper positioning of the infant's mouth on the breast. Also, if a mother with persistent sore nipples is using a lanolin cream, she should be assessed for a possible allergy to lanolin. Not being able to wear wool without discomfort is one indication of an allergy. At no time should the mother use plastic-backed pads in her bra cup. All materials that are in contact with the nipples should be dry, so frequent changes of bras are necessary, especially in the early weeks when leakage is common. Lowering the bra flaps allows the air to circulate, thus drying the nipples and promoting healing. Although it is generally best to offer both breasts at evey feeding, occasionally a mother with one very sore nipple will find it better to feed consecutively from one breast, giving the other nipple a few hours or half a day to improve. The sore breast, however, should not be permitted to become overfull, since this can lead to increased nipple soreness.

Another helpful suggestion for healing sore nipples is to experiment with position changes during feedings (Fig. 6-10.) The mother may sit upright at one feeding and lie down at the next. She may wish to cradle the baby in her arms in the usual manner at some feedings and use the "football hold" at others.

Correction of the causes of sore nipples should be followed by healing techniques, among which exposure of the breasts to the sun for short periods of time is extremely effective. If outdoor privacy is unavailable, a mother may sit in the direct sunlight near an open window or door. During rainy or cloudy seasons, an ultraviolet lamp is a good substitute. The following directions should be given to a mother using this type of light:

Sit approximately 4 feet from the lamp.

Expose the nipples 30 seconds the first day, then 1 minute twice a day on the second and third days. Occasionally it is necessary to use the lamp for a few more days, but never should the time be increased beyond 3 minutes.

Protect eyes with some type of shield.

Keep the lamp away from the rest of the household so the infant or other children will not accidentally become exposed to the light and possibly be sunburned.

The use of a wire tea-strainer inside the mother's bra will hold clothing away from the sore or cracked nipple and allow for circulation of air, thus encouraging more rapid healing. Plastic breast cups may also be worn for this purpose for a day or two, but care must be taken to remove the shield frequently to allow the circulation of air and to

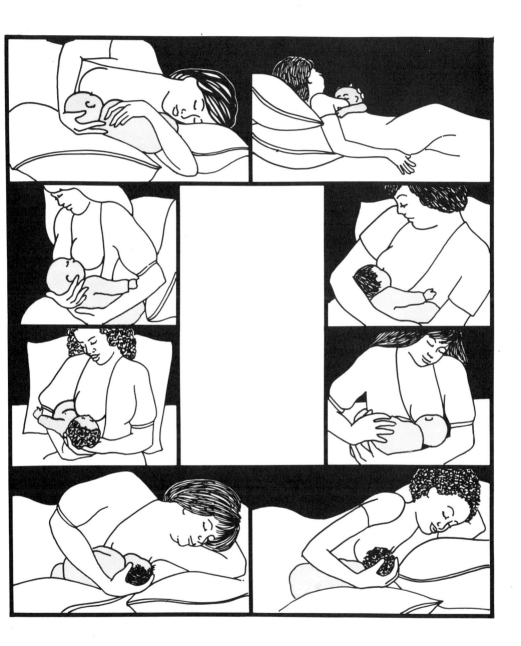

Fig. 6-10. Examples of breastfeeding position changes. (Courtesy Vis-u-lac Breastfeeding Teaching Aids.)

CHECKLIST FOR THE CARE OF SORE NIPPLES

_____ Allowing nipples to air after feeding?
_____ Using ointment? (Watch for possible allergic response with lanolin in sensitive individuals.)
_____ Positioning baby on nipple instead of areola?*
_____ Checking for thrush if persistent, extreme soreness with sudden onset?
_____ Rotating positions at successive nursings to change pressure points?
_____ Beginning breastfeeding on least sore side?
_____ Washing nipples with soap or antiseptic?* (Only clear water should be used.)
_____ Using plastic liners in bra?*
_____ Using a "bicycle-horn" pump?*
_____ Wearing a tight bra?*
_____ Pulling down bra flap when it has adhered to nipple?*
_____ If in extreme pain, hand expressing and offering milk by eyedropper, spoon, or syringe?

*Nurse should discourage or offer alternatives.

---

dispose of any milk that may have collected in the shields. Such shields should be sterilized by boiling daily.

Some authorities have recommended blow drying the nipples with a hair dryer, but the loss of natural moisture that this causes is probably more aggravating than helpful. A checklist is given above for helping damaged nipples.

Plugged duct

Complaints of tenderness, heat, and possibly redness in one area of the breast without a generalized fever lead the nurse to suspect that a breastfeeding woman has a plugged duct. Pathologic changes within the breast causing the "plug" are vaguely referred to in the literature as a stasis, clogging of milk, or "local accumulations of milk or dead cells that have been shed."[12] No one knows for sure. I can only describe the symptoms that are attributed to plugged ducts, or a caked breast, and suggest interventions and preventions.

Clinicians are aware of a higher frequency of plugged ducts during the winter. The reason for this is not clear, although it may be related to the restricting effects of winter clothing or simply the cold weather. This phenomenon bears investigation.

There also is some evidence that whereas some women are predisposed to developing plugged ducts, others never encounter it throughout multiple breastfeeding experiences. Another commonly mentioned difficulty with plugged ducts is that they can lead to mastitis, especially if ignored or untreated; however, a cause and effect relationship has never been substantiated.

Despite a lack of specific data on this problem, the following measures for self-care in treating a plugged duct are:
1. Continuing to breastfeed often
2. Applying moist heat to the area several times a day as soon as the symptoms become evident

3. Massaging the affected breast before feedings to stimulate the flow of milk, especially effective in a hot shower or bath
4. Changing positions of the infant during feedings to ensure emptying of all the sinuses and ductules in the breast

A constricting bra, skipped feedings, poor nutrition, and stress have all been implicated in the development of a plugged duct. Avoidance of these circumstances should be included in preventive teaching, especially for the woman who has a repeated problem. As we become more aware of the overuse, if not the misuse, of antibiotic therapy, it must be emphasized that there is no need for antibiotics for a plugged duct unless a fever and mastitis develop.

Skin problems

Thrush. When a mother has persistent sore nipples, thrush infection is likely. Thrush is caused by *Candida albicans* or other strains of yeast, also called *Monilia,* and it thrives on the warm moist areas of the infant's mouth and the mother's nipples. Thrush should be suspected if the mother has been breastfeeding without discomfort and then rapidly develops extremely sore nipples. In checking for thrush, inspect the woman's breasts for inflammation of the nipples and areola. The inflammation is usually quite striking, and the mother will complain of severe tenderness and discomfort during feedings. Also examine the child's mouth carefully for white patches surrounded by diffuse redness. However, the absence of symptoms in the child's mouth does not rule out thrush in the mother, since the infant can be asymptomatic. Infants and women who have received antibiotic therapy are more susceptible to thrush. A culture may be ordered by the physician to confirm the diagnosis. Treatment may consist of nystatin (Mycostatin) placed into the mouth with a medicine dropper or swabbed over the mucosa, gums, or tongue, or swabbing with an aqueous solution of 1% to 2% gentian violet. For less severe cases of thrush, a home treatment in which the infant's mouth and mother's nipples are swabbed with a baking soda solution (1 tsp to 1 cup water) is effective.[24] Along with using topical agents, the mother should expose her nipples directly to the sun twice a day. The sunlamp treatments previously described are also helpful in reducing the irritation and soreness, especially if direct exposure to the sun is impossible. Afterward the mother should apply a nipple cream to prevent dryness. The mother may also have a monilial infection in the vagina, and simultaneous treatment of this is advisable.

Other problems. Infrequently a whitish, tender area (or "bleb") develops on the upper areola that looks like milk that has somehow gotten under the epidermis and triggered an inflammatory response. Persistent and very painful during feedings, it can remain for several days or weeks and then spontaneously heal by a peeling away of the epithelium over the affected area. In a few cases, a sterile needle aspiration may be necessary to draw out the fluid. With ice packs, an analgesic to relieve discomfort, and a topical antibiotic, breastfeeding can continue and healing is rapid.

From time to time, erythematous rashes appear on the breast during lactation. Presumably they are spawned by frequent skin contact with the infant. Since these rashes are transient and responsive to treatment at home by keeping the area clean and dry and by exposing it to the sun, medical interventions are rarely needed. However, when the problem is persistent and characterized by erythematous papules and scaling plaques on the breast and other areas, especially the scalp, elbows, and knees, a medical referral should be made to determine the possibility of psorisis. Treatment with topical steroids or keratotic agents is effective in clearing psoriasis lesions, Before feedings, however, the medication must be wiped off.

When extremely painful vesicular lesions appear on the areola, a herpes viral infection may be present. Further discussion and photographs of breast herpes appear on pp. 129-131.

Breast nodules and changes

What if a breastfeeding mother develops a lump or nodule in her breast? Warnings by the American Cancer Society have made American women keenly aware of any breast lumps, and the mother discovering one is usually anxious and perhaps frightened. Although a breast lump in a breastfeeding woman is most often a galactocele or lacteal cyst caused by plugged milk within the ducts, it should be carefully watched. A galactocele is usually tender and will atrophy rather rapidly and disappear in a matter of days.

If it does not resolve or reduce in size, refer the mother to a physician, preferably an experienced gynecologist or surgeon, for an examination. A known breast mass (by palpation) can be evaluated further by ultrasound to determine whether it is fluid filled (cystic and benign) or solid (possibly malignant). Because of the tissue density of the lactating breast, mammography is often inconclusive.

Fibroadenoma, a benign tumor, is a common type of breast nodule in women of childbearing age. Some surgeons use needle aspiration to confirm the diagnosis and reduce the size of a fibroadenoma but allow it to remain without surgery at least until lactation is over and the child is weaned. Cystic breast disease is also a possibility, although it usually occurs in older women. If it is a cystic mass, as determined by sonography, a needle aspiration can be done, avoiding a breast biopsy. If surgical removal is necessary for any benign breast mass, it can usually be done on an outpatient basis with the mother resuming breastfeeding within a few days after surgery. Although the area will be tender, breastfeeding is less uncomfortable than the discomfort from engorgement, or listening to the cries of an unhappy child.[23]

For the mother with persistent benign breast disease, some dietary changes may alleviate the problem. Reducing or eliminating the consumption of caffeine (coffee, tea, cola, chocolate) has been found to be effective, particularly with cystic breast disease.[5] Likewise, cystic breast problems have responded to vitamin E supplements.[14]

However remote, there is a possibility of the tumor or nodule being malignant. Breastfeeding does *not* prevent breast cancer, although some studies support the hypothesis that it is protective.[17,20] For a woman who is susceptible to breast cancer, prolonged breastfeeding may at least delay its occurrence.

For a long time it was widely taught that pregnancy and lactation aggravated the course of mammary cancer; however, studies[34] have long ago disproved this, and many women who have had a mastectomy now breastfeed with subsequent pregnancies. Although breastfeeding must necessarily be more frequent with only one breast, the infant usually gains weight satisfactorily.

Questions raised several years ago about cancer-causing viral particles in human milk and their transmission to the infant have been resolved. There is no increased incidence of breast cancer in female infants who have been breastfed.[27,29] There is, however, some evidence[13] that years later, following an experience of the infant rejecting the breast without apparent reason, a woman may be more likely to develop breast cancer in the rejected breast. In such cases close surveillance is probably needed.

Bleeding from the breast when no nipple soreness or cracking is evident should indicate to the practitioner the possibility of an intraductal papilloma. Usually no mass or tumor is palpable, and there is moderate pain and discomfort. Often the bleeding stops spontaneously without any treatment, but if bleeding continues, the woman should be medically evaluated and followed closely. In any case, reassure the mother that the infant is not harmed by the intake of small amounts of serosanguineous discharge.

Breast augmentation and reduction

The ability to breastfeed following cosmetic surgery depends on the type of surgery and the removal of breast tissue. Silicone implants for augmenting breast size should not affect milk production, since the lobes and ductal system remain intact; however, there may be a loss of sensation if the nerve to the nipple and areola has been severed. This can be surgically avoided.[10] Silicone injections, which are now against the law in the United States, cause considerable scarring and thus interfere with lactation.

In breast reduction, the extent of the secretory tissue that has been removed determines whether or not lactation is possible, at least for producing enough milk to sustain the needs of the infant. One mother who had surgery successfully used a Lact-Aid Nursing Trainer to supplement her supply.

PROBLEMS RELATED TO GENERAL HEALTH
Rehospitalization of mother

Rehospitalization of a mother after she has gone home following delivery is a traumatic experience for all members of the family. A mother faced with separation from her infant, whether brief or prolonged, is a mother in crisis. For the breastfeeding mother and her infant it is essential that ongoing, intimate, and regular contact be maintained. During a postpartum illness, the baby should be allowed to room-in with the mother or at least be brought to her for breastfeeding at frequent intervals during her hospitalization.

Infections

Hepatitis. Whether or not breastfeeding is contraindicated in women who have been diagnosed as having hepatitis virus B (HBV) should be determined only after careful medical evaluation. Although isolation precautions must be taken in the hospital setting and the infant given hepatitis immune globulin, there is no reason why the infant should be separated from his mother, since the risk of transmission is greatest during pregnancy (transplacentally) and at birth.[25] Breastmilk is not an important mechanism of transmission. If the mother contracts hepatitis after delivery, the infant will, of course, already have been exposed during the incubation period. Whether the small likelihood of transmission of the HBV through the breastmilk outweighs the benefits of the antibodies and cell-mediated immunity against the virus in breastmilk is still being debated. However, denying the infant antibody protection available to him from his mother's milk during continued intimate contact with the mother is certainly a questionable practice.

Herpes simplex. The number of genital herpes simplex (HSV) infections in women is increasing so rapidly, it deserves more attention from the nursing profession. Information on mode of transmission, recurrence, follow-up care, and personal hygiene is essential for nurses.[2] Herpesvirus, type 2, has its most serious consequences during pregnancy and in the neonate. The infant, if he is well, may breastfeed and be with the mother in the room; however, scrupulous hand washing, gowning, and covering of any lesion must be done to prevent possible cross-contamination.[6] The mother does not need to wear rubber gloves while breastfeeding. Treatment is usually directed toward symptomatic relief and prevention of secondary infection, since there is no known cure. Povidone-iodine on the lesion may be helpful, and topical analgesic ointments can ease pain. Also, acyclovir, a new antiviral drug (ointment), has been shown to shorten initial infections of genital herpes.[2a]

Herpesvirus, type 1, is generally associated with herpes infections that occur above the waist. The common cold sore or "fever blister" on the lip is an example, but other areas of the body can be involved, including the breast nipple and areola. Although breast herpesvirus seems only a recent problem and there are no well-documented cases at the time of this writing, I have worked with two mothers who were diagnosed as having herpesvirus lesions on the areola (Figs. 6-11 and 6-12). Both women complained of extreme pain when breastfeeding, and both were advised to wean by their physicians. In one case, the child was taking only breastmilk at 5 months of age, and the mother chose to continue breastfeeding despite her physician's advice. The child and the mother remained well, and the lesions cleared in about a week. The other mother decided to wean her 17-month-old child.

Despite the lack of other information on breast herpes, it is assumed that it should be treated like any other type 1 herpes lesion and that breastfeeding probably could continue as before unless the pain becomes unbearable for the mother. Theoretically, antibodies in the milk should help protect the child against developing the infection. A culture should be done to verify the causative organism.

Urinary infections. Urinary infections are usually caused by a gram-negative bacteria and treated successfully with antimicrobial agents, particularly sulfa drugs. Nursing concerns in regard to breastfeeding center on the effect of the medication passing to the infant. Although the physician should use caution in prescribing a sulfa medication to a mother with an infant under 1 month, beyond the newborn period there is no risk to the healthy infant. Only an insignificant fraction (less than 1%) of a commonly used drug, sulfisoxazole (Gantrisin), is excreted in a mother's milk.[21] With repeated infections, preventive measures such as showers instead of baths and good personal hygiene should be taught by the nurse.

Alterations in endocrine and metabolic functioning

Diabetes mellitus. The woman with diabetes not only can breastfeed her infant but should be encouraged to do so. In addition to the known advantages of breastfeeding, it helps fulfill her need to feel like a "normal" mother. The diabetic woman usually needs less insulin while lactating than before she became pregnant. Nonetheless, blood glucose levels are affected by lactation and vice versa, with special implications for the nursing care of these mothers.

Any insulin-dependent pregnant woman is considered a high-risk obstetric patient. During pregnancy the blood glucose levels should be kept below 130 mg/dl most if not all of the time. During labor, delivery, and for some time after delivery, blood glucose levels must be closely monitored while she receives insulin in intravenous dextrose and

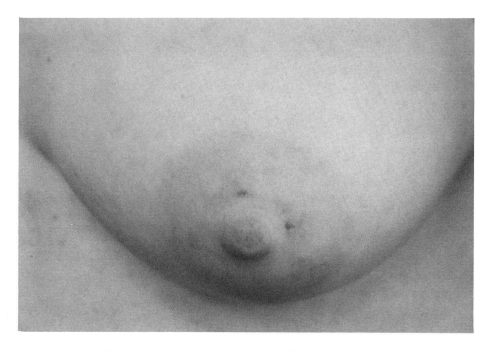

Fig. 6-11. Vesicles of herpes simplex virus on upper areola.

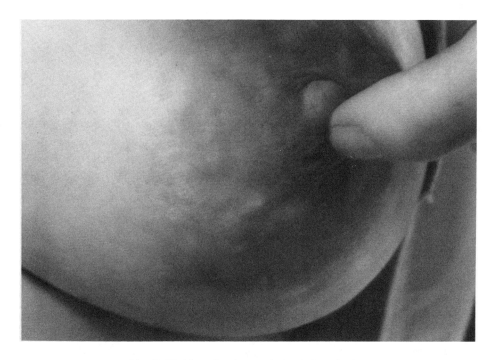

Fig. 6-12. Ulcerative herpes lesion below nipple.

Ringer's solution, carefully regulated by an infusion pump or the Biostator. Cesarean deliveries are much more likely for the diabetic at the present time. Despite the technology that is needed to bring her and her infant safely through childbirth, breastfeeding should begin as soon after birth as possible.

During the immediate postnatal period, sudden but normal hormonal changes cause drastic fluctuations in blood glucose levels. Hypoglycemia can be expected immediately to 5 to 7 hr after delivery.[26] In addition, lactose excretion in the urine drops to low levels 2 to 5 days after birth and then rises rapidly. These sudden metabolic shifts require close monitoring and recording.

Lactose is reabsorbed from the breast and is normally excreted in the urine; therefore nurses and mothers should be aware that in testing the urine after delivery, the presence of lactose may cause a false-positive test if copper-reducing urine testing (Clinitest) is used. Testape or Diastix, which measures only the glucose, should be used instead. Once physiologically stable, the patient can return to subcutaneous injection of insulin or to a portable infusion pump. Portable infusion pumps, although they are expensive and not yet widely available, have been successfully used. The pump strapped to a waist, arm, or leg automatically injects the correct insulin dosage throughout the day.

The Ames Glucometer or Dextrometer system is a usually reliable method of testing blood glucose that can continue to be used by the mother at home along with urine testing. By keeping a daily record of blood glucose levels and glycosuria, the mother can self-monitor day-to-day changes. Once the blood glucose stabilizes, it is generally lower during lactation, and less insulin is required than if the mother were not breastfeeding. Given the continuous conversion of glucose to galactose and lactose during milk synthesis, sometimes only half the insulin required before pregnancy is needed during lactation.

An advantage of working with diabetic women is their keen awareness of their body functions and the importance of diet. More than the average woman, they are knowledgeable about physiology and are quick to notice changes that forewarn problems. The most frequently asked question by these mothers is whether or not elevated blood glucose levels affect the amount of sugar (in this case, lactose) in breastmilk. It should be explained that the breast acts as a filter, screening out excess glucose in milk synthesis.

Any sudden drop in blood glucose appears to affect milk production because of the secretion of epinephrine that accompanies hypoglycemia. An example is the mother whose blood glucose suddenly dropped to 19 mg/dl 8 days following a cesarean birth. For the next 24 hours, which were spent in the hospital, she was unable to express any milk using an electric pump; but in the following days after returning home, she began to rebuild her milk supply.

The potential for mastitis and breast abscess during lactation should be no greater for the well-controlled diabetic mother than for other breastfeeding mothers.[15] Any infection will quickly raise the level of blood glucose, and self-care teaching must emphasize recognizing early symptoms of mastitis (see Chapter 7) and seeking prompt treatment while continuing to breastfeed. Diabetic mothers also risk *Monilia* (yeast) infection of the vagina and nipples if blood glucose levels are elevated. Prevention of this problem involves careful control of blood glucose, drying the nipples after breastfeeding, and awareness of early symptoms of thrush such as redness and soreness.

As her child begins to wean, the mother must again make alterations in her diet and insulin to compensate for a decrease in milk production. If weaning is gradual, there are fewer problems and adjustments.

Hypothyroidism. A lack of sufficient thyroid hormone production (hypothyroidism) over time results in symptoms of dry, thickened skin, thinning hair, and for women, menstrual difficulties. In addition, the client often has poor appetite, extreme fatigue, and depression. When the thyroid deficiency is not known, these problems are often attributed to postpartum hormonal changes and changes in life-style (notably, constant care of the infant) and go undiagnosed—at least for a time.

Pertinent to the lactating woman with hypothyroidism is a reduced milk supply. When her infant suddenly and completely weaned, a mother who has subsequently known to have hypothyroidism said she "never experienced any fullness in the breasts . . . it was as though I'd dried up overnight".[22] These complaints, possibly coupled with the infant's failure to gain weight satisfactorily on breastmilk, should always alert the nurse to the possibility of thyroid deficiency, and the mother should undergo further medical diagnostic evaluation. If replacement therapy of thyroid extract with crystalline sodium levothyroxine (Synthroid) or other thyroid preparation is adequate, the relief of symptoms as well as an increase in the milk supply can be quite dramatic. The daily replacement dose of thyroid is 0.1 to 0.3 mg of sodium levothyroxine or equivalent doses of other thyroid preparation.

Hyperthyroidism. An excess of thyroid hormone is characterized by loss of weight despite an increased appetite, nervousness, heart palpitations, and a rapid pulse at rest. A well-developed case of hyperthyroidism with exophthalmos (bulging eyes) is called Graves' disease. The ability to lactate does not appear to be affected, although the mother's nervousness may complicate her ability to cope with the day-to-day caretaking of her infant.

Diagnostic tests using radioiodine for evaluating thyroid function are contraindicated for breastfeeding women. Radioiodine taken into the body for testing is excreted in the milk, and breastfeeding must be temporarily interrupted for at least 48 hours. This imposes difficulties for the family that should be avoided. The mother should be aware that alternative tests can be used. Indeed radioiodine is rarely needed now because of other specific tests of functioning such as the radioimmunoassay for thyroxine. Measuring the activity of the thyroid is safer for the lactating woman if done in vitro (within the test tube) using T_3T_4 instead of in vivo (within the body) testing such as scanning or uptake testing using radioactive material.

A conservative approach to an apparent thyroid problem is best because occasionally a woman will develop an enlarged thyroid gland during lactation, which spontaneously atrophies later. Rather than risk drugs, surgery, or radioactive tests when there are few or no other symptoms interfering with functioning, some physicians prefer to defer immediate treatment while closely monitoring T_4 and TSH levels.

If needed, propylthiouracil (PTU) given orally is the treatment of choice for the lactating mother with hyperthyroidism. Although the infant should be closely monitored, PTU appears to have little effect on the thyroid functioning of the infant,[18] but it still should be used with caution. If monitoring indicates thyroid suppression, the physician can order a daily replacement dosage of 0.025 to 0.1 mg of sodium levothyroxine (or equivalent) for the infant.[39]

Malabsorption. Any chronic condition that interferes with the absorption of nutrients by the mother can affect lactation to some extent.

Although many women with Crohn's disease (ileitis) or cystic fibrosis or who have had elective intestinal bypass surgery have breastfed their children, their nutritional state must be constantly monitored. Rapid weight loss seems to be common. In one case the mother lost 3.4 kg (7.5 lb) in 5 weeks while breastfeeding.[38] Analysis of her milk revealed normal sodium and chloride concentration but elevated total protein and a low fat content. Another women with Crohn's disease lost 9.1 kg (20 lb) in 3 months and eventually stopped breastfeeding. Nevertheless, a woman with a malabsorption deficient should be encouraged to breastfeed and be given careful nutritional guidance and ongoing evaluation. Using a multidisciplinary approach with the help of a nutritionist, a dietary plan with supplements makes it possible for many of these women to breastfeed for long periods of time.

Dysfunctional uterine bleeding

Uterine bleeding may occur in the lactating woman after the normal lochia has ceased (2 to 3 weeks). In the early weeks this may be due to placental fragments retained in the uterus that can also inhibit breastmilk secretion.[32] Relaxation of the uterus rarely occurs in the breastfeeding woman, since the oxytocin released by the sucking infant causes the uterus to contract. Later bleeding may be due to the irregular onset of hormonal function and lack of ovulation. An early miscarriage is possible, but only rarely could a tumor of the uterus be responsible.

If bleeding is excessive, prolonged, or unexplained, curettage of the uterus is usually necessary to make a diagnosis. Often this procedure is curative in itself. Occasionally hormones, either estrogens or progesterone or a combination of both, may be necessary to control bleeding.

Anxiety always accompanies excessive bleeding. Nursing interventions should relieve the mother's anxiety and assist in determining the cause of the bleeding while maintaining breastfeeding. She should be referred to a gynecologist for an immediate appointment or, if the bleeding is especially severe and a physician is not available, taken to the emergency department. Because leaving her alone only increases her fear, the nurse or someone else should stay with her until she can be medically evaluated. If a dilation and curettage (D and C) is necessary, many hospitals offer services involving minor surgery on an outpatient basis, which reduces the time of mother-infant separation.

If hormonal therapy is advised, its risks and benefits must be considered in relation to continued breastfeeding. In this case the mother may want to seek another medical opinion for other options. The nurse can act as a sounding board in assisting her in making this decision.

Control of fertility

Lactation unquestionably lengthens the interval between births by extending postpartum amenorrhea. When breastfeedings are unrestricted without the use of supplements, the return of ovulation can be delayed up to a year or in some cases longer. This contraceptive protection provided by lactation, although substantial, is not absolute. Consequently, couples with a breastfeeding child require assistance in learning about the return of fertility and the options of fertility control if an early subsequent pregnancy is unwanted.

Identifying the resumption of ovulation following birth is difficult in both breastfeeding and nonbreastfeeding women. Formerly it was thought that the first one or two menstrual cycles following delivery were anovulatory. More recent information shows, however, that many women ovulate before the resumption of the menses,[4] making it difficult to pinpoint and thus avoid pregnancy. Even so, only about 3% to 10% of lactating women, including those who use supplemental feedings, become pregnant before menstruation resumes.

In presenting methods of controlling fertility, it should be pointed out that any method used during lactation should be chosen on the basis of both its efficacy and its effect on lactation.

Oral contraceptives. That the use of an estrogen-progestin oral combination suppresses lactation is well documented. Therefore it should not be recommended for breastfeeding women.[35] Nearly all the numerous studies conducted on the combined form of oral contraceptives corroborate that these contraceptives reduce milk yield and shorten lactation. In addition, the exposure of the infant to steroidal hormones over a long time has the potential for long-term harmful effects.

Progestin-only oral contraceptives—either by pills or by injections—have less of an effect on lactation, although the amount of certain nutrients in the milk decreases. Also progestin-only contraceptives are less effective than the combination type and are likely to be associated with irregular uterine bleeding.

Considering these risks and the cumulative risks of using oral contraceptives that involve virtually every organ system, the nurse should strongly discourage their use by breastfeeding women and offer other fertility control methods.

Intrauterine contraceptive devices (IUDs). IUDs have no systemic effects on lactation and are an effective (95% to 99%) method of preventing pregnancy. IUDs may in fact increase the duration of breastfeeding by stimulating the uterus, thus increasing the level of oxytocin. The disadvantages of IUD usage are the potential for increased menstrual flow, dysmenorrhea, spotting, and spontaneous expulsion.

Mechanical barriers. Like the IUD, the diaphragm and condom have no effect on lactation. Diaphragms, although effective (17 pregnancies/100 women at 1 year of use) when used correctly and consistently, are not preferred by women at the present time. The reasons for this are somewhat unclear, but complaints center on inconvenience of inserting and removing the device and the disruption of coital foreplay.

Condoms are particularly suitable as a contraceptive during the interim of lactation amenorrhea when ovulation is less likely to occur and thus complete protection is less crucial. The failure rate of condoms is high (3 to 36/100 women at 1 year of use). However, when the condom is used with a spermicidal foam, its effectiveness approaches that of oral contraceptives.

Natural methods. Natural fertility control is based on observable physiologic changes that occur during the ovulatory-menstrual cycle. Four methods are recognized[11]: calendar rhythm, ovulation, basal body temperature, and symptothermal. The calendar rhythm method consists of calculation of fertile days and is based on the assumption that ovulation occurs on day 14 ± 2 before the onset of the next menstrual period. The ovulation (Billings) method recognizes that there are unique changes in the cervical mucus immediately before and during ovulation when the "fertile" mucus becomes clear and slippery and stretches easily without breaking. In using the basal body temperature method, the time of ovulation is predicted by a drop in basal body temperature before ovulation and then a slight elevation of temperature for 1 to 3 days. The symptothermal method combines all these methods using a chart to plot the day-to-day changes to determine ovulation.

To be effective, these natural methods require a high level of motivation, close monitoring of the changes that herald the onset of ovulation and, along with the sex partner, a willingness to refrain from intercourse during the fertile period. They work most effectively when both partners are involved. Aside from religious beliefs, dedication to a natural life-style and self-responsibility make these natural methods popular among breastfeeding women in this country.

Epilepsy

Epilepsy can be so well controlled by medications that seizures are rarely a problem for the lactating mother. However, nurses need to know about the effect of these medications on the breastfed infant. Common medications are phenytoin (Dilantin), carbamazepine (Tegretol), primidone (Mysoline), and phenobarbital. Phenobarbital and carbamazepine are generally considered safe for the breastfeeding mother to use. Although phenytoin and primidone have been taken by breastfeeding women without any ill effects on the infants, these drugs, primidone particularly, should be used with caution. In the unusual case in which the mother has seizures, either psychomotor, focal, petit mal, even grand mal, breastfeeding is in no way contraindicated. Dropping or harming the infant during a seizure is no more probable during breastfeeding than it is during bottle-feeding. Usually a prodromal warning (aura) warns of an impending seizure, and the mother is able to take safety precautions to protect her infant by[3]:

1. Having a playpen available on each level of the house so she can quickly place the baby inside when a seizure is imminent.
2. Padding the arms of the rocker or chair where she usually breastfeeds with extra pillows and cushions for protection.
3. Placing guardrails padded with pillows around her bed if she customarily takes her infant to bed to breastfeed.
4. Attaching a tag stating that she has epilepsy, along with pertinent information, to her baby, the stroller, or baby carrier when she is away from home.

Altered competency

Postpartum depression. Hardly any problem is more distressing to all concerned than a mother suffering from postpartum depression or a psychosis. If she needs constant observation, there is the threat of hospitalization and separation, since the psychiatric units of most urban hospitals do not allow the infant. In this situation, nurses can be advocates for changing state laws and for relaxing hospital restrictions that unnecessarily place an additional hardship on the family. Denying the disturbed woman access to her infant imposes a justifiable paranoia in addition to whatever thought disorder is already present. Unfortunately, when postpartum depression or a psychosis occurs, the maternal-infant bond is being formed. Every effort should be made to foster this crucial bond and breastfeeding as well, since, according to Waletzky[36]:

> Body contact with the breast-feeding infant is also soothing. In addition, breast-feeding, aside from its psychological, nutritional and medical benefits for the baby, can enhance maternal identity and self-esteem, which is especially important for the new mother who has suffered a mental illness.

Moreover, Waletzky continues,

> When the infant stays with the mother, the mothers recover faster, have a lower relapse rate, and are more likely to look after their babies upon returning home.

Maternal depression can have a dramatic effect on the infant. Following a suicide attempt by his mother, a 12-month-old toddler suddenly refused any nourishment other than what he received from breastfeeding. All attempts to entice him into eating foods he had formerly enjoyed were firmly refused for several months. Presumably, he sensed that becoming totally dependent on his mother for food would ensure her continued presence.

Since psychotropic drugs may be needed, the risks and benefits of any particular agent must be carefully evaluated. Although many of these medications do not pass into the breastmilk in sufficient quantities to harm the infant, clearly the last word on prolonged high doses is not yet in.

Excepting phenelzine sulfate (Nardil), antidepressants appear to be relatively safe for short-term therapy. Chlorpromazine (Thorazine), a major tranquilizer, actually increases the milk production by blocking the prolactin-inhibitory factor. Since it passes through the milk in insignificant quantities, chlorpromazine is the drug of choice for manic disorders in breastfeeding mothers. Lithium, which is widely prescribed for manic-depressive states, is controversial for breastfeeding[1]; therefore, considering the benefits of continued breastfeeding, its use and thus possible weaning should be closely scrutinized. Diazepam (Valium), one of the most widely used drugs in the United States, is poorly metabolized by the neonate and should be avoided. Diazepam, however, is used for mild psychiatric disorders not for serious postpartum depression, and whenever possible, counseling and psychotherapy should be offered in lieu of drug therapy. The hazards of a drugged and drowsy mother in interacting with and caring for her infant are of no small consequence.

No information is available on the effects of electric shock therapy (EST) on lactation. It usually does, however, interrupt the menstrual cycle, which indicates a possible impact on lactation.

Maternal addiction. The overriding question in the case of a breastfeeding, drug-addicted mother is her ability to function and provide adequate care for her infant. Fears of an unstable life-style, child abuse, and neglect have been overrated, according to one study,[33] which showed that these children's mental and psychomotor development fell into normal limits up to 2 years of age when their mothers were under care and supervision. Although the drug-dependent mother needs more guidance and help, denying her maternal rights and responsibilities must be seriously questioned. Others[19] feel the addicted mother is a poor risk for parenting even if she is receiving help; however, the desire to mother and breastfeed can be a powerful motivation to stay off drugs. Generally, if the mother has been detoxified and is narcotic free, she should be encouraged if she desires to breastfeed. A woman on an average methadone maintenance will theoretically excrete only about 57 μg/day in her first 5 weeks, which is considered a trace amount not harmful to her infant[33] and may actually minimize withdrawal symptoms in the infant.

Withdrawal symptoms in the infant—tremors and hypertonicity—are not sufficient reason to separate the mother and baby during the hospital stay. *This* mother, more than any other, benefits from bonding through early and frequent contact with her infant.

Although not considered addictive, marijuana is so widely used today that questions concerning its use while breastfeeding frequently arise. Laboratory studies on animals show impairment of DNA and RNA formation and structural changes in the brain cells of the animal nursling.[30] On the other hand, there is yet no evidence that the primary active substance of marijuana passes into human milk, although it appears likely. There have been anecdotal reports of drowsiness in breastfeeding infants after their mothers smoked marijuana.

Despite the well-publicized warnings by health professionals against it, marijuana, like alcohol, is now an accepted recreational drug. Thus the dilemma: should a woman then be advised to not breastfeed if she refuses to give up her recreational use of marijuana? There are no easy answers. The optimal situation is for her body to be free of all drugs while breastfeeding, including marijuana. However, if the mother refuses to stop using marijuana, it is probably better for her to continue breastfeeding while using marijuana on a recreational basis rather than to wean and bottle-feed.

Medications

In addressing the problem of medicating the mother, the first concern is with the pregnant woman. Many drugs are contraindicated in pregnancy, since some readily cross the placenta and cause damage to the fetus. The importance of avoiding all drugs that are not essential to the mother's life and health is now well recognized. The situation is different for the breastfeeding mother: the situation changes and the infant is able to metabolize and excrete drugs, especially after the first week of life. It remains important, however, to evaluate the mother's real need for the drug before encouraging her to take it for minor ailments or for discomfort that will rapidly subside without drug therapy.

Most medications taken by the mother are found to some degree in breastmilk; a few are not. The chief conern is the effect the drug, in the amount found in mother's milk, will have on the infant.

When prescribing a medication for the breastfeeding woman, some physicians will invariably prescribe weaning as a precaution because they are unsure of the effect of the drug on the breastfeeding infant. With the availability of drug information today, some guidelines have been established, although considerably more research needs to be done. Studies thus far are primarily derived from retrospective data and anecdotal reports, as there are obvious limitations to conducting in vivo research, and laboratory procedures and testing protocols for studying drug excretion are problematic and expensive.

Although it has been assumed by some that a drug that is safe for the fetus in utero is invariably safe for the breastfeeding infant, this assumption has been shown not to be universally true. The infant's own regulatory and excretory mechanisms are not well developed in the early weeks after birth, whereas the fetus has the detoxifying and eliminatory systems of the mother available to him. It is important, therefore, to evaluate the risk/benefit ratio of each drug taken in pregnancy when its use is to be continued after delivery. The degree to which maternal medications pass into the milk depends on the ionization, pH, and solubility of the agent in fat or water. However, passage of medication into the milk and its potential effect on an infant is only one variable; the child's age and health, the frequency of feedings, and the length of time a medication is taken are others.

Because an infant is a dynamic, changing organism, what is true for him at one time may not be applicable in the following weeks or months. Developing enzyme systems, along with the lipid (blood-brain) barrier, are not yet fully functional. This prevents full detoxification, acetylation, or oxidation of chemicals in the milk during the first week or so of life for the well neonate and much later for the premature infant. Later development of these systems will enable the infant to handle with ease the medication that would have previously triggered harmful consequences. Sulfa drugs are commonly in this category.

Although some differences of opinion exist among various authorities about specific drugs, there is general agreement that most drugs given to the breastfeeding mother cause no harm to the infant. The drug list given in Table 6-3 is a guideline for determining whether and under what conditions a mother may take a specific drug. As noted, there are conflicting studies on some drugs and a lack of data on others. Since a physician must be involved in the administration of many drugs, the guide should be used by the nurse in conjunction with medical opinion. Rather than use the drugs noted as contraindicated on the guide and wean, every possible effort should be made to find an alternative therapy for the mother whose baby is breastfeeding.

Weaning the infant, even temporarily, is invariably undesirable because it brings physical and psychologic stress to both mother and child. The client with a physical problem sufficient to require medication suffers more when her problem is compounded by painfully engorged breasts and a disconsolate infant. The infant who is even temporarily weaned risks infections and may develop allergies from artificial formulas. What follows is an extreme example of the possible sequela when breastfeeding is interrupted because of medication.

Diagnosed as having a urinary infection and given a sulfonamide medication, a breastfeeding mother was told to discontinue breastfeeding for the duration of the therapy (10 days). Already discouraged from having pumped while her infant was jaundiced earlier, at this point she felt overwhelmed and decided to give up breastfeeding entirely. Two days later the physician's office called to say the urine culture was negative but that she should continue taking the drug as a precautionary measure. Shortly after, vomiting, diarrhea, and later eczema developed in her infant as the parents and physician desperately switched from one formula to another to find one the infant could tolerate. Periods of apnea became a problem, and the infant was placed on a home apnea monitor between hospitalizations. Ultimately, complications developed and an ileostomy was done. Desperate, this mother began relactation while collecting fresh breastmilk donated by women in the area, and eventually she was able to sustain the infant on her milk. At 5 years of age, this child is now reasonably healthy but still cannot tolerate milk and is allergic to many foods.

Can there be any question about the importance of nursing interventions and the suggestion of possible alternatives when medications threaten continued breastfeeding?

TABLE 6-3

Nursing guide to drugs and breastfeeding

Drug	Safe to use?			Comments
	Relatively safe	With caution	Contraindicated	
Analgesics				
Acetaminophen (Tylenol, Datril)	X			
Codeine	X			May use for short-term analgesic.
Meperidine (Demerol)	X			May use for short-term analgesic.
Methadone	X			Avoid excessive doses.
Morphine		X		May use for short-term analgesic. Long-term use may be addicting to infant.
Propoxyphene (Darvon)	X			
Salicylates (aspirin)	X			Caution in first week of life. Observe prothrombin time in infants and administer vitamin K if warranted.
Anticoagulants				
Coumadin (dicumarol, warfarin)	X			Caution if mother on high doses or if infant to have surgery.
Heparin	X			
Phenindione (Hedulin)			X	Causes prolonged prothrombin time in infant.
Anticonvulsants				
Carbamazepine (Tegretol)	X			
Phenobarbital	X			Observe for drowsiness in infant if mother on large doses (>100 mg).
Phenytoin (Dilantin)		X		Avoid large doses.
Primidone (Mysoline)		X		Monitor infant for drowsiness and prothrombin time.
Antihistamines and decongestants				
General (diphenhydramine [Benadryl], bromopheniramine [Dimetapp], promethazine [Phenergan], tripelennamine [Pyribenzamine], methdilazine [Tacaryl], trimeprazine [Temaril])	X			Use alternate drug if decrease in milk supply noted or if infant becomes irritable or drowsy.

Data compiled from Lawrence, R.: Breastfeeding: a guide for the medical profession, St. Louis, 1980, The C.V. Mosby Co.; O'Brien, T.E.: Am. J. Hosp. Pharm. **31:**844, 1974; Pagliaro, L.A., and Levin, R.H.: Problems in pediatric drug therapy, Hamilton, Ill., 1979, Drug Intelligence Pub., Inc.; White, M., and White, G.: Vet. Hum. Toxicol. **1**(suppl.):23, 1980 (available from La Leche League International); Wilson, J.T., et al., et al.: Drug excretion in human milk, Clin. Pharmacokinet. **5:**1, 1980.

TABLE 6-3—cont'd

Nursing guide to drugs and breastfeeding

Drug	Safe to use?			Comments
	Relatively safe	With caution	Contraindicated	
Antimetabolites				
Methotrexate		X		Excreted in breastmilk in very small amounts but only cases reported used low doses. Drug potentially very toxic.
Antineoplastics				
General (melphalan [Alkeran], cyclophosphamide [Cytoxan], cytarabine [Cytosar], busulfan [Myleran])			X	
Antimicrobials				
Aminoglycosides (amikacin [Amikin], gentamicin [Garamycin], kanamycin [Kantrex], tobramycin [Nebcin], Streptomycin)	X			
Cephalosporins (cefazolin [Ancef], cephradine [Anspor], cephalexin [Keflex], cephalothin [Keflin], cephradine [Velosef])	X			
Chloramphenicol (Chloromycetin)			X	Possibly toxic.
Clindamycin (Cleocin)	X			
Erythromycin (Ilotycin, Ilosone, Erythrocin)	X			
Penicillins Amoxicillin	X			
Ampicillin	X			
Oxacillin (Prostaphilin)	X			
Penicillin G, benzathine	X			
Penicillin G, potassium	X			
Metronidazole (Flagyl)		X		Avoid if infant under 6 months of age. Use alternate drug, if possible.
Nitrofurantoin (Furadantin)	X			

Continued.

TABLE 6-3—cont'd

Nursing guide to drugs and breastfeeding

Drug	Safe to use?			Comments
	Relatively safe	With caution	Contraindicated	
Antimicrobials—cont'd				
Nystatin (Mycostatin)	X			
Sulfonamides (sulfisoxazole [Azo Gantrisin], sulfame-thoxazole [Bactrium, Gan-tanol], mafenide [Sulfamy-lon])		X		Use only after infant is 1 month of age.
Tetracyclines (tetracycline [Panmycin], oxytetracy-cline [Terramycin], doxy-cycline [Vibramycin], deme-clocycline [Declomycin], minocycline [Minocin])		X		Avoid large dosages and long-term use. May possibly stain teeth and inhibit bone growth.
Autonomic drugs				
Atropine	X	X		Avoid if possible. Studies are conflicting. May inhibit lactation and/or cause toxic symptoms in infant.
Ergotamine (Cafergot)			X	Risk of ergotism in infant. May also suppress lactation.
Methocarbamol (Robaxin)	X			
Neostigmine (Prostigamin)	X			
Propantheline bromide (Pro-Banthine)	X			
Scopolamine (hyoscine)	X			
Cimetidine (Tagamet)		X		Effect unknown. Use alternate therapies.
Bronchodilators				
Aminophylline (theophylline)		X		Observe for irritability and insom-nia in infant.
Epinephrine	X			
Cardiovascular drugs				
Digitalis (Lanoxin, digitoxin)	X			
Hydralazine (Apresoline)		X		No data available.
Methyldopa (Aldomet)	X			
Propranolol (Inderal)	X			
Quinidine	X			
Reserpine (Serpasil)	X			Observe infant for nasal stuffi-ness, lethargy, and for diar-rhea.

TABLE 6-3—cont'd

Nursing guide to drugs and breastfeeding

Drug	Safe to use?			Comments
	Relatively safe	With caution	Contraindicated	
Central nervous system drugs				
Alcohol	X			Use in moderation.
Barbital (Veronal)		X		Avoid use if possible. Sedative effect in infants.
Bromides			X	Consider alternate medication.
Caffeine		X		May cause irritability if mother takes large amounts.
Chloral hydrate (Noctec, Somnos)	X			Observe for infant drowsiness.
Dextroamphetamine (Dexedrine)	X			No evidence of stimulation in infants. Not excreted.
Indomethacin (Indocin)		X		Avoid, especially in neonatal period.
Prochlorperazine (Compazine)	X			
Thiopental sodium (Pentothal)	X			
Diagnostic drugs and tests				
Barium	X			
Radiopharmaceuticals ^{67}Ga		X		Interrupt breastfeedings for 24 hr
^{131}I ^{125}I		X		Interrupt breastfeedings for 48 hr and test milk before resuming feedings.
^{99m}Tc		X		Interrupt breastfeedings for 24 hr
X-rays	X			
Diuretics				
Acetazolamide (Diamox)	X			
Furosemide (Lasix)	X			
Spironolactone (Aldactone)	X			
Thiazides (cyclothiazide [Anhydron], chlorothiazide [Diuril], hydrochlorothiazide [Hydrodiuril], chlorthalidone [Hygroton])	X			Observe for dehydration and electrolyte imbalance in mother.
Hormones				
Androgens (fluoxymesterone [Halotestin, Ultandren, Oratestryl], methyltestosterone [Oreton-Methyl, Metandren])			X	Suppress lactation.

Continued.

TABLE 6-3—cont'd

Nursing guide to drugs and breastfeeding

Drug	Relatively safe	With caution	Contraindicated	Comments
		Safe to use?		
Hormones—cont'd				
Contraceptives, oral (estrogen-progesterone combination) (norethynodrel [Enovid], norethindrone [Loestrin, Norinyl, Norlestrin, Ortho-Novum], ethynodiol [Ovulen])			X	Diminish milk supply. Change milk composition. Reports of gynecomastia in male infants.
Corticosteroids (dexamethasone [Decadron], prednisone, hydrocortisone [Solu-Cortef])		X		Avoid large doses and long-term use.
Corticotropin (ACTH)	X			
Epinephrine	X			
Insulin	X			Destroyed in GI tract.
Thyroid preparations (levothyroxine [Synthroid], liothyronine [Cytomel])	X			Increase lactogenesis if mother is thyroid deficient.
Laxatives				
Agar	X			
Bisacodyl (Dulcolax)	X			
Cascara		X		May cause diarrhea in infant.
Castor oil	X			
Magnesium sulfate (Epsom salt)	X			
Milk of magnesia	X			
Mineral oil	X			
Phenolphthalein		X		May cause diarrhea in infant.
Senna	X			
Psychotropic drugs				
Antidepressants Phenelzine sulfate (Nardil)			X	Inhibits lactation.
Tranylcypromine (Parnate)	X			
Tricyclics (amitriptyline [Elavil], desipramine [Norpramin], imipramine [Tofranil])	X	X		Use with caution for long term (>1 mo) administration. Watch for signs of sedation, anticholinergic side effects.

TABLE 6-3—cont'd

Nursing guide to drugs and breastfeeding

	Safe to use?			
Drug	**Relatively safe**	**With caution**	**Contraindicated**	**Comments**
Psychotropic drugs—cont'd				
Major tranquilizers	X			
Phenothiazines (thioridazine [Mellaril], piperacetazine [Quide], mesoridazine [Serentil], trifluoperazine [Skelazine], chlorpromazine [Thorazine])				
Haloperidol (Haldol)	X			Not known. No reports.
Minor tranquilizers				
Benzodiazepines				
Chlordiazepoxide (Librium)	X			May use after infant is 1 week old.
Diazepam (Valium)			X	Use alternate drug when possible.
Meprobamate (Equanil, Miltown)	X	X		Monitor infant closely.
Lithium		X	X	Conflicting data.
Miscellaneous drugs				
DPT	X			
Nicotine		X	X	Heavy smoking may decrease milk supply and cause nausea and vomiting in infant.
Poliovirus vaccine	X			
Potassium iodide		X		May cause goiter in infant.
Propylthiouracil		X		Monitor infant closely for thyroid function.
Rh immune globulin (RhoGAM)	X			
Rubella vaccine		X		Does not affect infant through milk, but *never* should be given if mother susceptible to pregnancy.
Smallpox vaccine	X			

Environmental contaminants

In recent years consumers and health professionals alike have become increasingly aware of the potential for damage resulting from indiscriminate and irresponsible use of pesticides and other contaminants. Exposure to environmental contaminants is the fate of all of us, breastfeeding mothers and infants, as well as older children, adults, men, and women alike. And, in small amounts, some of the contaminants appear in the breastmilk of mothers—as in milk of cows, goats, and other mammals.

Nothing is to be gained by discontinuing breastfeeding because of the presence of possible contaminants in human milk. There has been reported to date little evidence of either short- or long-term ill effects on the infant from pollutants in mother's milk.[8] On the contrary, the risk for the infant to ingest lead, a pollutant with known toxicity, is much greater when he is fed formulas that could be prepared with lead-contaminated tap water.[28]

Internationally known scientists have attested to the benefits of mother's milk, and they urge that all infants be provided with the protection against allergy, obesity, and bacterial and viral infections that mother's milk uniquely provides. Therefore the risk/benefit ratio is heavily weighted in favor of breastfeeding even when known contamination is present.

SUMMARY

In summary, prenatal assessment is a key nursing responsibility for preventing breastfeeding problems later on. The number of technologic or lactation aids given in this chapter can be useful adjuncts to breastfeeding, but they must be used wisely and cautiously so as to not interfere with the physiologic patterns of feeding at the breast. Breastfeeding women as well as nurses are not exempt from the lure of catchy devices.

Although not exhaustive, the maternal self-care deficits given here represent a cross-section of situations the nurse practitioner will find in working with breastfeeding women. Last, our Brave New World necessitates a discussion of drugs and contaminants, a pervasive element of our society, and their relationship to the child who takes nourishment at the breast.

REFERENCES

1. Anath, J.:Side effects in the neonate from psychotropic agents excreted through breastfeeding, Am. J. Psychiatry **135**:801, 1978.
2. Bahr, J.E.: Herpesvirus hominis type 2 in women and newborns, M.C.N. **3**:16, 1978.
2a. Beltoli, E.J.: Herpes: facts and fantasies, Am. J. Nurs. **82**:924, 1982.
3. Brewster, D.P.: You can breastfeed your baby . . . even in special situations, Emmaus, Pa., 1980, Rodale Press, Inc.
4. Buchanan, R.: Breastfeeding: aid to infant health and fertility Control, Popul. Rep. [J] **4**:49, 1975.
5. Cheek, W.: Benign breast lumps may regress with diet, J.A.M.A. **241**:1221, 1979.
6. Committee on Fetus and Newborn, Committee on Infectious Diseases: Perinatal herpes simplex virus infections, Pediatrics **66**:147, 1980.

7. Cotterman, J.: Intensive preparation for inverted or retracting nipples, Keeping Abreast J. **1**:330, 1976.
8. Doucette, J.S.: Is breastfeeding still safe for babies? M.C.N. **3**:345, 1978.
9. Evans, R.T., Thigpen, L.W., and Hamrick, M.: Exploration of factors involved in maternal physiological adaptation to breastfeeding, Nurs. Res. **18**:28, 1969.
10. Farina, M.A., Newby, B.G., and Alani, H.M.: Innervation of the nipple-areola complex, Plast. Reconstr. Surg. **66**:497, 1980.
11. Fogel, C.I., and Woods, N.F.: Health care of women: a nursing perspective, St. Louis, 1981, The C.V. Mosby Co.
12. Goldfarb, J., and Tibbetts, E.: Breastfeeding handbook, Hillside, N.J., 1980, Enslow Publishers.

13. Goldsmith, H.S.: Milk rejection sign of breast cancer, Am. J. Surg. **127:**280, 1974.

14. Gonzalez, E.R.: Vitamin E relieves most cystic breast disease, may alter lipids, hormones, J.A.M.A. **244:**1077, 1980.

15. Guthrie, D.W., and Guthrie, R.A.: Nursing management of diabetes mellitus, ed. 2, St. Louis, 1982, The C.V. Mosby Co.

16. Hoffman, J.B.: A suggested treatment for inverted nipples, Am. J. Obstet. Gynecol. **66:**346, 1953.

17. Ing, R., Ho, J.H., and Petrakias, N.L.: Unilateral breastfeeding and breast cancer, Lancet **2:**124, 1977.

18. Kampmann, J.P., et al.: Propylthiouracil in human milk: revision of a dogma, Lancet **8171:**736, 1980.

19. Kantor, G.K.: Addicted mother, addicted baby: a challenge to health care providers, M.C.N. **3:**281, 1978.

20. Kaplan, S.D., and Acheson, R.M.: A single etiological hypothesis for breast cancer? J. Chronic. Dis. **19:**1221, 1966.

21. Kauffman, R., O'Brien, C., and Gilford, P.: Sulfisoxazole secretion into human milk, J. Pediatr. **97:**839, 1980.

22. La Leche League International: News **18:**69, 1976, The League.

23. La Leche League International: Nursing after breast surgery, La Leche League News **22:**10, 1980.

24. La Leche League International: The womanly art of breastfeeding, Franklin Park, Ill., 1981, The League.

25. Lawrence, R.: Breast-feeding: a guide for the medical profession, St. Louis, 1980, The C.V. Mosby Co.

26. Miller, D.L.: Birth and long-term unsupplemented breastfeeding in 17 insulin-dependent diabetic mothers, Birth Fam. J. **4:**65, 1977.

27. Miller, R., and Fraumenti, J.: Does breastfeeding increase the child's risk of breast cancer? Pediatrics **49:**645, 1972.

28. Miller, R.W.: Carcinogens and drinking water, Pediatrics **57:**462, 1976.

29. Morgan, R.W., Vakil, D.V., and Chipman, M.L.: Breastfeeding, family history and breast disease, Am. J. Epidemiol. **99:**117, 1974.

30. Nahas, G., and Panon, W., editors: Marihuana: chemistry, bio-chemistry, and cellular effects, New York, 1976, Springer-Verlag, New York, Inc.

31. Neifert, M.R.: Personal communication, July 1981.

32. Neifert, M.R., McDonough, S.L., and Neville, M.C.: Failure of lactogenesis associated with placental retention, Am. J. Obstet. Gynecol. **140:**477, 1981.

33. Ostrea, E.M., Chavez, C.J., and Stryker, J.C.: The care of the drug dependent woman and her infant, Lansing, Mich., 1978, Michigan Department of Public Health.

34. Peters, M.V., and Meakin, J.W.: The influence of pregnancy on carcinoma of the breast, Prog. Clin. Cancer **1:**471, 1965.

35. Strauss, L.T., et al.: Oral contraception during lactation: a global survey, Int. J. Gynaecol. Obstet. **19:**169, 1981.

36. Waletzky, L.: Emotional illness in the postpartum period. In Ahmed, P., editor: Pregnancy, childbirth and parenthood, New York, 1981, Elsevier North-Holland, Inc.

37. Waller, H.: The breasts and breastfeeding, London, 1957, Heinemann, Medical Books.

38. Welch, M.J., Phelps, D.L., and Osher, A.B.: Breastfeeding by a mother with cystic fibrosis, Pediatrics **67:**664, 1981.

39. White, M., and White, G.: Breastfeeding and drugs in human milk, Vet. Hum. Toxicol. **1**(suppl:23, 1980.

ADDITIONAL READINGS

Applebaum, R.M.: The obstetrician's approach to the breast and breastfeeding (editorial), Reprod. Med. **14:**98, 1975.

Arena, J.M.: Contamination of the ideal food, Nutrition Today **5:**2, 1970.

Beasley, P.R., et al.: Breast-feeding and hepatitis B., Letter to the editor, Lancet 2 (7944):1089, 1975.

Bowes, W.A.: The effect of medications on the lactating mother and her infant, Clin. Obstet. Gynecol. **23:**1073, 1980.

Breastfeeding: aid to infant health and fertility control, Population Reports, Series J., No. 4, Washington, D.C., 1975, U.S. Department of Medical and Public Affairs.

Brown, M.S.: Controversial questions about breastfeeding, J.O.G.N. Nurs. **4:**15, 1975.

Brunner, L.S., et al.: Textbook of medical-surgical nursing, Philadelphia, 1970, J.B. Lippincott Co.

Caldwell, K.: Improving nipple graspability for success at breastfeeding, J.O.G.N. Nurs. **10:**277, 1981.

Countryman, B.A.: How the maternity nurse can help the breastfeeding mother, Franklin Park, Ill., 1977, La Leche League International, Inc.

Grassley, J., and Davis, K.: Common concerns of mothers who breastfeed, M.C.N. **3:**347, 1978.

Howie, P.W., et al.: How long should a breast feed last? Early Hum. Dev. **5:**71, 1981.

Knowles, J.A.: Drugs excreted into breastmilk. In Shirkey, H.C., editor: Pediatric therapy, ed. 6, St. Louis, 1972, The C.V. Mosby Co.

Kushner, R.: Breast cancer, New York, 1975, Harcourt Brace Jovanovich, Inc.

Murdaugh, A., and Miller, E.L.: Helping the breastfeeding mother, Am. J. Nurs. **72:**1420, 1972.

Nichols, M.G.: Effective help for the nursing mother, J.O.G.N. Nurs. **7:**22, 1978.

Otte, M.J.: Correcting inverted nipples: an aid to breastfeeding, Am. J. Nurs. **75:**454, 1975.

Rees, D.: Good news for "innies," up front facts, Keeping Abreast J. **1:**46, 1976.

Riker, A.P.: Successful breastfeeding, Am. J. Nurs. **60:**1443, 1960.

Vorherr, H.: Drug excretion into breastmilk, Postgrad. Med. **56:**97, 1974.

White, M.: Medications for the nursing mother, Franklin Park, Ill., 1976, La Leche League International, Inc.

Wilcox, P.M.: Benign breast disorders, Am. J. Nurs. **81:**1644, 1981.

Mastitis

JAN RIORDAN

Nurses who practice in an outpatient clinic setting have the opportunity to work with and help breastfeeding women who develop mastitis. On the other hand, hospital nurses do not see women with mastitis often, since it usually develops after the postpartum hospital stay, except rarely when the infection progresses to the point at which hospitalization is required. However, this is usually unnecessary with timely and effective interventions.

Very little information on mastitis is available in the nursing literature. When mastitis does appear, it is only briefly discussed. This is particularly unfortunate, because it is usually the nurse who first speaks with the calling mother whose symptoms might be the early indicators of mastitis. It is the nurse who usually does the immediate health teaching that can make a difference in preventing an infection from developing to an abscess, especially if the mother mistakenly thinks she should stop breastfeeding. As Newton and Newton[11] point out, "the care of the woman with this disease often falls between the obstetrician, the pediatrician, and the surgeon." Functioning as a primary health-care provider, the nurse is in a position to help by reason of her general knowledge and experience.

CLINICAL COURSE OF MASTITIS

The initial symptoms of puerperal mastitis are fatigue and a flulike, muscular aching. If a breastfeeding mother calls into the clinic or office complaining that she has the "flu," the first consideration of the nurse is to rule out a breast infection.

Typically, fatigue and muscular aching are followed by fever, a rapid pulse, and the appearance of a hot, reddened, and tender area on the breast. There appears to be an inverse correlation between localized symptoms and fever—that is, the more tender and reddened the breast, the less likely it is that a high fever will occur. Presumably, the immune defenses in the infected area, the leukocytes and lymphocytes, are effectively walling off the infection, as evidenced by redness or swelling, and a systemic hyperthermic response to fight the infection is not needed. Although the inflammation is usually unilateral and in one area, mastitis can occur bilaterally in more than one area of the breast. The infection can also affect milk composition: an elevation of sodium and chloride in the milk from an infected breast has been noted in one report.[1] Mastitis usually occurs in the first 5 weeks after delivery, and symptoms last from 2 to 4 days, followed by resolution. The best treatments of preventing abscess formation and hasten-

TABLE 7-1 _____

Bacterial isolates from breastmilk during sporadic puerperal mastitis

Bacterium	Infected breast (N-48)	Contralateral breast (N-45)
Staphylococcus epidermidis	32	27
S. aureus	23	17
α-Hemolytic *Streptococcus*	4	6
Hemolytic *Streptococcus*, neither group A nor group D	3	2
Diphtheroids	2	2
Group A β-hemolytic *Streptococcus*	1	0
Enterococcus	1	0
Nonhemolytic *Streptococcus*	0	1
Lactobacillus	0	1
No growth	0	4

From Marshall B.R., Hepper, J.K., and Zirbel, C.C.: J.A.M.A. **233**:1377, 1975.

TABLE 7-2 _____

Bacterial isolates and colony counts from the breastmilk of 19 lactating women without mastitis

Bacterium	Right breast		Left breast	
	No. of positive specimens	Colonies/ ml of milk	No. of positive specimens	Colonies/ ml of milk
Staphylococcus epidermidis	10	100-50,000	12	300-5,000
Diphtheroids	5	100-5,000	2	1200-5000
α-Hemolytic *Streptococcus*	4	300-5,000	5	400-10,000
Nonhemolytic *Streptococcus*	2	800-50,000	1	6800
S. aureus	1	100	0	—
No organism	6	—	4	—

From Marshal, B.R., Hepper, J.K., and Zirbel, C.C.: J.A.M.A. **233**:1377, 1975.

ing recovery are continued breastfeeding, the application of moist heat, forced fluids, judicious use of antibiotics and bed rest.

The most common infecting organism in the breast according to the medical literature is a staphylococcus. Only rarely is a streptococcus involved.[13] Table 7-1 shows the various types of bacteria found in cultured milk during mastitis, and Table 7-2 shows that similar bacteria can be isolated from the milk of women who do not have mastitis, leaving little doubt that the breast of every lactating mother is at some time exposed to pathogenic bacteria. The entrance of the pathogen and establishment of an infectious process appear more complex than its simple presence. Probably more important are the antecedent conditions that facilitate the infection.

TYPES AND INCIDENCE

Before the advent of antibiotics and short hospital stays following delivery, puerperal mastitis was divided into two types: one that occurred in epidemic form and one that

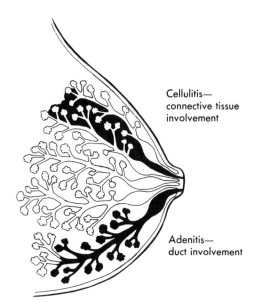

Cellulitis—
connective tissue
involvement

Adenitis—
duct involvement

Fig. 7-1. Mastitis primarily involving connective tissue between ducts (cellulitis) and in the ducts (adenitis).

developed sporadically away from the hospital. Because of short hospital stays, the epidemic form is now seldom seen. Still many cases are thought to be hospital acquired, especially those that occur within the first few weeks after delivery.

As shown in Fig. 7-1, mastitis has been classified into two types according to the location in the breast and the clinical features. Gibberd[5] has described these two types as (1) cellulitis and (2) adenitis. A third type, subclinical mastitis, has also been described.

Cellulitis is thought to involve the interlobular connective tissue as a result of the introduction of bacteria through cracked nipples, usually in the early weeks of breastfeeding. The woman develops a fever, often with chills, malaise, and headache. The infected breast may develop a warm, reddened, circumscribed area that is extremely tender. The formation of pus seldom occurs in cellulitis, especially with prompt treatment. In adenitis the ducts of the breast are infected, and the clinical symptoms are less severe. Sometimes more than one duct is involved, and suppuration is more likely to be seen. In both conditions abscess is less common if breastfeeding is continued.[6, 10] If an abscess does occur, which is rare, it appears as a localized, indurated white area just under the surface of the skin that is very tender and warm to the touch. Medical intervention with antibiotics and possibly incision and drainage will be needed. With an abscess, a temporary interruption in breastfeeding (with pumping and discarding the milk) can be followed by resuming breastfeeding. An electric breast pump minimizes discomfort and further trauma. Only rarely does the infection progress to the point at which there is a purulent dischrge from the breast. In this case the mother can continue to express from the affected breast and breastfeed on only one side for about a week. When the symptoms clear, she should resume feedings from both breasts.

With the third type of infection, subclinical mastitis, the milk colonizes *S. aureus,* but the woman remains free from symptoms other than an occasional low-grade fever when there is adequate drainage from the breast without stasis.[2]

How common is mastitis? Data from various sources cite a variance from 1% to 10%.[4, 8, 10] However, the duration of breastfeeding of the mothers studied is not specified, and no published data on the incidence of mastitis in long-term lactation are available.

PREVENTION IN THE HOSPITAL

There is strong evidence[11] that the common vector for virulent staphylococci strains picked up in maternity and nursery units is a nose or throat carrier among the staff. In preventing these staphylococci, usually *S. aureus,* from colonizing in the infant or the mother and causing mastitis, the identification and exclusion of personnel with staphylococcal infections and stringent handwashing are, of course, paramount for nursing care. Just as important for infection control is early breastfeeding. If, in the first minutes of life, the mother gives her baby her own mixture of strains of respiratory organisms, such as the staphylococcus, these maternally provided strains grow and populate the infant's respiratory and gastrointestinal tracts and prevent the growth of the hospital strains of staphylococcus, which are more likely to be virulent. Klaus and Kennell[7] liken this process to a lawn planted with grass that resists the growth of weeds after the grass has had a good start. This phenomenon, called bacterial interference, has been used successfully in clinical settings[9, 14] to prevent *S. aureus* from spreading by directly inoculating the nares of infants with a benign strain of staphylococcus. The implication for nursing care in preventing mastitis and staphylococcal skin infections in the infant by putting the baby to breast early and often is clear.

MEDICAL INTERVENTIONS

The severity and type of mastitis determine whether antibiotic therapy is needed. Mastitis is largely self-limited; therefore, in view of warnings against the overuse of antibiotics, practitioners should guard against routinely prescribing them for mastitis, particularly if the infection appears to be resolving on its own. If antibiotic therapy is indicated and started early and breastfeeding is continued, the infection is usually under control within 48 hours. The drugs of choice are semisynthetic antistaphylococcal penicillins such as dicloxacillin, oxacillin, nafcillin, and cloxacillin, which are not excreted in the milk.[15] Because many staphylococci strains have become resistant to ampicillin, it is not recommended.[3] In severe or prolonged mastitis, culturing the milk is indicated; however, it often proves impractical for the immediate problem, since the infection is usually under control before the results of the culture and sensitivity test are available.

SURVEY
Methodology

To collect more data on mastitis I surveyed women attending La Leche League meetings in Wichita, Kansas, over a period of 1 month in 1980. Questionnaires with eight forced-choice items and one open-ended item were constructed for the survey. Since breast problems run the gamut from plugged ducts to caked breasts, for purposes of the survey mastitis was defined as fatigue accompanied by an inflammation of the breast, tenderness, redness, and a temperature of 38° C (100.4° F) or higher. Respondents who qualified as having mastitis according to these criteria were asked to indicate on breast diagrams the breast side (right or left or both) and the location of the infection. For respondents who had more than one case of mastitis three diagrams were given, including a question asking if the repeated infection occurred with the same infant. Other items included the postpartum month of occurrence, physician contact, hospitalization, and duration of symptoms. The open-ended question asked about antecedent conditions that might have caused the mastitis.

Results

Despite the limitations of this study, which was on a select population, the results are informative (Table 7-3). Of 100 women surveyed, 26 reported having had mastitis, some more than one time, for a total of 46 cases.

Although not statistically significant, mastitis occurred more frequently on the left breast (56.5%) than on the right (36.9%). Most areas of infection were distally located in the outer half of the breasts. I do not have an explanation for this. Although in any 1 month the highest incidence of mastitis was during the first month (26%), the survey led me to suspect that mastitis is not uncommon after 6 months. The survey also demonstrated that mastitis can frequently go unreported: 21 out of the 46 cases of mastitis did not involve physician contact. The reasons are not clear, but it may be that these women, all of whom were in contact with La Leche League, had sufficient information in recognizing and treating the problems themselves. Thus they chose to forego medical intervention, particularly if the mastitis was not severe and was responding to home treatment. Also, most people do not go to their physician for the flu; after a day or two, when the mother realizes it is a breast infection, her symptoms are likely to have subsided, and she forgoes seeking her physician's help.

The survey revealed certain antecedent conditions that were consistently reported by mothers who developed mastitis. These are described, along with reasons why they are important.

TABLE 7-3
Characteristics of mastitis in 46 cases

Characteristics	No.	%
Site		
Right breast	17	36.9
Left breast	26	56.5
Bilateral	3	6.5
Contacted physician	25	54.3
Took antibiotic	21	45.6
Recurrence with same baby		
Once	10	21.7
Twice	4	8.6
Occurring after delivery		
First mo	12	26.1
2-6 mo	22	47.8
Beyond 6 mo	12	26.1
Hospitalization required	0	0

Frequency of feedings. A sudden change in the number of feedings usually leads to overdistention. If the number is reduced for any reason, milk collects in the ducts with stasis; on the other hand, if the number of feedings suddenly increases and then decreases, the effect is the same as in the case of a mother who reported: "We were on vacation 1000 miles from home. After driving for 2 days with exclusive breastfeeding, we arrived at our destination and the feedings were cut back quite a bit. The infection started a few days after this." Accompanying an increase in the frequency of feedings is the potential for engorgement or overdistention of the breast.

Overdistention/engorgement. Four-hour hospital feeding schedules increase milk stasis by overdistention. Thus the likelihood of breast infections is greater than when the mother and infant have free access to one another for unrestricted feedings. Such schedules could rightfully be called iatrogenic.

During the later months of lactating, a number of other conditions can lead to overdistention, such as these related by our respondents:

- My baby began sleeping longer and my breasts got overfull.
- I breastfed too long on one side, not emptying the other breast because of my favorite position while sleeping.
- I worked one afternoon, missed a feeding, and did not express any milk.
- I breastfed from the right breast three times in a row before using the left breast, the one that was infected.

In one case when a mother was plagued with repeated mastitis, I found her infant was sleeping through 10 hours at night—an unusual circumstance. When she awakened in the morning, her breasts were always hard and sore. As soon as she began waking up her infant for a night feeding, she had no more problems with mastitis.

Stress. The effect of stress on the individual's immune defense system is well known, and I will not elaborate on it here. What is important is that half the women responding to the survey stated that they were under some sort of stress before mastitis occurred. These mothers were stressed from overwork or lack of sleep and described themselves as exhausted by circumstances above and beyond the normal stresses of taking care of any infant, for example: "I was doing too much—just starting to get out with my first baby and trying to get ready for our first Christmas."

Cracked or fissured nipples. Quite obviously, a breakdown in the epidermis provides an avenue of entry into the breast tissue. Self-care suggestions, such as proper positioning in prevention of sore and cracked nipples, given elsewhere in this text, can prevent nipple tissue breakdown and hence the infection. But what about women who develop mastitis and have no soreness and cracking? Only a small number of the respondents described soreness or fissuring before mastitis. It appears that mastitis, like most other diseases, is multifactorial in origin and more than one antecedent condition is usually present before the infection can occur.

Constriction. Several respondents reported that they were wearing a tight, constricting bra just before the infection started. A tight bra produces the same stasis as overdistention—only its pressure is from outside the body. A face-down sleeping position also has a constricting effect.

Trauma. Bruising and trauma to the breast tissue may trigger the proliferation of a pathogenic organism that might otherwise lie dormant. Trauma to the breast is as widely varied as trauma to other areas of the body. For women with other small children, it is frequently an inadvertent blow to the breast by an older child: "My other daughter kicked my breast hard during the night and I woke up sore and sick with an infection," recalled one mother.

Other factors. Other conditions, such as anemia, poor nutrition, the premenstruum, and a high salt intake have been implicated in mastitis, particularly if the women have repeated infections.[16] These should be noted in the nursing assessment and history, and the mother should be instructed in self-care for preventing future infections.

NURSING INTERVENTIONS

A mother with mastitis feels ill and discouraged. She asks, "Why does this have to happen to me?" and she may contemplate immediate weaning. This is the time when she needs mothering herself, a role that the nurse can assume to reassure her that the infection will pass with time and treatment and that to stop breastfeeding will only increase the risk of a worse infection. "Tender loving care" will go a long way in helping her through this difficult time. She will also need specific advice. The following lists the cardinal elements in a short-term, self-care plan for the mother with mastitis.

1. *Rest in bed.* The mother's taking the baby to bed with her will minimize her effort in caring for and feeding the baby. Arrange for help with the household.
2. *Continue breastfeeding.* Frequent feedings, day and night, as often as the baby will take the breast, will prevent stasis in the ducts and promote healing.
3. *Apply heat to the affected area.* Moist heat is better than dry heat in relieving discomfort; wet and warm small towels wrapped in plastic wrap are easily obtainable for use.
4. *Monitor the body temperature.* This should be done orally every 4 hours to evaluate the progress of the infection.
5. *Maintain fluid intake.* Most mothers are thirsty but not hungry during the acute phase. Fresh fruit juices and water should be at their bedside.
6. *Continue taking the prescribed antibiotic.* This should be done for the full recommended course of prescription, even though the symptoms have subsided.

A long-term plan for self-care in mastitis should also be used. My survey showed that a considerable number of mothers develop mastitis more than once during the course of lactation. Therefore certain mothers may be prone to infections, and prevention is important. Review with the mother all the possible factors that preceded and may have contributed to mastitis, such as not alternating breasts, improper positioning that led to sore and cracked nipples, overdistention, and stress as discussed earlier. Encourage her to seek medical help early if and when symptoms occur again. This point is of considerable consequence, since so many mothers do not consult their physicians. Establishing a follow-up counseling system that puts her in contact with experienced breastfeeding mothers, such as those in La Leche League, reinforces and supplements nursing services.

SUMMARY

In summary, the temporary distress of mastitis need not interfere with ongoing breastfeeding, although the mother needs support, sympathy, and information on self-care. In addition, antibiotics may be needed, although mastitis is usually self-limited.

Teaching should include identification of causes, thus helping to prevent further infections. Above all, breastfeeding should continue unless an abscess necessitates temporary interruption.

REFERENCES

1. Conner, A.E.: Elevated levels of sodium and chloride in milk from mastitic breast, Pediatrics **63:**910, 1979.
2. Ezarati, J.B., and Gordon, H.: Puerperal mastitis: causes, prevention and management, Nurse-Midwifery **24:**3, 1979.
3. Fleiss, P.M.: Discussion on mastitis and acute and chronic illness. In Lawrence, R., editor: Counseling the mother on breastfeeding, Report of the Eleventh Ross Roundtable on critical approaches to common pediatric problems, Columbus, Ohio, 1980, Ross Laboratories.
4. Fulton, A.A.: Incidence of puerperal and lactational mastitis in an industrial town of some 43,000 inhabitants, Br. Med. J. **1:**693, 1945.
5. Gibberd, G.F.: Sporadic and epidemic puerperal breast infections, Am. J. Obstet. Gynecol. **65:**1038, 1953.
6. Kimball, E.R.: Breastfeeding in private practice, Northwestern University Medical School Bulletin **25:**257, 1951.
7. Klaus, M.H., and Kennell, J.H.: Maternal-infant bonding: the impact of early separation or loss on family development, St. Louis, 1976, The C.V. Mosby Co.
8. Leary, W.G.: Acute puerperal mastitis: a review, Calif. Med. **68:**147, 1948.
9. Light, I.J., et al.: Use of bacterial interference to control a staphylococcal nursery outbreak, Am. J. Dis. Child **113:**291, 1967.
10. Marshall, B.R., Hepper, J.K., and Zirbel, C.C.: Sporadic puerperal mastitis: an infection that need not interrupt lactation, J.A.M.A. **233:**1377, 1975.
11. Newton, M., and Newton, N.: Breast abscess: result of lactation failure, Surg. Gynecol. Obstet. **91:**651, 1950.
12. Pritchard, J.A., and MacDonald, D.C.: Williams' obstetrics, ed. 16, New York, 1980, Appleton-Century-Crofts.
13. Schreiner, R.L.: Possible breast milk transmission of group B-streptococcal infection (letter to the editor), J. Pediatr. **91:**159, 1977.
14. Shinefield, H.R., et al.: Bacterial interference: its effect on nursery-acquired infection with *Staphylococcus aureus,* Am. J. Dis. Child **105:**646, 1963.
15. White, G.J., and White, M.: Breastfeeding and drugs in human milk. American Academy of Clinical Toxicology, Vet. Hum. Toxicol. 23(suppl.):1, 1980.
16. White M.: Breast infections, La Leche League International, Spirit of South California and Nevada, p. 8, Spring 1975.

ADDITIONAL READINGS

Devereaux, W.P.: Acute puerperal mastitis, Am. J. Obstet. Gynecol. **108:**78, 1970.

La Leche League International, Inc.: Sore breast: what, why and what to do, Franklin Park, Ill., 1975, The League.

Miller, M.A., and Brooten, D.A.: The childbearing family: a nursing perspective, Boston, 1977, Little, Brown & Co.

Théberge-Rousselet, D.: The treatment of mastitis in nursing mothers, Can. Nurse 72:32, 1976.

The ill breastfeeding child

JAN RIORDAN

The self-care deficit that exists when the breastfeeding child or infant is ill is best met when the nurse supports and makes every effort to help the mother and family to continue breastfeeding. Recovery is much faster and less stressful in the security of the mother's arms and breasts, a foundation that absorbs the shock of pain, injury, and fear. A screaming, hysterical toddler is transformed into a soothed, pacified one within seconds after he is placed on his mother's lap and vigorously begins to breastfeed. The advantages of the antiinfective and nutritional components of his mother's milk make continued breastfeeding even more urgent, if it is at all possible.

Without question, breastfeeding infants and children are less likely to become ill and be hospitalized.[4, 8] Despite increased resistance to infections and fewer allergies, however, breastfed chidren do become ill. Also, breastfeeding obviously cannot protect against genetically transferred deficits or accidents, although it can have ameliorating effects. Since nurses are generally involved in direct care during hospitalization, I shall explore the psychosocial considerations of caring for the breastfeeding child and the family in the hospital, although the concepts are applicable to nurses in medical offices and community health centers.

DIFFERENCES OF THE BREASTFEEDING CHILD

Subtle differences emerge when caring for an ill infant who is completely breastfed as opposed to one who is bottle-feeding or breastfeeding only part of the time. The latter, for instance, will take a feeding from caretakers other than his mother, the nurse, or the father; however, an infant fed solely at his mother's breast for a few months often refuses the bottle. The breastfed infant has become conditioned to sucking patterns that differ widely between breast and bottle and has also come to expect many other sensory experiences at feeding time—the close warmth of his mother's body and breast, the direct en face gazing, playful pats, and stroking are all part of breastfeeding.

Unrestricted breastfeeding means that the mother is with her infant most of the time and is more involved in his direct care during hospitalization. Since she may be hesitant with the hospital staff, fearing that she might be considered overprotective or overindulgent, the mother needs the reassurance and confidence that she is indispensable to the child's recovery. As one nurse kidded a mother, "You're his milk supply, we've got to keep you around!" Like any mother of a sick child, she can also feel vulnerable and out of control. After all, the nurses know what they are doing, and she is "just" the mother.

Regression during illness is universal with children. In the breastfed child, regression, a positive coping mechanism, takes form in his need to breastfeed more often than before. Many times this behavior is the first sign that something is wrong before other symptoms of the illness appear. A child well on his way to weaning, perhaps only breastfeeding before bedtime, suddenly reverts to feeding several times or more during the day when he becomes ill. If he is already on solid foods, he often refuses them, exclusively breastfeeding as he did in early infancy. Because he continues to take in small amounts of easily digested breastmilk, his hydration and electrolyte balance are more likely to be maintained within normal limits, especially if he has fluid loss from vomiting or diarrhea. Weight loss is also minimized. Some infants even manage to gain weight with frequent breastfeeding during an acute illness. Because breastmilk passes from the stomach in about 2 hours, the usual 6 hours of fasting before surgery can be reduced to 4.

Once the infant is well again, he gradually picks up where he left off in his progression toward ultimate weaning and breastfeeds only as often as he did before he became ill. The child with free access to the comfort of his mother's breast recovers more rapidly both physically and emotionally from physical trauma or illness.

DEVELOPMENT

Assessing the child's developmental level and being able to apply a working knowledge of developmental patterns is as important as knowing the specifics of a child's health problem. Children vary greatly in their tempo of growth and development. Developmental age as opposed to the chronologic age of a child is a more accurate indicator, especially with an ill child who is regressing. Since a comprehensive discussion of normal physical and psychosocial development is not within the scope of this text, I refer the reader to the many available excellent nursing references that discuss in detail child development and the use of assessment tools such as the Bayley Scale of Infant Development, Denver Development Screening Test, and the Brazelton Neonatal Behavior Assessment Scale. I can say, however, that illness disrupts the progression of growth and development, which resumes itself after the crisis is over. Several theories (Table 8-1) of psychosocial development are particularly relevant to the ill breastfeeding child who is threatened with separation from his parents and care by strangers.

TABLE 8-1

Theorists, age, and stage in development

Theorist	Stage	Age
Freud	Oral gratification	Birth-18 mo
Bowlby	Separation anxiety	6 mo-2½ yr
Erickson	Trust vs. mistrust	Birth-18 mo
Erickson	Autonomy vs. shame	1½-3 yr
Piaget	Object constancy	After 8 mo
Emde	Stranger distress	8-12 mo

Separation anxiety

Aware of the sensory capabilities of an infant responding to his environment, the nurse can appreciate the losses and fears of any hospitalized child who is robbed of his familiar, comforting surroundings and is suddenly surrounded by strange people and frightening equipment. Those of us who practice in a pediatric acute care setting have observed the traumas of a child when his mother leaves even for a short time. As she goes out the door, anxious eyes follow her. Almost instantly the child's face is contorted by rage and he loudly cries, ''Mama, mama!'' He throws himself wildly about, kicking and screaming. Nothing that nurses try to do at this point brings solace. This behavior is the first phase of separation anxiety, a phenomenon emerging toward the middle of the first year, peaking from 13 to 20 months, and decreasing after the second birthday. Separation anxiety, according to psychoanalytic theory, is the painful effect of anxiety engendered by the threat of actual separation from a loved one. Bowlby[1] and later Robertson[16] delineated three phases of separation anxiety in young children (Table 8-2).

Protest. In an angry and yearning attempt to recover his mother, the child violently cries and throws himself about, kicking and screaming. He is angry at the world and at his mother for leaving him. He feels that she must be angry with him also, since she

TABLE 8-2

Coping behaviors of child 8 months and older based on stages of hospitalization

Protest	Despair	Denial	Mastery
Cries	Clings to familiar objects	Accepts staff as surrogate parent	Verbalizes fears
Screams, kicks, or bites	Withdrawn and inactive	Rejects parents	Verbalizes fantasies of environment and procedures/body or illness
Shuts eyes	Hopeless affect	Socializes with staff	
Tries to escape	Unresponsive verbally	Separates from parents with relative ease	Initiates communication with staff
Clings to mother or father	Makes no demands		Questions procedures
Tries to regain contact with mother and father	Sad facial expression	Does not cry	Talks comfortably about his illness
	Holds rigidly still	Apathy toward parents	
	Autoerotic behavior		Cooperates during procedures
Rejects staff's comforting measures	Autoaggressive	No verbalization of name and family	Explores environment
Aggressive to others	Thumb-sucking		Willing to share ''his nurse''
	Regressive behavior		
	Anorexic		Participates in own care
	Urinary frequency		Role plays with familiar toys
	Constipation or diarrhea (unrelated to illness)		Participates in play therapy
	Cries when parent is present		Interest in play with other children
			Talks about home and friends

From Bayles, P., and Olson, J.: Assessment of the child's adaptation to hospitalization and illness, Wichita, Kan., 1979, unpublished.

left him. According to the energy of the child, the care of the hospital staff, his developmental age, and the quality of his relationship with his mother, this phase lasts from a few hours to several days.

Despair. Gradually the child moves into quiet grieving and mourning as he begins to accept his fate. He shows little interest in his environment but suffers intensely; his expression is one of great sadness. Regressive behaviors such as thumb-sucking begin as the child turns inward for solace.

Detachment or denial. The child develops a defense mechanism to deal with his loss by detaching himself from the importance of his mother's love. He gradually begins to interact with the staff, going to anyone, eating well, and even appearing cheerful. This stage is often misinterpreted by nurses as adapting or ''settling in'' and charted as such. In actuality, it is coping with his loss by indiscriminate attachment to caretakers. When he is reunited with his mother, he appears uninterested and may appear not to recognize her.

Trust vs. mistrust

Fear of separation is less when the child is in charge of his environment, that is, when he crawls or walks away from his mother. This is consistent with Erickson's theory of development. According to Erickson,[6] the first year encompasses the time when confidence in having needs met and feeling physically safe results in the infant's either trusting or mistrusting his environment. Once trust, as opposed to mistrust, is established, the toddler moves into the next stage, in which autonomy must be mastered over shame and doubt. By then (1½ to 3 years), he walks, runs, and expresses himself orally, eagerly exploring his exciting new world, still needing reassurance by returning to his mother for ''emotional refueling.'' Breastfeeding for nourishment becomes breastfeeding for reassurance and comfort in this stage. The process of individuation, a realization that he is a separate individual, unfolds gradually as the child begins to assert control over his world.

Object constancy

Yet another theory interfaces with separation: object constancy, an intellectual development first described by Piaget.[14] Piaget suggests that the infant, before 8 months, lacks the ability for mental representations. For instance, when an object, such as a toy, is out of sight, it ceases to exist and the infant does not search for it. It is now quite certain that person permanency precedes object permanency in that infants *do* recognize their mothers long before 8 months and thus experience loss or anxiety of this all-important person when she is not present. Later on as the child broadens this ability to recognize a separate existence from his mother, he begins to tolerate brief periods of separation with a different caretaker. This ability roughly coincides with diminishing anxiety and with Erickson's establishment of trust progressing to the beginnings of autonomy.

Stranger distress

During the second half of the first year of life another developmental phenomenon appears: stranger distress. The infant, up to that time curious about everything in his environment including strangers, suddenly frowns, cries, and may even attempt physical escape when a stranger approaches. Only in the past 2 decades have distress reactions to strangers been extensively studied, and although limited information is available, the following data about stranger distress have been observed:[5] (1) it appears in all infants quite suddenly as early as 6 months but more commonly at 8 months and (2) it is more pronounced when the mother or primary caretaker is not present. As a consequence, illness and exposure to a variety of strangers and health-care workers is extremely disrupting to an infant of this age. Although stranger distress occurs about the same period of development as separation anxiety, it is a separate phenomenon. Since the proximity of his mother reduces the stranger distress, her presence is very beneficial. "Friendly"-appearing clothing, such as pastels and embroidery, worn by the pediatric staff may help to ameliorate the infant's distress, but by no means does it prevent his crying and avoidance behavior as the nurse approaches him—especially for the first time. How can nurses who are at first strangers to the child minimize this fear? First, we can take advantage of his attachment to his mother by relating to the mother first in the presence of the child. While we are interacting with his mother, the child is carefully observing her response to and acceptance of the "stranger" and will take cues from her. Even body position is important: turning slightly sideways away from the child to avoid en face contact while talking with the mother is less threatening to the child. Spitz demonstrates in one of his films that when the stranger approaches with his back to the child, the latter, instead of crying, becomes curious and will even reach out after a bit and tug at the stranger. Using a soft, low voice instead of a loud or high-pitched one is more pleasing to the child and facilitates his acceptance of this new person in his life.

Nursing and medicine have made great progress in recognizing and applying developmental theories to practice. The magnificent work by Bowlby[1] and Spitz[18] and later studies by Prugh[15] and Fagin[7] leave little doubt that lengthy separation from the parents, particularly the mother, is traumatic, the effects lasting months, years, or a lifetime. As a result, most hospital pediatric policies now encourage parents to stay with their children, sometimes admitting the parents with the child and allowing them to stay until the child goes home. Restricting parental visitation now is fortunately rare, yet it has been only a few years since restricted visiting was commonly practiced. A review of nursing literature during the 1950's shows many articles promoting unrestricted visiting and pediatric family-centered care in the years before the practice was widely adopted by hospitals during the 1960's. Hospital visiting restrictions before this time now seem in retrospect barbaric, particularly for the breastfeeding mothers and babies who were suddenly forced to wean. If hospitals were to regress to their previous restrictive policies, they would not only again impose the miseries of separation, but hospital staffing would have to triple to compensate, however inadequately, for the care the parents now give their children.

HOSPITALIZATION

Like any crisis, hospitalization can be a time for learning and growth despite its negative effects. Chances for a positive experience increase when the mother stays with her child, who finds security and comfort in breastfeeding. Much of the help we can give as nurses has less to do with specific techniques and more to do with being sensitive human beings.

The goal of self-care for the hospitalized infant or child is to minimize the discrep-

ancy between care provided at home and care given in the hospital setting and to maintain and strengthen family unity. Thus, for the child who is breastfed, feeding and nurturing patterns should approximate as closely as possible the situation before the onset of illness. Obviously, this is not always possible—surgery, diagnostic tests, and other therapeutic interventions are necessary obstacles—but the goal is still the same.

Nursing assessment

A complete data base and assessment help the nurse achieve the goal of minimizing the discrepancy of care and thus trauma to the child. Through the assessment phase of nursing, collection of both subjective and objective data is accomplished through interviewing and observation. Only by acquiring this information can the nurse give personalized and individualized care to families. One method to gain a data base on normal activity of daily living patterns before hospitalization is to have the mother or father complete a detailed questionnaire. This information, in addition to the interview and the information from the observation, increases the likelihood of meeting the individual needs of the family. If the child is breastfeeding, some appropriate questions that should be asked during the taking of the nursing history are: How often does he breastfeed at home? How do you usually feed him—sitting up or lying down? Does he take any solids or supplements? Is he accustomed to coming in bed with you at night for feedings? Some families choose to sleep in a "family bed," that is, in the same room with their infant or young children.[19] What is his favorite word for breastfeeding? If the breastfeeding child is old enough to talk, the family may use a favorite word for breastfeeding, such as "nummies," "yum-yum," "nursie," "snuggles," or "side." A family who called breastfeeding "night-night" enjoyed the reaction of relatives and friends when their "good" little girl asked to go "night-night" all by herself.[3] Keep these code words in mind the next time a breastfeeding toddler in your unit keeps demanding a "nursie"—he may not mean you, the hospital nurse. Acceptance of the normalcy of a breastfeeding walking and talking child is expanded on further in the chapter on weaning.

Parental stresses

Driving to and from the hospital from their home 100 miles away to alternate staying with their sick infant, a breastfeeding mother and the father try to cope from day to day. With three other children at home they can snatch only a few hours of sleep at a time. It is the third surgery for their infant, who was born with a congenital defect. Although their physician encourages them that the prognosis is good, the worry and strain seem endless. The mother expresses her milk with a pump when necessary, and her baby is able to breastfeed part of the time. Lately she can express only a few drops at a time, and she can barely feel a let-down. She wonders how long she will be able to continue.

All parents of ill children are in a stressful state, but consider the effects of chronic stress on parents who must deal with it over many months and perhaps years, such as the family described here. Selye[17] showed that in response to stress, the individual uses a complex system of defensive somatic reactions, which involve the pituitary and adrenal glands and result in heightened secretions of adrenocorticotropic hormone (ACTH) and glucocorticoids that ultimately affect every system of the body. I can say unequivocally that the mother under stress is affected physiologically as well as psychologically. The question then becomes, what effect does stress have on breastfeeding and what measures can the nurse take to help these parents through this stressful time?

When it becomes apparent that the child is ill and might have to be hospitalized, one of the first concerns of the mother is, "Can I keep on breastfeeding?" She has already recognized the unique healing effect of putting a child to breast when he is hurt or ill.

The mother's hormonal responses and let-down are vulnerable to brief stress, as shown by Newton,[12] who noted a significant reduction in the milk supply when a mother is subjected to brief episodes of pain or emotional disturbance; however, there appears to be an adaptive mechanism in lactation over longer periods of stress. Evidence for this mechanism is the numerous experiences of women who have successfully breastfed under prolonged adversity such as war and personal calamity. Given no choices, women during the London blitz continued to breastfeed their thriving infants while the bombs exploded overhead. Divorce, loss of a loved one, moving, or worry over her sick infant can all temporarily affect the mother's ability to lactate for a short while, but with continued sucking or pumping the milk reappears, providing that the mother is motivated to continue and is helped in the process.

Continuing to breastfeed, unless the child refuses or is too ill, brings a sense of normalcy in an otherwise highly stressful time. The mother needs reassurance that breastfeeding can continue or assistance if breastfeeding must be temporarily interrupted. Many medical centers have electric pumps available, or arrangements can be made for the mother to rent one. Hand pumps and hand expression are other alternatives. More information on lactation aids and direction on collection and storage of breastmilk are found in Chapters 9 and 12.

When the child must undergo surgery or other therapeutic intervention, particularly if it will be painful, encourage the mother to breastfeed as soon as possible afterward. It is hard to say who benefits most, the mother or the baby, when the sobbing child settles into his mother's lap for the comfort of her breast. What is readily apparent is the relief from stress for them both. A careful explanation of the procedure beforehand will also relieve the anxiety of the mother, and this relief is in turn transmitted to the child. Parents can handle nearly any treatment if they know what it will be. Of all our nursing interventions, anticipatory guidance is and shall always be one of the most effective.

But what about the father? During the stress of the child's illness, attention is focused on the mother and the ill child. Because his wife is breastfeeding, she will be the one spending the most time at the bedside. While his child is in the hospital, the father is expected to be the rock of Gibraltar, an anchor in a sea of distress. In addition to carrying on job responsibilities, he has the responsibility to keep things running at home, nurture and care for any other children, and spend as much time as possible at the hospital. Fathers are people, too, and their stresses are enormous.

These stresses lap over onto the marriage bond. When her sick child becomes the focus of her attention, other relationships and responsibilities are secondary for the mother. Some husbands, sensing this, withdraw emotionally until the crisis is over. Yet, for other couples, their mutual concern causes them to grow closer and draw emotional support from one another. Some parents feel guilty about having sex while their child lies ill. If it seems appropriate, point out that sexual enjoyment reinforces their bond together—a bond that strengthens them during this difficult period.

Unreasonable as such feelings may be, both parents may harbor feelings of guilt for bringing on the illness or for not recognizing how sick the child was in the early stages. Questions like "What have I done?" or "What should I have done?" torment them. It is easier for the breastfeeding mother who continues in close contact and participates in her child's recovery to deal with these feelings than it is for the father. Picking up cues about his feelings and encouraging him to talk about it helps and also provides the opportunity to reassure him that these feelings are normal. The therapeutic value of "talking it out" is significant enough to produce physiologic changes associated with stress reduction.[9] Hearing their own statements aloud releases the parents' tension and speeds resolution of their inner conflicts.

Hospitalization brings about a disruption of life-style and environment to the family tantamount to culture shock. A barrage of unfamiliar stimuli is thrust on them: infusion pumps that periodically sound an alarm, mist tents, and a constantly rotating staff of new faces all place tremendous stresses on the family.

Usually affable parents can be demanding and even hostile when anger becomes a by-product of stress and guilt. Although it can be difficult and even painful for nurses to deal with such parents, I would far rather work with concerned parents who assert themselves than with parents who are unconcerned or passive. Sympathetic listening and simple, understanding statements such as, "I can see you are upset," or "this is such a difficult time," can help the parents through this trying time. Nurses should be understanding, not defensive.

Some parents, many miles from home during their child's hospitalization, must arrange for sleeping accommodations in the area if both are not allowed to stay overnight at the hospital. One father of a child in my unit rode the bus for 6 hours one-way and back each weekend to visit his wife and baby in the hospital. If the stresses are severe and lengthy, the marital relationship may suffer. I have found the services of the hospital social workers to be tremendously valuable in helping parents deal with stress when their child is hospitalized.

Parents of hospitalized babies form their own self-care groups, another support system for parents that is seldom mentioned. Even mothers of two breastfeeding babies sharing the same hospital room can form a self-care group.

> I was nervous and upset when Meghan and I arrived at the hopsital but the staff made me feel right at home. I soon found out there were many other mothers staying with their children and we would get together in the parents' lounge after our children were sleeping to share our thoughts and try to unwind.[11]

Other mothers, especially if they are experienced and confident, prefer to be by themselves and appreciate the solitude.

Coping with siblings

Siblings are often the forgotten members of the family when attention and concern is on the sick child. In nursing, the concept of family-centered care extends to every person in the family, including the children at home, who frequently react to their brother's or sister's illness with anger, resentment, jealousy, and guilt.

The situation is especially difficult when an older child is hospitalized and a younger breastfeeding baby or toddler is at home. The mother is emotionally torn between being with her sick child and with her breastfeeding baby who also needs her. If the baby is one of breastfeeding twins or if the mother is breastfeeding both a walking child and a baby, the problem is further compounded. Older children at least have verbal communication as a means for coping; infants do not. Few hospitals allow siblings to visit in the unit because of the fear of transmitting infections; therefore, in this situation, suggest that the father or a close relative, such as a grandmother or aunt, stay at the bedside so that the mother can spend time at home without feeling that she is neglecting her sick child. Also encourage sibling visits with the mother in the lobby or other public area of the hospital and the dismissal of the child at the earliest possible moment.

Staying overnight

Rollaway beds, cots, or day beds, which can be used as a couch or chair during the day and made into a bed at night, are much preferred for parents staying overnight. Nothing heals stress as much as deep sleep that allows for rapid eye movement (REM) cycling and subconscious release of daytime fears and stress. Many breastfeeding families normally have a sleeping arrangement known as the family bed. Hardly a new concept, family beds in which parents and their children snuggled in with each other (Fig. 8-1) have been the norm rather than the exception in the history of mankind. For a baby or child customarily tucked in with his parent, being isolated in a crib by himself

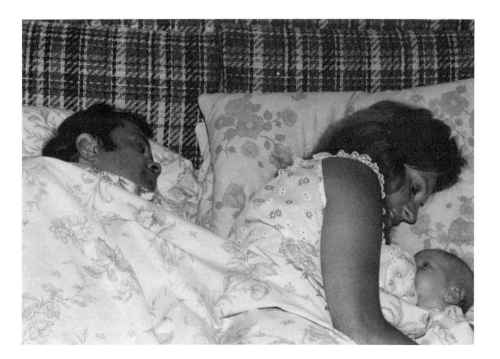

Fig. 8-1. "Family bed."

is a strange and frightening experience. Unless IV's or other therapeutic techniques interfere, there is no reason why a child accustomed to the closeness of his mother or father at night cannot be taken into the bed where his parent is sleeping. When parent and child are allowed to do so, night nurses rejoice—it makes their job much easier.

Beds for parents facilitate comfortable breastfeeding and simulate the home experience. When no bed is provided by the hospital, parents can be very inventive. One breastfeeding mother simply crawled in with her baby at night and pulled up the sides of the crib. To the astonished nurse making rounds in the morning she succinctly expressed her philosophy of health-care services: "I'm paying for this bed and I can darn well do what I want with it!"

At hospitals where parents sleep in lounge chairs with tilting backs, comfortable night feedings are difficult, if not impossible, no matter how small the child is. One mother complained: "If I tilted the chair back so I was comfortable enough to sleep, I couldn't turn to the side to breastfeed her, I had to sit up. Then when I sat up I couldn't sleep." When there are no comfortable sleeping arrangements available, suggest that the parents bring an air mattress or a lightweight folding cot or lawn chair that can be easily stored during the day. Breastfeeding mothers who are rooming-in with their sick child should also be provided with nutritious snacks and a water pitcher for their added nutritional and fluid needs, a justifiable "extra" since no formula cost is involved.

Emergency department admission

Staff nursing in emergency situations takes split-second reactions and demands a thorough background of a wide range of nursing knowledge. No one nurse, of course, can be expected to know everything. In addition, patients come and go quickly, transferred to other units of the hospital or dismissed without being seen again.

Unless the nurse has had personal experience with a breastfed infant or child, she is unlikely to understand all the needs of the family who come into the emergency unit with a child who is being breastfed. An example is a situation in which the mother, not the child, became very ill and overheard the harried nurse say: "If she had given that baby a bottle, we wouldn't be in this mess" when the infant first refused and later vomited bottle-feedings. Given that emergencies distort perceptions and magnify emotions, criticism by parents is not always a fair analysis of the situation, but there is a lesson for us here. How do we avoid insensitivity in nursing care when we are faced with a situation beyond our experience or understanding? Is it necessary to say that we need to look at the family's needs through the eyes of each family member? Perhaps it is. The best way is to actively support the mother and her family when an emergency threatens the symbiosis of a breastfeeding relationship. For some infants it has been the sole source of their nourishment.

In the case cited in the preceding paragraph, the comment of her co-worker so jarred another nurse in the unit that she developed an in-service program designed to acquaint the staff with the breastfeeding infant's special needs.

Home, the rebound effect

The child's response following hospitalization depends on the extent of trauma and separation he has undergone and his defenses to protect himself. Fagin[7] clearly indicates in her study of hospitalized children that when a mother rooms-in with her child, very little if any behavior changes occur on returning home.

Once home, the young child who has experienced a painful separation is likely to show changes from his normal behavior. He may at first even refuse the breast and show little interest in his mother or family, using withdrawal as a means of coping, or he may cry a great deal, wanting to be held and breastfed exceptionally often, vigorously protesting having his mother out of sight for even a moment. Nightmares and insomnia are common, and the child may even protest at having his picture taken if the camera reminds him of an x-ray machine.[2] Because the members of the family must also adjust, emotional upheaval is frequent during the first few weeks following hospitalization.

Short separations during hospitalization are usually inevitable; however, if a child feels safe and secure in his parent's love, trauma from the illness and temporary separations give way to restoration of trust after being reunited with his family. Helping the parents to recognize this is vital to nursing care of the hospitalized child. Inherent in any crisis is its potential for bringing families closer together with new awareness and appreciation of one another.

CHRONIC GRIEF AND LOSS

When the breastfeeding child is chronically ill or has a disabling defect, the disappointment, sorrow, and frustration of parents can be overwhelming. Instead of the perfect child expected during the pregnancy, there is an intense feeling of loss. If the child will require indefinite special care and attention, there is a persistent effect described by Olshonsky[13] as chronic sorrow. Unlike acute grief, which is limited in time, chronic grief is prolonged and recurrent. Through grieving, coping processes evolve, and parents can find satisfaction and even joy from their child: "The shock and numbness linger for days, even months. . . It is only after you have gotten over that first crisis that you begin to realize a life and soul have been given into your care."[10]

Breastfeeding has an ameliorating effect for both the child and the parents in chronic illness. The baby receives added protection from his higher risks of infection and also close contact and stimulation. Engendered in the parents, especially the mother, is the satisfaction of giving something special to her child that helps her deal with her feelings of loss. As a mother of a baby with Down's syndrome said: "As I looked back at Chad's first year, I'm sure that breastfeeding and that closeness that comes with it helped me to love and accept him just as he was. There were still lots of tears sometimes falling on my special baby as we rocked along, so alone, yet so close. I had many anxieties about the future."[10]

Magic milk syndrome

In the process of grieving, parents move through stages of adjustment. After the initial shock and emotional numbness, they reach a stage characterized by rationalization, denial, and sometimes a search for a magic cure.

If the baby is not being breastfed, a few frightened parents will desperately search for donated breastmilk in hopes that it will help cure their children. The unique properties of breastmilk are becoming so well known that it is sometimes perceived by parents to contain magic curing properties. There are, of course, cases in which breast-milk can help—allergies and metabolic disorders often respond well to breastmilk. In some circumstances it is lifesaving. In these situations in which the need is real and substantiated by a medical opinion, local lactating women, usually through La Leche League, generously give their milk. They usually ask, however, that the mother attempt to relactate so she can gradually begin giving her own milk to her baby. Breastmilk also can be obtained from milk banks throughout the country (Appendix C), although the cost over a long time is considerable.

The nurse's intervention at such times will depend on a realistic assessment of the child's problem. If giving breastmilk does seem like a reasonable intervention, she should put the parents in touch with the appropriate community resources and begin helping the mother with the relactation process. In cases in which breastmilk is not likely to help, gentleness and an understanding, caring attitude can guide the parents to the reality of the situation and to the awareness that breastmilk per se will not cure their child.

Empty cradle

The tremendous task of coping and somehow continuing with life must be faced by parents when their child dies. The first reactions of shock, disbelief, and denial are all the more intense when the death is unexpected, as with sudden infant death syndrome. Parents need to be able to express their feelings by crying, yelling and screaming, or just talking about how they feel.

Compassionate care assists closure after death. Giving the parents the opportunity to hold their child and to say good-bye helps this process. Afraid at first, one family changed their minds and cradled their dead baby in their arms. "Holding him is what helped us most to accept the death of our baby; it made us feel he was really our own. He smelled sweet and felt soft and we just stroked him and talked with him for awhile."

The focus of concern is often on the mother, and the father, who has had a signifi-cant, loving relationship with his child, is forgotten. The cultural stereotype of male stoicism belies his true feelings of shock, grief, and pain. Fathers need to grieve but sometimes require different kinds of outlets to express it.

As the shock subsides, acute mourning and bereavement are followed by a devel-oping awareness of the full impact of their loss. Guilt, silent or expressed, is an almost universal emotion during this period, and the parents examine their past misdeeds. Questioning the nurse about the possible effect of heredity on the disease is likely as their grief turns inward in the form of self-blame. Explanations of hereditary factors must be honest and factual, tempered with an understanding of what the parents are ready to accept.

Physical symptoms such as sleeplessness or a lack of appetite accompany the par-ents' feelings of loss and pain. Some parents describe feeling "dead inside" or having "a hole inside that nothing can fill." The breastfeeding mother must cope with the physical discomfort of breast engorgement for awhile and should be advised to pump her breasts once or twice for relief. Occasionally a mother continues to pump her milk for several weeks, donating it to a milk bank so that other children may benefit from it. Doing so is her way of coping by maintaining visible evidence of the existence of the lost child.

The worst part for the mother is the time when her husband returns to work and the family begins to function as before the child died. Something inside her cries, "Wait, I'm not ready!" In the process of detachment, memories that tie the mother to the child must be painfully revived before being painfully, slowly forgotten. Especially important to her is the acknowledgment that her child was special; she should never be denied the right to her sorrow. Statements like, "You can always have another baby" are no consolation to her loss of *this* baby. Verbalizing feelings of anger, fear, guilt, and anxiety helps her deal with these emotions and validate them.

Resolution can come only after the parents work through their grief. As preoccupation with memories lessens, they are able to establish new interests and develop new goals. "Time heals all wounds" is true in the sense that healing occurs with time, but the emotional scars and the times of feeling empty and lonely will endure as long as they live. Prolonged or abnormal grief is more often seen in the mother rather than in the father. This is more likely to happen if she has lost another significant person in her life and never resolved the loss or if she has emotional problems. If her child was chronically ill, a mother can miss this special mothering role that made her feel useful, important, and needed.

For many mothers, the peer support systems that previously helped them in parenting and breastfeeding change in their significance: now seeing breastfeeding mothers and their babies is a painful ordeal and the mother assiduously avoids them as a group, choosing one or two especially close peers with whom she can privately talk about her feelings and emotional pain. One of the community support systems available for parents during this difficult period is AMEND (Aiding Mothers Experiencing Neonatal Death). This group has trained counselors to individually help parents work through their grief.

SUMMARY

From my discussion of the ill breastfeeding child in this chapter, I can say that overall humane nursing approaches are more alike than different whether the infant is breastfed or bottle-fed. Yet there are unique considerations for helping the mother and child in maintaining the symbiosis inherent in breastfeeding. These special needs can be met by recognizing developmental stages, assessing family life-style, reducing parental stress, involving the mother in direct care of her child, and most of all minimizing separation. If the child dies, comprehending the impact of the parents' grief and the stages of adaptive coping requires special sensitivity and crisis intervention skills on the part of the nurse in helping the bereaved parents in their journey through pain toward an adaptive resolution of their loss.

REFERENCES

1. Bowlby, J.: Attachment and loss, vol. 2, Separation, New York, 1973, Basic Books, Inc., Publishers.
2. Brewster, D.P.: You can breastfeed your baby . . . even in special situations, Emmaus, Pa., 1979, Rodale Press, Inc.
3. Bumgarner, N.J.: Mothering your nursing toddler, Norman, Okla., 1980, privately printed.
4. Cunningham, A.S.: Morbidity in breast-fed and artifically-fed infants, J. Pediatr. **90**:726, 1977.
5. Emde, R., Gaensbauer, T., and Harmon, R.: Emotional expression in infancy, New York, 1976, International Universities Press, Inc.
6. Erickson, E.: Childhood and society, ed. 2, New York, 1963, W.W. Norton & Co., Inc.
7. Fagin, C.: The effects of maternal attendance during hospitalization on the post hospital behavior of young children, Philadelphia, 1966, F.A. Davis Co.

8. Fallot, M.E., et al.: Breastfeeding reduces incidence of hospital admissions for infections in infants, Pediatrics **65:**1121, 1980.
9. Foster, S.B.: An adrenal measure for evaluating nursing effectiveness, Nurs. Res. **23:**118, 1974.
10. Good, J.: Breastfeeding the Down's syndrome baby, La Leche League International, Franklin Park, Ill., 1980, The League.
11. La Leche League, International, La Leche League News, **20:**6, 1978.
12. Newton, N.: Maternal emotions, New York, 1955, Paul B. Hoeber, Inc.
13. Olshonsky, S.: Chronic sorrow: a response to having a mentally defective child, Social Casework **43:**190, 1962.
14. Piaget, J.: The construction of reality in the child, New York, 1954, Ballantine Books, Inc.
15. Prugh, D., et al.: A study of emotional reactions of children and families to hospitalization and illness, Am. J. Orthopsychiatry **23:**70, 1971.
16. Robertson, J.: Young children in hospitals, New York, 1958, Basic Books, Inc., Publishers.
17. Selye, H.: The stress of life, New York, 1956, McGraw-Hill Book Co.
18. Spitz, R.: Hospitalism: the psychoanalytic study of the child, New York, 1945, International Universities Press, Inc.
19. Thevenin, T.: The family bed: an age old concept in childrearing, Minneapolis, 1976, privately printed.

ADDITIONAL READINGS

Ainsworth, M.D., et al.: Patterns of attachment, Hillsdale, N.J., 1978, Lawrence Erlbaum Associates, Inc.

Brown, M.S., and Murphy, M.A.: Ambulatory pediatrics for nurses, New York, 1975, McGraw-Hill Book Co.
Countryman, B.: In hospital: the child and the family, Franklin Park, Ill., 1974, La Leche League International.
Fraiberg, S.: The magic years, New York, 1959, Charles Scribner's Sons.
Gibes, R.M.: Clinical uses of the Brazelton Neonatal Assessment Scale in nursing practice, Pediat. Nurs. **7:**23, 1981.
Gracely, K.A.: Parental attachment to a child with a congenital defect, M.C.N. **2:**38, 1977.
Kagan, J., Kearsley, R.B., Zelazo, P.R.: Infancy: its place in human development, Cambridge, Mass., 1978, Harvard University Press.
Klaus, M.H., and Kennell, J.H.: Maternal-infant bonding: The impact of early separation or loss on family development, St. Louis, 1976, The C.V. Mosby Co.
Kunzmon, M.S.: Some factors influencing a young child's mastery of hospitalization, Nurs. Clin. North Am. **7:**13, 1972.
Scipien, G.M., et al.: Comprehensive pediatric nursing, ed. 2, New York, 1979, McGraw-Hill Book Co.
Wong, D.: Bereavement: the empty mother syndrome, M.C.N., **5:**385, 1980.
Young, R.K.: Chronic sorrow: parent's response to the birth of a child with a defect, M.C.N. **2:**38, 1977.

Pediatric health problems and breastfeeding

JAN RIORDAN
EDWARD R. CERUTTI

Why devote an entire chapter to health problems of infants and children relating to breastfeeding when details of these problems can be easily found in other nursing textbooks? It is done here simply because the care of a breastfeeding infant differs from that of a bottle-fed one, and these differences in the ill breastfeeding child and his family mark them apart for special nursing consideration. Also, the crucial role of nursing in direct primary care of a child with a health problem often makes the difference between unnecessary weaning and continued breastfeeding. Despite its advantages, it is often assumed that breastfeeding must be terminated when a serious illness strikes. Even when breastfeeding continues, a disruption of the established patterns is inevitable. Nurses must know when and how to intervene effectively when a child's health is at stake.

The purpose of this chapter is thus to provide specific information on health problems that affect breastfeeding, although there are obviously far more pediatric health problems than those presented here. Lactation aids and technology will be an integral part of nursing interventions, but rather than repeat the information on pumps in Chapter 12 and the Lact-Aid Nursing Trainer in Chapter 13, we discuss here only a few that are also helpful during the crises of illnesses.

INFECTIONS

From the moment of birth, the infant is exposed to a variety of pathogens in his environment. Breastfeeding enhances the infant's immune system and helps to protect him against infection, but this protection is not complete, and nurses are sometimes called on to care for a breastfed child with an acute infection.

Fallot and coworkers[6] demonstrated significantly fewer hospital admissions for infants who were breastfed. Of those who were admitted with infections, none of the exclusively breastfed infants had a bacterial infection. As shown in Table 9-1, the most common types of infections in the breastfed infants were viral syndrome, upper respiratory infections, and nonbacterial or aseptic meningitis.

Flulike symptoms

Most gastrointestinal disturbances labeled intestinal "flu" are usually caused by a rotavirus or reovirus. Mothers of breastfed infants frequently report that although the

TABLE 9-1

Episodes of illness according to feeding mode at illness onset

Illness	Exclusively breastfed	Partially breastfed	Exclusively bottle-fed
Viral syndrome	4		15
Upper respiratory infection (URI)	4		13
Bronchiolitis			17
Transient expiratory stridor			1
Apnea*	1		2
Pertussis/probable pertussis†			7/2
Pneumonia			
Viral, interstitial‡	1		18
Aspiration			1
Otitis media		2	11
Gastroenteritis	1		8
Meningitis			
Aseptic	4	1	7
Bacterial‡		1	6
Sepsis			2
Bullous impetigo			1
Urinary tract infection			1
Abscess			
Cervical			1
Breast			1
Pneumonitis with conjunctivitis			1
Conjunctivitis			1
Thrombocytopenia§			1
TOTALS	15	4	117

From Fallot, M.E., Boyd, J.L., and Oski, F.A.: Pediatrics **65:**1121, 1980, copyright American Academy of Pediatrics, 1980.

*One case felt to be aborted sudden infant death syndrome (SIDS); two cases secondary to URIs.

†Two cases were partially treated with erythromycin prior to obtaining cultures, and cultures were reported as negative.

‡Includes one mortality.

§Etiology presumed infectious after other possible diagnoses were ruled out.

entire family develops flulike symptoms, the breastfeeding infant remains healthy. The interferon in breastmilk may play a role in protecting the infant against viral infections.

If a breastfeeding infant does develop flu symptoms, he may have a low fever, irritability, vomiting, and diarrhea for a few days. If he is willing to take anything by mouth, it should be breastmilk. Although many health professionals advise that even breastfed infants avoid milk products in the case of vomiting and diarrhea, this is a grievous error. Nurses can and should intercede when the mother has been given this advice. Because breastmilk is digested so rapidly, even the infant who is vomiting regularly will absorb some of the nutrients and fluid of the milk before it is regurgitated. Commonly suggested fluids, such as sodas or jello water, offer little in the way of nourishment and none of the immunities of breastmilk. After being told to interrupt breastfeeding because her infant was vomiting and had a mild fever, a mother who is also a nurse found:

He needed to breastfeed and refusing him for 24 hours would have been devastating. I walked him around to quiet him, waiting as long as I could between feedings. The breastmilk stayed down about 20 minutes before he vomited it up, but at least I felt like he was getting something.

All infants "spit up" occasionally and, of course, this does not necessarily mean the infant is ill. An infant with persistent vomiting, on the other hand, should be examined for other problems, such as pyloric stenosis, if an infection is ruled out.

The infant may have diarrhea with the flu; however, since the breastfed infant's stools are normally loose, there is a possibility of the "diarrhea" being a normal stool pattern. Any gastrointestinal losses, particularly diarrhea, involve losses of sodium and potassium along with water with the risk of dehydration and acidosis if the loses are extensive. Only in moderate to severe diarrhea is supplementing breastmilk with an electrolyte oral solution such as Pedialyte necessary, but this is rarely a problem in the breastfeeding child.

The parents, by observing their infant's general responsiveness, skin turgor, and urine output, can assess the sickness and hydration level of the infant. Normally six to eight diapers wet with urine in 24 hours is an indication of adequate hydration; however, frequent stools confuse estimates of urine output. If the mother reports symptoms of dehydration because of diarrhea and vomiting, fluids can be given with a spoon or dropper if the infant is too young to drink from a cup. She should also place the infant on his abdomen with his face to one side to prevent aspiration if he is regurgitating.

Respiratory infections

Infection of the respiratory tract, the most common cause of illness in infancy and childhood, is usually caused by a virus. Care is at home by the mother and family unless the child's symptoms worsen. In helping the breastfeeding mother of a child with a respiratory infection several points should be emphasized.

First, instead of the usual response of wanting to breastfeed more, an infant may be less interested in feedings and may even refuse the mother. Since infants are obligate nose breathers, blocked airway passages pose the risk of compromising their oxygen intake even more during feeding. To make it easier for the infant to breathe, the mother should feed him sitting up, holding him in an upright position as much as possible. For older infants and children, decongestant nose drops can be administered 15 to 20 minutes before the time he is expected to breastfeed. A less satisfactory way to clear nasal secretions is to gently suction them out by using a nasal infant aspirator or rubber ear syringe.

Second, the infant simply may not be hungry. Anorexia is often caused by respiratory infections in a toddler or small child, especially if he is coughing. If hydration is not a problem, he should be allowed to determine his own need for food. Once the acute symptoms are over in a day or so, his appetite returns. Until then the mother should pump or hand express.

If the infant or child has laryngeal involvement with hoarseness or a croupy cough, a vaporizer in the room or area where he sleeps both soothes and moistens mucous membranes. A cool-mist vaporizer is preferable and prevents a walking child from accidentally burning himself. If no vaporizer is available, an effective method for creating concentrated steam and temporarily relieving croup is for the parent, while safely hold-

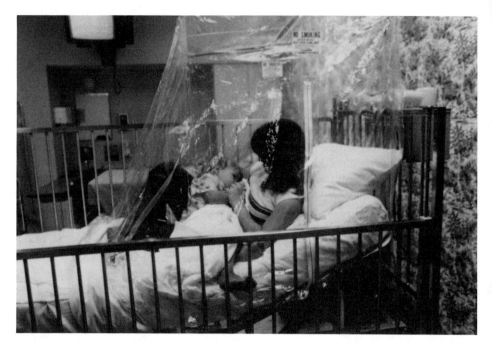

Fig. 9-1. Breastfeeding in a Croupette. (Courtesy La Leche League International.)

ing the child, to turn on hot water in the empty shower full force with the bathroom door closed. Warm wrappings will be needed afterwards to prevent the child from becoming hypothermic.

Pneumonia, if it develops in a breastfed child, is almost always viral, not bacterial, with the respiratory syncytial virus (RSV) responsible for most viral pneumonias. Antibiotic therapy is still used as a prophylaxis for viral infections despite the fact that the unnecessary use of antibiotics is now widely disclaimed. Hospitalization might be necessary, and the child should be placed in a Croupette to aid breathing.

Croupettes or mist tents impose a necessary, albeit therapeutic, isolation of the child from the parents, but there is no reason for it to interfere with breastfeeding if the child is well enough to be interested. Taking him out of the tent for brief periods of holding and feeding has more benefits than risks. Another alternative is for the mother herself to climb into the tent and have the side of the tent zipped to prevent loss of cool mist and oxygen. Many mothers have done it as shown in Fig. 9-1. Other than being nontraditional, it has no disadvantages (most mothers of sick babies could care less about their hairdos), and the mother's presence quiets a crying, unhappy infant who has little energy to spare.

Meningitis

When meningitis occurs in the breastfed infant, it is usually, but not always, aseptic or viral in origin. It can also be associated with other viral diseases such as enteroviruses, measles, mumps, or herpes. The range of clinical symptoms and their severity varies widely in meningitis, and they may be sudden or gradual in onset. Signs of meningeal irritation, nausea and vomiting, and abdominal pain often develop. There may be a maculopapular rash, which, with other acute symptoms, subsides and disappears within a few days.

According to one mother whose child developed meningitis on a family vacation, "We had no idea of just how sick he was, but I had a strong feeling that if we did not get him to a doctor he would die. He didn't have much fever, but he had stopped nursing and he no longer seemed to recognize his older brother and sisters. Every time I moved him he would cry."[14]

Since the child is usually hospitalized and has a spinal tap done for fluid culture, the presence of the mother and continued breastfeeding minimize the trauma of these procedures. Intravenous (IV) antibiotics are usually administered until bacterial meningitis can be ruled out. The mother will need help in careful handling of the IV site in moving her child to her breast. Infants are usually uninterested in breastfeeding for a day or two during the acute phase but then quickly resume it and breastfeed as eagerly as before.

Herpes simplex virus

Generally associated with maternal genital infection, herpes simplex virus, type 2, is the etiologic agent in most herpes infections in the newborn. The infant can be infected during delivery or when the virus ascends through the birth canal. Because of the increasing incidence of herpes simplex virus (HSV) infections, the nurse should be aware of the gravity of this problem and its implications for the breastfeeding couple.

The newborn infant with HSV is in serious jeopardy since his visceral organs, cardiorespiratory system, and central nervous system can be affected. When the disease is not evident at birth, the first signs may be nonspecific: irritability, convulsions, and lethargy are followed by vesicles on the skin or the oral mucous membranes, and the infant may not breastfeed well. Currently the outcome is poor; more than half these infants do not recover, and at least half the survivors have significant neurologic or ocular sequelae. However, vidarabine, only recently approved by the FDA, is a promising drug for treating HSV in neonates.

The most important means of controlling HSV infection in the infant is its prevention. A cesarean birth should be considered when the mother has a positive culture or a primary vaginal herpes lesion close to the time of delivery. Infection in the mother, however, does not warrant separation from the newborn, and rooming-in is an effective nursing intervention to isolate the infant; the mother can still breastfeed, but careful attention to hygiene is essential.[16] Before breastfeeding, the mother should thoroughly wash her hands and be covered with a clean sheet to prevent contamination. If the infant stays in the room, an Isolette rather than an open crib is also protective.

CONGENITAL PHYSICAL DEFECTS

When the child has myelomeningocele, a cleft palate, or any other abnormality that requires special care over a long period of time, the parents must adjust psychologically after the birth to the discrepancy between the ideal child wished for during pregnancy and the real child they have. For the mother who intended to breastfeed, the loss of a perfect infant is compounded by the possible loss of being able to feed her infant at her

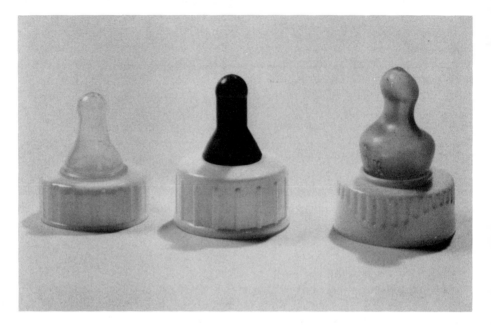

Fig. 9-2. Comparison of *(left to right)* standard rubber nipple, premature nipple, and NUK orthodontic nipple. (Courtesy Charles Cooley.)

breast, and sensitivity to these feelings is essential for nurses. The potential for breastfeeding depends on several variables: the extent of the problem, the mother's level of motivation to breastfeed, and the help she receives.

Sometimes the infant is so ill that the parents are told he may not survive. Should nurses in this case encourage the mother to go through the trouble of establishing and keeping a milk supply when she may not have the infant for very long? Experience leads us to believe that she should and that doing so makes her feel she has done everything possible for her infant. Moreover, grieving, if the infant does die, occurs more normally when the mother has attached herself emotionally to the infant when he is alive. The giving of herself through her milk enhances attachment and bonding as much as looking at him and touching him.

With the medical technology now available, most infants with congenital abnormalities survive and go on to live relatively normal lives. During the first months after birth, if hospitalization, surgery, or the infant's weakness interfere with normal breastfeeding, the mother must depend on other means to stimulate her milk supply and remove her milk. To do this, she needs specific information on what pumps or lactation aids are available and how she can obtain the one most suitable for her. Any time temporary bottle feedings are necessary, the NUK orthodontic nipple is preferable to a regular nipple. Designed to closely resemble a human nipple, it requires tongue movement and mandibular action similar to breastfeeding, thus facilitating the transition to the breast. Fig. 9-2 compares the NUK nipple with other commonly used rubber nipples.

In working with this mother, whose self-esteem has already been undermined, the nurse must make every effort to avoid stimulating any further feelings of failure. Therefore all words and actions should be carefully chosen. One such mother was devastated after being told, ''We've never seen anything like this before'' when she was unable to express any milk from the hospital electric pump. Already having a child that was different, she could not tolerate being different again, although for other mothers the remark would probably have gone unnoticed. For this mother, maintaining her milk supply until she could breastfeed directly was a way of retaining normalcy in her relationship with her infant. Ironically, the pump was later found to be faulty.

Neurologic and neuromuscular defects

Because the suck-swallow reflexes are neurologically mature at birth, full-term healthy infants usually have little difficulty in establishing a pattern of satisfactory sucking. The neurologically damaged child, however, is different.

Any neurologic deficit that affects neuromuscular function carries the risk that the child will have a decreased sucking ability. Feeding at the breast requires vigorous muscle action for drawing the milk out from the lactiferous sinuses. Sucking and swallowing, as well as breathing, are integrated under medullary (brainstem) control. When this control is impaired, the normally tense muscles involved in these functions become dystonic and flaccid. As a result, feeding, either by breast or by bottle, can be difficult and frustrating. Despite the problems, a number of determined women with the help of their physicians and nurses and others have breastfed, developing techniques through trial and error that overcame these initial problems. When the mother's attempt to breastfeed in this circumstance does not succeed, she should in no way be made to feel that she is a failure.

Down's syndrome. Children with Down's syndrome (trisomy 21), along with varying degrees of mental retardation, also have muscular hypotonia, which affects muscular development and thus their ability to suckle. A large protruding tongue, usually not evidenced at birth, is another deterrent to breastfeeding, yet a large number of babies with Down's syndrome are successfully and completely breastfed. Some of these parents have told others about their experience to help them overcome initial feeding difficulties.[9] One mother learned that by inserting her finger between the roof of her baby's mouth and tongue in an upside-down position and then turning it right side up, to correct the upward tongue thrust, the infant was prevented from placing his tongue above instead of below the nipple. She repeated this procedure several times before each feeding to condition her infant's sucking reflex for breastfeeding.

Another method to stimulate sucking is to place a few drops of milk in the infant's mouth at the start of the breastfeeding. The infant automatically swallows and follows with a reflexive suck. Any number of devices can be used to accomplish this: the Lact-Aid Nursing Trainer has the advantage of automatically controlling the infusion of milk once the sucking has started; however, first the mother must squeeze the Lact-Aid Nursing Trainer bag to express a few drops into his mouth to get him started. Another, less expensive, way is to draw up the milk into a tuberculin syringe and slowly infuse a few milliliters, carefully observing for swallowing before adding more. Better yet, attach a small (No. 8 French) feeding tube to a syringe and place the tip of the tube into the corner of the infant's mouth (Fig. 9-3). Although the photograph shows the mother alone, it is safer and more convenient to have another person available to help.

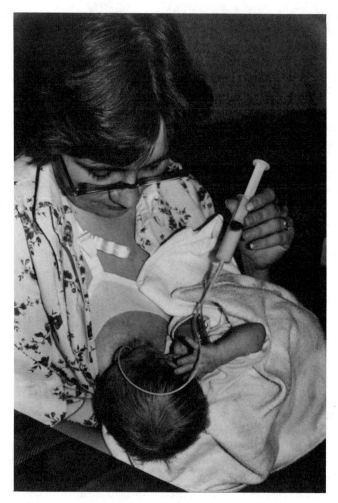

Fig. 9-3. Using syringe connected to small-gauge feeding tube to stimulate sucking.

Other suggestions to give to the mother of an infant with Down's syndrome or those with sucking problems are:

1. Hand express a few drops of milk into his mouth to arouse his interest or brush the nipple across his cheek to stimulate his rooting reflex. Placing a thumb under the baby's bottom lip or the chin encourages bilabial closure and suction.

2. Awaken him to feed frequently. Since the baby with Down's syndrome is sleepy and placid, his normal cues for feeding, such as crying and restlessness, cannot be relied on, and the mother must watch the clock for feedings if weight gain is to be maintained. Use the jackknife or Valsalva procedure to awaken him if it seems necessary. To do this, hold him in a supine position, supporting the shoulders and head with one hand and the legs with the other. Then bring his knees toward his head as far as possible, trying to touch the infant's nose (Fig. 9-4). Repeat several times to increase his circulation and stimulate his alertness.

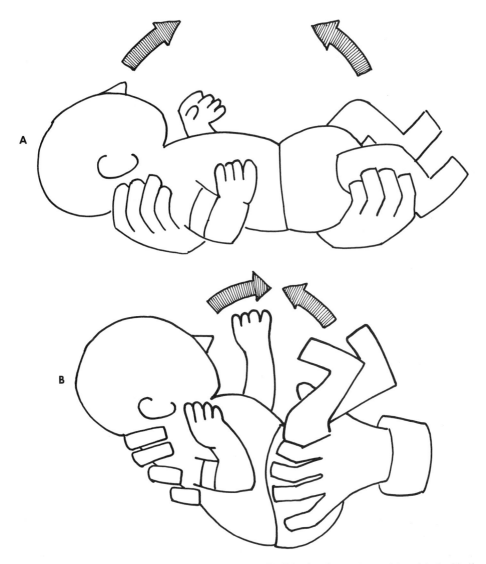

Fig. 9-4. A, Holding infant for Valsalva maneuver. **B,** Bringing knees toward head in jackknife position.

3. Stimulate the infant with frequent touching, exercising his extremities in a patterned sequence, carrying him, and talking, varying voice pitch and intonations. In short, play, laugh, and have fun with the baby. The infant with Down's syndrome has increased respiratory secretions; therefore the same activities that stimulate the infant's sensory system also help postural drainage, preventing pooling of mucus. Gentle suctioning of his nose and mouth with a bulb syringe may be necessary.
4. Hold the baby in an upright position as much as possible while feeding on the breast. First, swallowing is easier with the force of gravity rather than against it, and second, body alignment in a sitting position facilitates the passage of food.

Myelomeningocele. Abnormalities along the neural axis occur often enough to warrant their discussion in relation to breastfeeding. With successful surgical interventions many of these infants are able to function and fully participate in life, including being able to breastfeed.

In myelomeningocele, a segment of the spinal cord and meninges protrudes through a defect in the bony spine, usually in the lumbosacral region. The infant may have some weakness or complete flaccid paralysis of the legs, as well as bladder and bowel control dysfunction later on. The important aim of early nursing care is to prevent infection of the sac and to preserve the muscular and neurologic functions. Surgical correction to close the opening is done as early as possible, preferably in the first 24 to 48 hours. If the defect is extensive, one or more surgical procedures are done later using skin flaps.

Since the infant is in the intensive care unit during the critical period, parents should be encouraged to feel they have access to their infant and whenever possible should help in caretaking. If the mother is able to feed the infant by breast, the nurse should stay with her during the first several feedings, especially helping her to carefully pick up the infant and position him on the breast while protecting the sac or the surgery site from any pressure. A normal feeding position can be used with the mother's elbow rotated around a protective device (Fig. 9-5) to avoid pressure on his back. The infant can also be fed with the mother lying side by side with him on the bed. Feedings should be brief at first to conserve the infant's energy. Since the infant cannot be burped or bubbled in the normal way, gently rubbing him between his shoulders or rocking on a firm surface helps to release any ingestion of air.

If brainstem impairment is involved, the mother may not be able to breastfeed for a long time, if ever. Yet maintaining her milk supply to be given to the infant is immensely rewarding to her. Here is one example.

After a happy, normal birth, one mother, Marsha, was told that her baby had a myelomeningocele and would be transferred to another town to the regional perinatal center. Hand pumping for a few days and later switching to an electric pump, she began breastfeeding her infant daughter when she was able to travel and stay at the medical center. According to Marsha, "In spite of the IV, monitor wires, and not being able to touch her lower back, I felt very much at home." Several formula feedings were also given to her baby before it was discovered that the infant had a severe swallowing dysfunction from brainstem impairment. Shortly after the infant developed aspiration pneumonia, she was put on the respirator and fed intravenously. Marsha continued to pump her breasts several times a day. When the infant was able to start gastric tube feedings, she was given breastmilk, sometimes mixed with formula and sometimes alone. Marsha stayed with her most of the day and night, recalling, "The two things I had to offer during her struggle were breastmilk and a mother's touch. Giving her my milk was the one thing I was actively doing for her. The touching came with many hours of stroking and patting her little body to let her know she had a family who loved her." Although this child, because of the severity of her problems, was never able to feed directly from her mother's breast, most infants with a myelomeningocele can breastfeed. Another mother, of an 11-month-old baby, readmitted to my unit for surgery, had missed very few breastfeedings since the baby's birth and therefore had an ample supply of milk. Moreover, she was confident she could do it, having breastfed an older child. Her husband, one of nine children who were all breastfed, was entirely supportive.

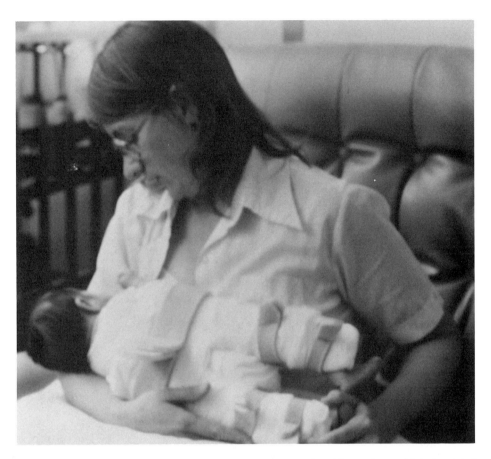

Fig. 9-5. Plastic bifurcated splint protects myelomeningocele site while mother and infant comfortably breastfeed.

Hydrocephalus. Hydrocephalus, which sometimes occurs with myelomeningocele, is an accumulation of fluid in the intracranial cavity because of an interference in the flow or absorption of cerebrospinal fluid. In communicating hydrocephalus, the infant has normal communication between the ventricles and the subarachnoid space; in the noncommunicating type, the infant's brain has a partial or complete block between these two areas. The circulation of the cerebrospinal fluid is blocked at some point within the ventricular system, preventing its flow to the subarachnoid spaces.

As the fluid distends the ventricles, the infant's head enlarges, and the sutures begin to separate with bulging fontanels. The "setting sun" sign of the eyes from the intracranial pressure, a high-pitched cry, muscle weakness, and severe neurologic defects occur if the hydrocephalus is already advanced at birth or is allowed to progress. Surgery should be performed as soon as the diagnosis is made. The surgical treatment is by means of a shunt to bypass the obstruction point and drain the cerebrospinal fluid to another area, usually the peritoneum, where it will be absorbed and finally excreted.

The infant with hydrocephalus requires careful nursing care, and the parents need

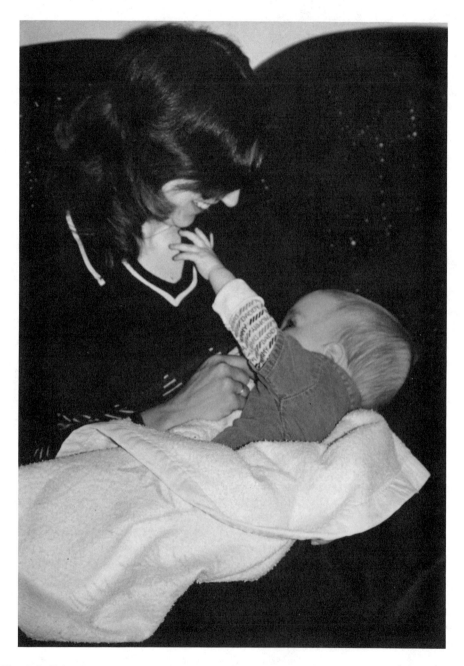

Fig. 9-6. This infant, born with hydrocephalus, is completely breastfed at 6 months and is developmentally normal. A shunt was performed 9 days after birth.

emotional support. Breastfeeding is often possible, and with early treatment many children can lead normal lives (Fig. 9-6). Care must be taken positioning and supporting the infant's head, and feeding lying down with his head supported by a pillow is probably the most comfortable position for the infant with advanced hydrocephalus. To prevent regurgitation, feedings should be frequent and on demand. When there is severe brain damage and breastfeeding has not been possible, some mothers of hydrocephalic infants have pumped their milk, deriving the satisfaction of still being able to give their infant their milk in a gavage tube or bottle.

Congenital heart defects

Congenital heart defects range from infants free of symptoms to those with severe defects, in which any exertion such as breastfeeding can cause cyanosis and early signs of congestive heart failure. For many infants. congenital heart defects are not severe enough to interfere with breastfeeding, and the nurse should encourage it for these infants as she would for any other. Frequently there are so few symptoms that the problem is not recognized until later in life.

A serious problem, however, can cause the infant to suck poorly and tire easily at the breast. He may begin with vigorous sucking, pulling away after a few minutes to rest. Typically the hungry infant will again grasp the breast, and the cycle is repeated.[19] After a time, an inadequate intake of breastmilk leads to failure to gain weight. Medical interventions with drug therapy such as digitalis can alleviate a lack of oxygenation and increase cardiac output. Often corrective surgery is indicated in one or several stages.

With a more severe defect, the infant can show early signs of heart failure, becoming cyanotic with fast respirations (tachypnea) and pulse rate (tachycardia). While she is holding her infant, the heartbeat may be so prominent that the mother is aware of it. Any of the symptoms described, along with auscultation of abnormal heart sounds or palpation of a thrill or unequal femoral pulses, leads the nurse to suspect a cardiac defect. The child should be immediately referred to a pediatrician for subsequent diagnostic testing to determine whether a defect is present and what type it is.

There are several points to remember in helping the breastfeeding mother. First, encourage her to feed frequently in an upright position for short periods of time to avoid distending the infant's stomach and impeding his breathing capacity. If the infant is distressed during feeding, pumping some of the milk and feeding it through a Lact-Aid Nursing Trainer to him at the same time he is feeding at the breast will reduce his exertion. Corrective or palliative surgery such as pulmonary banding can dramatically improve the infant's condition.

When surgery is performed, feeding at the breast when oral feedings can be resumed reduces the trauma of the surgery and hospitalization. The infant in Fig. 9-7 resumed full-time breastfeeding 6 days following surgery. If the child is too ill to hold or feed, arrange for the mother to stay close to her baby so she can have eye contact and reach out and touch him.

Infants with severe congenital heart defects and cyanosis are more susceptible to infections such as colds or sore throats. For this reason, these babies should be breastfed to give them the immunity that they desperately need. Of course, this immunity is not absolute; these children can still get upper resiratory infections or otitis, but they are much more benign and fewer in number. Therefore, even when breastfed, the infants should be protected from exposure to infection.

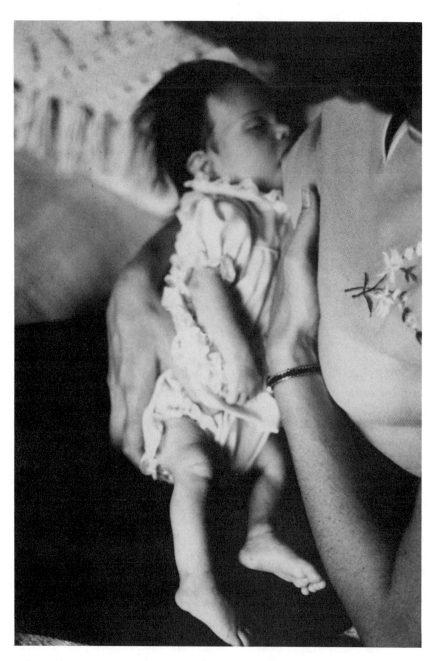

Fig. 9-7. Infant with patent ductus arteriosus and coarctation of aorta at breast. Photograph taken before corrective surgery.

Oral and gastrointestinal defects

Esophageal reflux (chalasia). Rarely, a breastfeeding infant will develop persistent, nonprojectile vomiting because of a laxity of the cardiac sphincter and lower esophageal muscles. This problem is more pronounced in formula-fed infants, presumably because the stomach digests formula or cow's milk more slowly and less completely than breastmilk.

Vomiting generally starts within a week after birth, especially when the infant is lying down. A barium swallow x-ray examination can confirm the diagnosis of esophageal reflux. The condition tends to be self-limited after several months and is minimized if the mother breastfeeds the infant in an upright position, keeping him upright for a short time after the feeding. Because some of the feedings are lost through vomiting, they need to be more frequent to compensate for the loss, maintaining hydration and ensuring adequate caloric intake.

Understandably, an infant's constant regurgitation is very upsetting to the mother, and she needs to have her self-confidence restored. The nurse helps by reassuring her that the problem is in no way related to her breastfeeding, but on the contrary, is helped by it.

Tracheoesophageal fistula. In the most common form of esophageal anomaly, tracheoesophageal fistula (T-E fistula), the upper end of the esophagus ends in a blind pouch with a fistula connecting the lower segment of the esophagus to the trachea. An infant with unexplained episodes of cyanosis, choking, and increased mucus secretion is suspect for this problem. Checking for this anomaly is done by gently passing a catheter into the esophagus and aspirating for gastric secretions. In some hospitals this is done routinely on all infants, although such a practice is dangerous and should be questioned by nurses. If gastric content cannot be determined and other symptoms are present, medical attention should be obtained at once. If the diagnosis is confirmed by x-ray examination, surgery is performed to connect the esophagus by end-to-end anastomosis.

Postoperatively, the infant is placed in an Isolette with his head elevated. He should have continuous low suction by sump tube in the esophageal pouch and intermittent low suction to the gastrostomy tube. Until the infant can take oral feedings, the mother can maintain lactation by pumping or hand expressing. Her milk should be saved and frozen according to the storage guidelines in Chapter 13. If temporary bottle-feeding is necessary to test for feeding tolerance, a NUK nipple and her milk should be used, since human milk is a physiologic fluid and less irritating than glucose water.

As soon as the suture line begins to heal, the mother can breastfeed while simultaneously feeding him her milk through the gastrostomy tube. Oral feedings are extremely important, since any infant not fed by mouth for a long time often has developmental problems during early childhood. Usually it takes a few days before the infant begins to breastfeed enthusiastically.

Imperforate anus. An imperforate anus in an infant is often initially detected by the nurse during the first assessment as she tries to take a rectal temperature. There are several types of this anomaly, ranging from no opening at all to a normal appearing rectum ending in a blind rectal pouch just above the opening, which is only confirmed by careful examination and a diagnostic x-ray examination. Treatment is reconstruction of the anal opening with surgery. In postoperative nursing care, the area around the surgical repair site should be kept clean and dry to promote healing. As soon as peristalsis returns, the infant can be fed from his mother's breast. The normally loose stools of the breastfed infant lessen the risk of constipation with subsequent breakdown of the surgical area and local infection.

Following her infant's surgery for a high, imperforate, anal defect that included a temporary colostomy, one mother was encouraged by her physician to resume breastfeeding 2 days later. When the infant suddenly developed Ritter's disease (toxic epidermal necrolysis) and had to be rehospitalized, she continued to breastfeed and alternately pump her milk for tube feedings. A few months after recovering, the infant underwent pull-through surgery to bring the colon back down to the anal opening with anoplasty. Solids were deliberately delayed to avoid any undue pressure until the colostomy was completely closed at 8 months. This child continued to breastfeed until he weaned himself at 18 months.

Pyloric stenosis. Pyloric stenosis, a hypertrophy of the pyloric sphincter, is more commonly found in white male infants. The symptoms usually appear after the first few weeks of life when the infant begins projectile vomiting after every feeding. Rapid dehydration and electrolyte imbalance become a real threat. During and following a feeding, it is possible with side lighting to see peristaltic waves that pass from left to right, and an olive-shaped tumor (the hypertrophic pylorus) can be palpated in the right upper quadrant of the abdomen.

Surgery can be delayed until the infant is rehydrated and the electrolyte imbalance restored. Breastfeeding has to be temporarily interrupted for a day or so after surgery. The mother should be advised to feed with only one breast and for a short time at first to prevent overfilling. The infant must be handled very carefully, "as if he were made of crystal"—using an infant seat for a few days helps to stablize his position during feeding.

Cleft lip and palate. Cleft lip and palate are congential malformations characterized by incomplete fusing of the central processes around the upper jaw and lip. The clefting may involve only the lip, may extend into the hard and soft palate, and may be unilateral or bilateral. The general classifications are:

    CL: Lip only
    CLP: Both the lip and palate
    CP: Hard and soft palate only

Cleft lip and cleft palate each account for 25% of the malformations; clefting of both of these structures is found in 50% of all cases.[25]

Surgical repair of the lip is done before the palate—usually within 2 months. Early surgery is favored to enhance bonding and attachment to a more "normal" infant whose appearance is closer to the ideal baby that the parents expected during the pregnancy. Surgical closure of the palate between 6 months and 3 years of age takes advantage of normal palatal changes in development.

The nurse will work most frequently with cases involving both the lip and the palate. Although it can be done, few mothers of children with cleft palates are encouraged to try breastfeeding or to even maintain lactation to give their milk by bottle or other means. Because nurses work so closely with these mothers, they are the key professionals able to offer them the opportunities to breastfeed. If a mother is strongly motivated to breastfeed, willing to try different techniques, and aware of some of the problems she will face, she can breastfeed, even though the definition of breastfeeding may alter from its usual meaning. Mothers who pump their milk for their infants are in fact breastfeeding mothers because they are providing their child with the milk produced by their bodies. In working with a mother who pumped and fed her infant her milk for 4 months, both she and I considered her to be a breastfeeding mother. The infant was never able to feed in the usual way at her breast, but she was extremely proud to see her infant grow and thrive on her milk.

If the infant has unilateral cleft lip with only minor alveolar ridge deficiency and no palate involvement, he will probably be able to breastfeed with only minor difficulties. However, he must find a way to form a satisfactory seal with his mouth and nose defect. Mothers of these infants have found that by holding their infant inward, pressing the cleft as tightly to the breast as possible, and placing a thumb or index finger over the cleft, enough suction is created for the infant to effectively milk the breast. Even when this technique is used, the infant must develop strong muscles and jaw capabilities to withdraw the milk.

When the hard and soft palate are involved in the cleft (CP and CLP), feeding at the breast is more difficult. Since there is a direct space into the nasal cavity, the infant must quickly gulp his food between breaths to prevent regurgitation through his nostrils. This is not possible unless the milk flows easily and quickly into the back of the oral cavity where it can be swallowed rapidly.

Establishing the suction necessary to keep the nipple in the infant's mouth is another consideration; an intact palate coming in contact with the base of the tongue builds up enough suction to produce a vacuum that keeps the nipple and areola in place. However, active suction by the infant during breastfeeding probably plays only a small part in the sucking process. The milk is forcibly ejected by the let-down reflex under hormonal influences and is thus actively "delivered" into the infant's mouth. During feedings, the infant's lower jaw, by alternate lowering and raising, reduces the pressure in the mouth and presumably exerts a suction. When the jaw is raised, the tongue presses on the lower surface of the nipple to reduce it to about half its previous width. When necessity demands it as in the case of the cleft lip, the infant is amazingly adaptive. Radiographic observations on an infant with a bilateral cleft lip showed that during sucking the tongue is grooved longitudinally, and a peristaltic wave moving backward obliterates the groove, presses on the nipple, and expresses the milk from it.[11]

One mother started breastfeeding her twins without realizing that one of them had a cleft in the soft palate. The infant cried constantly from hunger and could only drink the milk already let-down in the breast. After discovering the cleft, the mother noticed that by milking the breast with his gums and tongue, the child could suck effectively when the breasts were full and hard. "Then we discovered that the only purpose of the suction was to draw in and keep the nipple in her mouth. I found that by placing my index finger on the top edge of my areola and my middle finger on the bottom, I could press my nipple out between these fingers; it would protrude as if it were full of milk. I held the nipple in her mouth during the whole feeding as much as I would a bottle and its nipple."[10] After 4 months of using this technique, supplementation was no longer necessary and the mother was able to breastfeed completely.

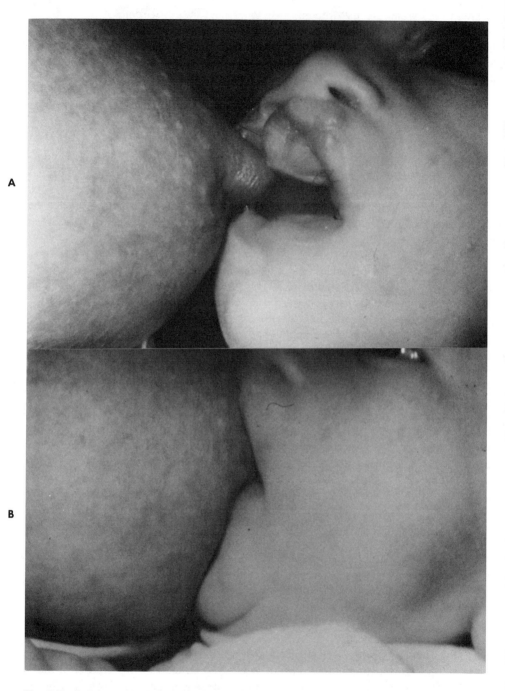

Fig. 9-8. A, Infant with cleft lip and complete cleft of hard and soft palates. Palatal obturator in place. **B,** Same infant at breast. (**A** and **B** courtesy David Barnes, D.D.S.)

Another woman[4] was determined to breastfeed or at least try, even after a stern 20-minute lecture from her physician as to why she could not breastfeed her infant who had a bilateral cleft lip and complete clefts running through the entire hard and soft palate. In short, the infant had no palate. First stimulating her milk supply by hand expression, electric pump, and occasionally breastfeeding a friend's baby, this mother found she was able to breastfeed by using the following techniques:

1. She held her infant sitting up directly facing her, with infant's legs spread on either side and his head lightly tilted backward. Lying down, the flow of milk under gravity caused the milk to run out through his nose, causing him to choke.
2. She pushed her breast into his mouth as far as possible. In this way, her breast sealed off the cleft.
3. She stroked her breast at the beginning of the feeding to let down. She reported, "When it did, he thought he had done it!"
4. She stimulated a normal sucking-chewing movement by placing her fingers under his jaw and firmly pushing up and down. The infant soon caught on and initiated the sucking movements himself, which became stronger as time went on.

A palatal obturator, a plastic dental plate appliance devised by her dentist, covered the cleft palate and immediately improved the sucking (Fig. 9-8). This child, who breastfed until he was 1 year old, is now in school. Unlike other children born with a cleft palate, he has no speech problems and enunciates well. The mother and the school speech therapist feel that this is due to the powerful muscle action developed during breastfeeding.

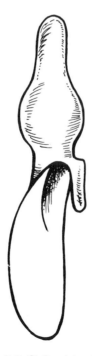

Fig. 9-9. Cleft palate nipple.

During the intervals between experimentation with different methods of feeding, pumping maintains lactation. Unless the mother is very efficient in hand expression, an electric pump is recommended because of the ease with which it stimulates the breast over a longer time with minimal energy. Meanwhile, the infant can be fed breastmilk by using various methods. Some parents find that a small spouted cup works well. Others favor an eyedropper, a rubber-tipped syringe, a pipette, or a NUK nipple turned upside down so that the outlet faces away from the cleft.[17] Recently the Lact-Aid Nursing Trainer has been used successfully for infants with cleft palates.[7] A cleft palate nipple made by the Bittner Company resembles the elongated soft so-called Lamb's nipple used by veterinarians (Fig. 9-9). This nipple fits onto a regular bottle cap to feed pumped breastmilk. The Beniflex Nurser is another alternative for feeding breastmilk.

DENTAL CARIES

As a result of a few isolated reports of breastfed infants with dental caries in the dental literature in recent years, a brief discussion of this problem is warranted, especially for nurses working in ambulatory pediatrics.

Breastfeeding has been unjustifiably blamed for the development of caries. There are several arguments that must be made. First, as the numbers of breastfeeding toddlers increase, it is reasonable to expect that some of them will develop dental disease, especially after the introduction of solids that in our society so often contain sugar, overt or covert. It is generally conceded that increased sugar consumption is related to the incidence of dental decay.

Second, the nutritional state of the mother before and during pregnancy plays a large part in the formation of dentition in the child's primary teeth. It is also thought to be an inherited trait; therefore it could be argued that some breastfed children develop caries not because they were breastfed but in spite of it.[26]

Last, overall, breastfed children have less dental decay than those who are fed otherwise.[22] Consider the mechanical differences between breastfeeding and bottle-feeding. Drawn deep into the child's mouth, the nipple rests at the junction of the hard and soft palate during breastfeeding, posterior to the child's teeth. Removing milk from the breast requires active effort by the infant, the active suck always being automatically followed by a swallow. Both prevent the teeth from being bathed in pooled milk. By contrast, the milk from a bottle flows out spontaneously with only the slightest pressure into the anterior part of the mouth, permitting stagnation of the milk on and around the teeth.[1]

In spite of these differences and arguments, dental health in no way should be neglected just because the child is breastfeeding. Teaching and guidance to parents should include optimal prenatal nutrition, restriction of refined carbohydrates in the child's diet (including fluids he drinks from a cup), the use of fluoride when the amount in the water supply is inadequate, regular brushing as soon as the primary teeth erupt, and dental visits after about 2 years of age.

METABOLIC DYSFUNCTION
Inborn errors of metabolism

Two rare disorders, phenylketonuria and galactosemia, are briefly discussed here because of their effect on breastfeeding. Phenylketonuria (PKU) is an inherited metabolic disorder associated with mental retardation. Because of liver enzyme deficiency, the affected child is unable to metabolize the essential amino acid phenylalanine, one of the 20 amino acids necessary for growth. Accumulation of high levels of phenylalanine in the infant appears to prevent normal development of the brain and central nervous system.

Testing for PKU, mandatory in most states, is usually done by using the Guthrie method: blood is drawn for testing from a heel stick in the neonate just before the infant's discharge from the hospital. In the case of a home birth, it should be done in the physician's office. The first test may be false-negative before higher levels of phenylalanine have had a chance to develop and be detected; therefore the test should probably be repeated later. Even then there are problems with reliable testing. Many false-positive tests have caused extreme concern and immediate weaning, only to be found inaccurate later. Therefore it is recommended that infants treated with a phenylalanine-restricted diet be challenged with a phenylalanine load between 3 and 6 months to reconfirm the diagnosis.

Until recently, medical intervention for breastfeeding infants with PKU was immediate weaning, thereby controlling phenylalanine levels, since the amount of breastmilk taken by the infant could not easily be measured. Since the infant requires some phenylalanine in his diet (20 to 30 mg/kg/day), limited breastfeeding is now considered possible without the harmful sequelae of brain damage. The following quotation from a United States Public Health Service pamphlet is evidence of this changing approach:

> It is our belief that continued nursing of the PKU infant is feasible. Mature breastmilk is low in phenylalanine (41 mg/dl) compared with whole cow's milk (159 mg/dl) and infant formulas such as Enfamil (73 mg/dl) and Similac (75 mg/dl). The phenylalanine requirement of some infants with PKU may be as high as 75 mg/kg of body weight/day. Thus, once control has been established, an infant may be able to consume up to 20 ounces of human milk daily to meet his/her phenylalanine requirement. However, Lofenalac must still be included in the diet to provide adequate kilocalories and nutrients.[24]

The key to preventing harmful buildup of phenylalanine in the breastfeeding infant is careful dietary management using Lofenalac, a casein-free hydrolysate from which 95% of the phenylalanine has been removed. Levels should show blood levels remaining below 10 mg/dl. Table 9-2 shows the recommended daily amounts of phenylalanine, protein, and energy needs for infants with PKU.

How the breastfeedings and the Lofenalac feedings are alternated is individually determined. As part of a PKU team, the nurse will find that it is better for one mother to offer the Lofenalac before the feeding, whereas it is better for another to give it after the breastfeeding. Still another will substitute Lofenalac for one or two breastfeedings a day, pumping her breasts in lieu of the feedings to maintain her milk supply. Because weighing the infant before and after feedings at the breast is important to determine the amount taken by the infant, the family will need an accurate pediatric scale at home.

The Lofenalac should be given with a NUK nipple, if given by bottle, to prevent nipple confusion. Using a Lact-Aid Nursing Trainer filled with Lofenalac while breastfeeding has not worked well, since it tends to clog the unit.

Another hereditary metabolic condition, galactosemia, occurs once in about every 85,000 births. A rare disorder of the metabolism of galactose-1-phosphate, galactosemia

TABLE 9-2 _____

Recommended daily amounts of phenylalanine, protein, and energy for infants with PKU

Age (mo)	Phenylalanine (mg/kg/day)	Protein (gm/kg/day)	Energy (kcal/kg/day)
0-3	58 ± 18	4.4	120
4-6	40 ± 10	3.3	115
7-9	32 ± 9	2.5	110
10-12	30 ± 8	2.5	105

From United States Department of Health and Human Services: Guide to breastfeeding the infant with PKU, DDHS Pub. (HSA) 79-5110, Washington, D.C., 1980, Bureau of Community Health Services.

is an enzyme deficiency that is transmitted as an autosomal recessive trait. With galactosemia, the liver enzyme that changes galactose to glucose is absent, and as a result the infant is unable to metabolize lactose. Any intake of galactose results in liver dysfunction and disease.

These infants appear normal at birth but soon start having feeding difficulties. Vomiting and poor weight gain follow. Without treatment, cerebral impairment and lethargy appear at first, followed by mental retardation. Galactosemia is one of the few cases that demands immediate and total weaning, since breastmilk has a high lactose content. All milk and galactose-containing foods must be eliminated from the diet and the infant placed on special galactose-free formula. Nurses should give dietary guidance and reassure the mother that by holding and stroking during bottle-feedings she can meet the needs of her infant.

Congenital hypothyroidism

Congenital hypothyroidism (cretinism) is due to an inborn lack of thyroid secretion because of an absent thyroid gland or because of inborn enzymatic defects in the synthesis of thyroxine. It is a common endocrine problem of childhood, and the clinical symptoms can appear in the first weeks or months of life. Uusally the symptoms of hypothyroidism become noticeable in 3 to 6 months. Before this time we often hear parents praise their "good" baby because he cries so little. After 3 months, classic symptoms of myxedema appear: coarse, brittle hair, anemia, a large protruding tongue, a short wide forehead, and lack of skeletal growth.

Does breastfeeding protect the infant with congenital hypothyroidism? There is conflicting evidence as to whether the breastfed infant is somewhat protected because human milk provides thyroid hormone to compensate for the hormonal deficit.[5,15] Despite the possible protective effects of breastmilk, an infant with this problem will need replacement therapy with desiccated thyroid gland while he continues to breastfeed and following weaning.

Celiac disease

Often called malabsorption syndrome or gluten enteropathy, celiac disease is characterized by changes in the intestinal mucosa or villi that prevent the absorption of foods, mainly fat. The mucosal damage appears to be from a sensitivity to the gluten factor of protein found in wheat, rye, oats, and barley. There is also some evidence that cow's milk allergy is implicated in gluten intolerance.[2] Although the exact cause is yet unknown, elimination of gluten in the diet results in dramatic improvement of symptoms.

The breastfeeding infant will gain adequate weight and show no symptoms of the disease until solids containing gluten are introduced into his diet. Then the clinical symptoms are insidious and chronic. Because fat is not absorbed, the infant's stools become frothy in appearance, foul smelling, and excessive. Deficiencies of the fat-soluble vitamins (A, D, K, and E) appear; and if the disease progresses without treatment, abdominal distention and general wasting are evident.

There are two general nursing considerations in working with the family. First, the child's diet must be modified and vigorously maintained to exclude gluten, thus improving food absorption and preventing malnutrition. The optimal time for nutritional guidance is when the child is in the hospital and can receive specific food plans from the nutritionist. The mother must be able to recognize foods with hidden amounts of gluten and read label ingredients carefully.

The second consideration is to encourage continued breastfeeding, which provides optimal nutrition to the infant and helps delay symptoms. If the family is planning to have more children, breastfeeding should be encouraged for subsequent pregnancies as well, since celiac disease tends to occur in several members of the family.

Cystic fibrosis

Cystic fibrosis, a congenital disease manifesting itself as a chronic generalized dysfunction of the exocrine (mucus-producing) glands, occurs once in every 1500 to 2000 births. The glands of the affected child produce abnormally thick and sticky secretions that block the flow of pancreatic digestive enzymes, clog hepatic ducts, and impede the movement of cilia in the lungs. The increased sodium chloride in the child's sweat provides an important diagnostic clue: the family reports that the child tastes salty when kissed.

In spite of a voracious appetite, the infant fails to gain weight. When he begins to eat cereals and solids, the stools become bulky, more frequent, foul smelling, and frothy. Pulmonary complications are almost always present, and the child suffers persistent, severe respiratory infections because of retained mucus.

Care primarily involves protection from respiratory infection by postural drainage, aerosol therapy, medications such as expectorants and antibiotics, and dietary supplements. There is no need to interrupt breastfeeding. In fact, breastfeeding should continue on demand and as frequently as possible. Many infants will develop symptoms of cystic fibrosis only after breastfeeding is stopped. In milder forms of the disease, breastmilk appears to be actually protective. To replace those that the child is not producing, pancreatic enzymes should be added in powdered form to small amounts of pureed food that the child especially likes and given by spoon. Aqueous preparations of fat-soluble vitamins A, D, E, and sometimes K should be given daily. Supplemental oral salt may also be necessary in hot weather.

Hypoglycemia

In the healthy newborn, hypoglycemia is generally defined as a blood glucose level below 30 mg/dl. The nurse is responsible for direct analysis of blood glucose concentration with a heel stick using Dextrometer system or Dextrostix. Since testing is prone to error, any questionable readings should be rechecked in the laboratory before instituting therapy.

Hypoglycemia in the neonate is the result of depeletion of glycogen caused by a number of conditions such as a long, difficult labor, toxemia, or diabetes of the mother. Respiratory distress, hypothermia, and erythroblastosis also increase the infant's use of blood glucose, thus reducing his stores of glycogen. Especially susceptible are premature or small-for-gestational-age (SGA) infants who have deficient subcutaneous fat and liver glycogen stores. Because they are expected to have lower levels of blood glucose, 20 mg/dl and below is used as the criterion for hypoglycemia in these infants. Many authorities disagree with this lower criterion, believing that these infants are no less (and may be more) susceptible to brain damage than normal infants.

Early and frequent feedings at the breast help prevent hypoglycemic depressions of glucose. The higher protein levels in colostrum have a more stabilizing effect on blood glucose levels than does glucose water. Since hypoglycemia usually occurs soon after birth, some supplements may be necessary until the mother's milk supply is established.

In severe hypoglycemic states, IV infusions of 10% to 25% dextrose solutions may be ordered by the physician; however, in infants of diabetic mothers, hypertonic solutions should only be given with extreme caution, since glucose will stimulate insulin release and result in rebound hypoglycemia. Throughout therapy the rate of infusion must be carefully controlled using an infusion pump, and blood glucose levels must be monitored to prevent circulatory overload and hyperglycemia. If a fragile and easily displaced infusion line in the scalp necessitates temporary interruption of breastfeeding, it can be resumed when the infant's condition stabilizes.

ALLERGIES AND FOOD SENSITIVITIES

It is widely recognized that breastfed infants and children are much less susceptible to allergies from food. Nurses, especially those in pediatric settings, know that this advantage of breastfeeding is not to be taken lightly. The infant becomes fussy and miserable and possibly develops eczema, and the parents' frantic search for a formula he can tolerate is an unnecessary emotional and economic burden to the family.

Allergies, altered adverse reactions to a foreign substance or antibody, are accompanied by immunologic changes—notably a rise in IgE—however, a lack of definitive laboratory tests makes verification difficult.

Infants develop any number of allergic reactions, and each has an individual way of responding. For instance, from the same food one infant will develop diarrhea, colic, or gastrointestinal problems; another responds through his central nervous system and becomes irritable or hyperactive; a third can have a dermatologic symptoms such as urticaria or eczema. The list of allergy symptoms is long; in addition, the child may have rhinitis, otitis media, coughing, asthma, conjunctivitis, nausea, vomiting, lack of appetitie, and frequent respiratory infections. Dark circles under the eyes ("allergic shiners") are also a common indicator of allergy. Because foods belonging to the same botanical group have similar antigens, they can trigger a similar allergic response in the same child. Onions, for instance, along with garlic, leeks, and asparagus all belong to the same botanical family; allergy to one may mean allergy to the others.[21]

Many factors in the environment other than food can trigger allergic responses; environmental inhalants, pollens, and contact allergies are common and need to be considered as well as food allergies—particularly if the infant or child is completely breastfed. Rashes can be caused by chemicals in laundry products, lanolin, lotions, dyes, synthetic fabrics, or (if the child has been outside), grass or poison oak or ivy.

The introduction of solids into the infant's diet often marks the first sign of food allergies. However, if solids are not given until after 6 months, the infants's enzyme system is mature and he is much more prepared to tolerate potential sensitizing proteins in his diet; thus potential food allergies are delayed, and when they do appear, they are lessened. Even so, each new introduction of foods should be watched and low-antigenic foods selected.

Most importantly, allergies are usually inherited; 40% to 80% of individuals with allergies have a family history. Therefore a complete nursing history is vital to the total assessment. Identifying the cause is akin to doing detective work, so in addition to determining family allergies, take a careful, detailed history of food intake for clues to the causes of the child's allergies.

Allergies while breastfeeding

Now and then, even infants who are completely breastfed and are receiving no solids develop allergic symptoms that appear to be from something they have ingested. In this case the infant is probably reacting to foods or substances taken in by the mother that are being transmitted through the breastmilk.[8] Vitamins, dyes, or additives consumed by the mother could be causing the problem; however, the most common allergic-producing offenders are cow's milk and milk products. Realizing that her baby was fussiest after breastfeeding, a mother contacted her La Leche League leader, who suggested the mother stop drinking milk. Almost immediately the infant's fussiness stopped. If this mother were to start drinking milk again, her daughter would again become noticeably unhappy after breastfeeding.[13]

Common offenders

In addition to cow's milk, the most common offending foods that tend to produce allergic responses in Western cultures are chocolate, cola, corn, citrus fruits, egg white, peas and beans (legumes), tomato, wheat, cinnamon, and artificial food colors.[20] This list does not preclude other possible offenders, such as shellfish, pork, beef, onion, nuts, and many others. In other areas of the world the list reflects commonly eaten food as it does in ours. In Japan, soy and fish are culprits. There may also be a combined effect in which eating more than one potentially allergic food triggers allergies that would not have occurred with eating just one alone. The onset of the allergic response occurs anywhere from half an hour to a day later. Often it is within the first hour after eating the offending food.

Sensitivities

Health-care professionals are now beginning to realize that some individuals, including young children, have adverse reactions to food without the typical IgE response changes. This is called food sensitivity or "hidden food allergy." Children with food allergies may develop new sensitivities to foods they eat regularly. A fast pulse rate after eating can mean a sensitivity. Eliminating the certain foods to which the individual is sensitive can bring about relief from the more subtle reactions of sensitivity, such as headaches or fatigue.

Elimination and challenge of suspected foods

If no single offending food can be identified and possible environmental causes of allergy symptoms have been ruled out, an elimination diet may be used. If it is to be of any value, however, it has to be carefully followed and clearly spelled out—written instructions are the most helpful. While they are on the diet, scrupulous label reading on packaged foods by the parents avoids inadvertent eating of foods that should be eliminated (Table 9-3).

Providing that the elimination diet brings relief, the allergy should be "challenged" by reintroducing the suspected foods, one at a time, into the diet. Starting with small amounts and gradually increasing the suspected food in about a week's time, the parents watch for any signs of the allergy developing again. To definitely establish the offending food or foods, a challenge should be done two or more times.

TABLE 9-3

Types of food and food ingredients most commonly associated with allergic reactions and examples of hidden sources of these foods

Food type	Possible hidden sources
Milk in any form	Bread, pudding, cream soups, most bakery products, sherbet, some gravies, many mixes, butter, margarine, some hot dogs and bologna
Eggs, especially egg white	Mayonnaise, breaded foods, cakes, cookies, custard, some ice cream, noodles, noodle soup, meatloaf, spun soybean protein used in meat analogs, candies, meringue
Wheat, sometimes other small grains	Bakery products, breaded foods, pasta, many soups, some puddings and gravies, mixes, stuffing, some hot dogs and bologna, some textured vegetable protein
Citrus fruit, especially oranges	Some fruit desserts, some types of punch
Kola nut family	Chocolate, cocoa, cola beverages
Corn	Corn cereals including hominy and grits, Cracker Jacks, corn chips and other corn snack foods, tortillas, and certain other Mexican foods; foods containing refined corn products such as corn syrup, corn starch, corn flour, corn oil may cause problems in persons allergic to corn
Legumes	Peanut butter; foods containing soy protein, soy flour, or perhaps soybean oil; assorted soups; licorice
Tomato	Meatloaf, stews, and other prepared dishes
Spices, especially cinnamon	Catsup, baked goods, candy, chewing gum, various prepared dishes
Food colors, especially tartrazine (FD & C Yellow No. 5)	Soft drinks, candy, pudding, frosting, colored breakfast cereals, and other artificially colored foods; many medications
Nuts	Candy, bakery products, granola
Fish, meat, bananas	Identity is usually apparent

From Suitor, C.W., and Hunter, M.F.: Nutrition: principles and practices, Philadelphia, 1980, J.B. Lippincott Co.

Finally, the most effective prevention of allergies in infants is complete breastfeeding for the first 6 months and gradual introduction of solid foods, one at a time, observing for any symptoms of allergy. Delaying solids for more than 6 months in infants who are highly allergic to a variety of foods is safe, providing the hemoglobin level is monitored at intervals. Usually the hemoglobin remains high because of the efficient absorption of the iron in breastmilk; however, the mother must be prepared to breastfeed often to provide the necessary calories that otherwise would have been provided by solids.

SUDDEN INFANT DEATH SYNDROME (SIDS)

One of about every 300 to 500 live-born infants[3] worldwide dies suddenly, usually in his sleep without apparent cause. Put to bed without any indication that something was wrong, save perhaps a slight cold, the child later is found lifeless. Suddenly, without warning, the parents' beautiful baby has been taken from them and their lives are irrevocably changed.

Research studies and proposed theories on causes of SIDS have raised more questions than they have answered. At one time breastfeeding was thought to protect the infant against SIDS. Now there is increasing evidence that although it may offer some slight protection, it is not preventive.

Current theories of cause are sudden, acute respiratory viral infection; unknown metabolic errors; occlusion of the infant's airway[23]; laryngospasm; neurologic abnormalities[12]; and defect in the central regulation of respiration. Episodes of a "near miss" for sudden infant death are being extensively studied.[12] In near misses for SIDS, the parents report finding the infant apneic, pale, or cyanotic and requiring vigorous stimulation or resuscitation. This infant should be placed on an apnea monitor, since a second apneic episode is not uncommon.

Community health nurses, specially prepared to work with families who have lost a child through SIDS, are an invaluable resource for helping the parents. The breastfeeding mother, in addition to her emotional anguish, has painful, engorged breasts, full of milk for the child who is no longer there. One of the many therapeutic aids given by the nurse at this critical time is helping her with physical relief of her engorgement. White, Professional Advisory Member of La Leche League International, suggests that the mother restrict salt but not fluids and express only as much milk as is needed for comfort until it is reabsorbed. A slight fever during the period of milk reabsorption may be expected.

While counseling the parents, the nurse must make them aware that the risk of SIDS happening again with another child is probably only slightly greater[18] and that nothing could have been done to prevent it from happening. To reinforce these points and give them more information, printed materials on SIDS for parents are available from local chapters or the National Foundation.*

CONCLUSION

Discontinuing breastfeeding is rarely necessary for the child with a health problem, although feeding patterns may have to be modified. Too often, however, weaning is

---

*National Foundation for Sudden Infant Death, Inc., 1501 Broadway, New York, N.Y. 10036.

automatically taken for granted, and once the infant is weaned a new cycle of health problems, especially allergies, can appear.

Each family will be unique. The experience of one situation can never be duplicated; therefore the tasks of nurses in helping the family with a breastfeeding sick child require versatility and a firm knowledge of the nature of the health problem. Just as important is recognizing the psychologic needs of the breastfeeding child and his family, especially the mother. Nursing interventions also require awareness of devices that aid lactation and how they can be obtained. Support must come from the health-care team, not just one or two, so there must be communication among the staff for continuity of care. Informing the parents about every aspect of the health problem and including them in decision making create mutual respect and a working relationship between the nurse and the family.

REFERENCES

1. Abbey, L.M.: Is breastfeeding a likely cause of dental caries in young children? J. Am. Dent. Assoc. **98:**21, 1979.
2. Bahna, S.I., and Heiner, D.C.: Allergies to milk, New York, 1980, Grune & Stratton, Inc.
3. Bergman, A.B.: Sudden infant death, Nurs. Outlook **20:**777, 1972.
4. Birdwell, P.: Personal communication, Aug. 1981.
5. Bode, H.H., Vanjonaek, W.J., and Crawford, J.D.: Mitigation of cretinism by breastfeeding, Pediatrics **61:**12, 1978.
6. Fallot, M.E., Boyd, J.L., and Oski, F.A.: Breastfeeding reduces incidence of hospital admissions for infections on infants, Pediatrics **65:**1121, 1980.
7. Frantz, K.: Paper presented at Conference on Special Situations: Helping the Breastfeeding Mother, Wichita, Kan., April 1979.
8. Gerrard, J.W.: Allergy in breastfed babies to ingredients in breast milk, Ann. Allergy **42:**69, 1979.
9. Good, J.: Breastfeeding the Down's syndrome baby, Franklin Park, Ill., 1980, La Leche League International.
10. Grady, E.: Breastfeeding the baby with a cleft of the soft palate, Clin. Pediatr. **16:**978, 1977.
11. Jenkins, G.N.: The physiology and biochemistry of the mouth, ed. 4, London, 1978, Blackwell Scientific Publications.
12. Korobkin, R., and Guilleminault, C.: Neurologic abnormalities in near miss for sudden infant death syndrome, Pediatrics **64:**369, 1979.
13. La Leche League International, Inc.: La Leche League News **21:**25, 1979.
14. La Leche League International, Inc.: La Leche League News **20:**83, 1978.
15. Letarte, J., et al.: Lack of protective effect of breastfeeding in congenital hypothyroidism, Pediatrics **65:**703, 1980.
16. Nurses' Association of the American College of Obstetricians and Gynecologists: Infection control for the obstetric patient and the newborn infant, Technical Bulletin 9, March 1981.
17. Nursing Mothers' Association of Australia News: Breastfeeding and cleft palate, p. 12, June 1980.
18. Peterson, D.R., Chinn, N., and Fisher, L.D.: The sudden infant death syndrome: repetitions in families, J. Pediatr. **97:**265, 1980.
19. Shor, V.Z.: Congenital cardiac defects: assessment and case finding, Am. J. Nurs. **78:**256, 1978.
20. Speer, F.: Food allergy: the 10 common offenders, Am. Fam. Prac. **13:**106, 1976.
21. Suitor, C.W., and Hunter, M.F.: Nutrition: principles and practices, Philadelphia, 1980, J.B. Lippincott Co.
22. Tank, G., and Storvick, C.A.: Caries experience of children of one to six years old in two Oregon communities, J. Am. Dent. Assoc. **70:**101, 1965.
23. Tonkin, S.: Sudden infant death syndrome: hypothesis of causation, Pediatrics **55:**650, 1975.
24. United States Department of Health and Human Services: Guide to breastfeeding the infant with PKU, DHHS Publication (HSA) 79-5110, Washington, D.C., 1980, Bureau of Community Health Services.
25. Whaley, L.F., and Wong, D.L.: Nursing care of infants and children, St. Louis, 1979, The C.V. Mosby Co.
26. White M.: Breastfeeding and dental caries, La Leche League News **20:**53, 1978.

ADDITIONAL READINGS

Babson, S.G., Pernoll, M.L., and Benda, G.I.: Diagnosis and management of the fetus and neonate at risk: a guide for team care, ed. 4, St. Louis, 1980, The C.V. Mosby Co.

Brewster, D.P.: You can breastfeed your baby—even in special situations, Emmaus, Pa., 1979, Rodale Press, Inc.

Crook, W.G.: You and allergy, Jackson, Tenn., 1980, Professional Books.

Filston, H., and Izant, R.: The surgical neonate, New York, 1978, Appleton-Century-Crofts.

Foman, S.J.: Infant nutrition, ed. 2, Philadelphia, 1974, W.B. Saunders Co.

Larter, N.: Cystic fibrosis, Am. J. Nurs. **81**:527, 1981.

Marlow, D.R.: Textbook of pediatric nursing ed. 5, Philadelphia, 1977, W.B. Saunders Co.

National Foundation for Sudden Infant Death: Facts about sudden infant death syndrome, New York, The Foundation.

Pillittera, A.: Nursing care of the growing family, Boston, 1977, Little, Brown & Co.

Wilson, E.: Guide for the celiac, Jersey City, N.J., 1975, American Celiac Society.

10

Jaundice

RICHARD A. GUTHRIE

Few other problems of the newborn, particularly the full-term newborn, have a greater deterrent effect on breastfeeding than does jaundice. More infants have breastfeeding discontinued in the early newborn period because of jaundice than for any other single reason. This practice is the more tragic because it is unnecessary. Discontinuing breastfeeding because of jaundice often results from a failure of the health-care team to properly understand and use the principles of normal physiology. Understanding is particularly important for the maternity or pediatric nurse, since she is the one who gives continuous care to the mother and her infant and can favorably affect the course of breastfeeding.

A professor of mine began each lecture with a slide that said, "Before we can understand the abnormal, we must first understand the normal." I thought then in my inexperience that this was a trite statement, but the older and more experienced I become, the more truth I see in it. We in the health professions continually make mistakes because we do not understand the variations of normal. This is eminently true with jaundice in the newborn. For this reason I begin this chapter with a discussion of the normal physiology of bilirubin metabolism.

NORMAL PHYSIOLOGY OF BILIRUBIN

Jaundice in anyone is the accumulation of bilirubin in the tissue, especially the skin, where it is visible as a yellow pigment. In the older child or adult, jaundice is always a pathologic condition—not so in the newborn. Let me explain why. In the fetus, respiration occurs via the transfer of maternal oxygen to the fetus through the placenta. Maternal blood, by the time it reaches the placenta, is relatively low in oxygen. For this reason the infant develops a high red blood cell count with a high hemoglobin content so that he will have more oxygen-carrying capacity in his blood. Babies are often born with a hemoglobin level of 20 gm/dl or more, in contrast to a normal adult level of 10 to 14 gm/dl. Hemoglobin can have either a low or high affinity for oxygen. If affinity is low, the pickup of oxygen is less, but the release of the oxygen to the tissue is greater. The hemoglobin the baby makes is fetal hemoglobin, which has a low affinity for oxygen. Since fetal hemoglobin does not pick up oxygen well from the placenta (low affinity) and placental blood has a low O_2 concentration, there is a need for more of it.

Adult hemoglobin, on the other hand, has a high affinity for oxygen. It can pick up oxygen well but cannot release it to the tissue. In the older infant, child, or adult an enzyme called 2,3-diphosphoglycerate (2,3-DPG) handles this problem. In peripheral tissue, 2,3-DPG enters the hemoglobin molecule, where it changes the affinity of hemoglobin for oxygen, displacing the oxygen that then is available to the tissue for use.

The development of 2,3-DPG and the advent of an oxygen-rich environment in the air-breathing lung eliminates the need for fetal hemoglobin and for the high fetal hemoglobin level. As the newborn now needs only a hemoglobin level of 10 to 12 gm/dl and as the bone marrow switches to making red blood cells with adult rather than fetal hemoglobin, there is a need to rid the body of excess fetal hemoglobin containing red blood cells.

Ridding the body of unneeded red blood cells is the function of the reticuloendothelial (RE) system of the spleen. In the spleen the old cells are filtered out and destroyed, releasing the fetal hemoglobin. Since free-circulating hemoglobin can damage certain tissues, especially the kidneys, it is further acted on by the spleen before release.

Hemoglobin is a complex molecule consisting of heme, globin, and iron. The first step in its degradation is to split the globin releasing the iron. Globin returns to the circulation and is of no concern to us in this connection, and iron returns to the bone marrow where it can be reused for new hemoglobin synthesis. But it is the heme molecule with which I am concerned here and that causes jaundice through the creation of (indirect) bilirubin.

This compound, indirect bilirubin, is fat soluble and thus cannot be dissolved and carried in the water-soluble blood. To be excreted, fat-soluble bilirubin must be conjugated with compounds that make it water soluble for excretion in the bile and urine. The task of making bilirubin water soluble is carried out by the liver.

The problem is how to get the fat-soluble bilirubin from the spleen to the liver. This is accomplished by conjugating the fat-soluble bilirubin in the serum with albumin and other carrier proteins that are water soluble. In the liver the indirect bilirubin is detached from the albumin and transported into the liver cells, where it is then conjugated with other water-soluble proteins for excretion. Most of the bilirubin is conjugated with glucuronic acid to form bilirubin-glucuronide (direct-reacting bilirubin) and excreted in the bile. A small amount of direct bilirubin enters the circulation and is excreted in the urine.

Bilirubin in the bile is carried to the gut, where it is converted to a yellow compound, urobilinogen, by the bacteria. It is this compound that gives the stool its yellow color. Some urobilinogen is reabsorbed from the gut and recirculates to the liver for reexcretion or goes to the kidney, where it is excreted in the urine.

The conjugation of indirect bilirubin by the liver to form direct bilirubin is accomplished by a series of enzymes, the most important of which is glucuronyl transferase. This enzyme conjugates the glucuronic acid to the bilirubin. A complete deficiency of this enzyme results in a rare, serious disease called the Crigler-Najjar syndrome. Infants with this deficiency are severely jaundiced and remain so for life.

Physiologic jaundice

The mild jaundice of normal newborns, often called "physiologic" jaundice, results from an exaggeration of some of the factors of the normal process of hemoglobin degradation. Primarily it results from the very rapid breakdown of excess fetal hemoglobin and from the inability of the liver to excrete rapidly the excess bilirubin because the glucuronyl transferase enzyme is somewhat sluggish in the first few days of life. Thus the combination of the breakdown of a large red cell mass and the sluggish excretion of bilirubin by the liver results in an accumulation of indirect bilirubin in the serum. Some of the bilirubin becomes deposited in the skin as a yellow pigment, thus producing physiologic jaundice of the newborn. For yet unknown reasons, full-term American Indian, Japanese, Chinese, and Korean neonates develop a more severe form of physiologic jaundice than do white neonates.[3]

CLINICAL ASPECTS OF JAUNDICE

Most jaundice of the newborn, or "physiologic" jaundice, is thus the natural result of a normal physiologic process. This process, the replacement of red cells and bilirubin, is present in all living beings but becomes exaggerated in the newborn because of the initially high hematocrit and sluggish disposal mechanism. Of these factors, the high hematocrit and rapid dissolution of the excess red cells are the most important. Characteristically, physiologic jaundice begins on the second or third day of life, reaches a peak on the fifth to seventh day, and then slowly recedes. Indirect serum bilirubin rises on the second or third day to a peak of 7 to 12 mg/dl but seldom exceeds 15 mg/dl. There is no scientific evidence that bilirubin levels below 20 mg/dl in the first 3 days of life and less than 25 mg/dl thereafter have any harmful effect on full-term infants.

Usually, the sclera of the eyes first appear yellow, followed closely by yellowing of the face and trunk. The extremities are next to yellow, and finally the palms and soles are affected. Indeed this sequence of progressive yellowing of the skin can be used as a rough approximation of the serum bilirubin. In assessing jaundice, clinical yellowing should not be used as a substitute for laboratory determinations of bilirubin but can be used as a guide as to when to begin laboratory determinations and how frequently to obtain them.

As a rough rule of thumb:

Scleral icterus	Bilirubin about 3 mg/dl
Face	Bilirubin about 5 mg/dl
Early trunk	Bilirubin about 5 to 7 mg/dl
Complete trunk	Bilirubin about 7 to 10 mg/dl
Spread to extremities	Bilirubin about 10 to 12 mg/dl
Extremities yellow—palms and soles clear	Bilirubin about 12 to 15 mg/dl
Jaundice of palms and soles	Bilirubin about 15 mg/dl

By careful nursing observation of the progress of jaundice, some blood samplings can be avoided, saving infant trauma and parental money.

The clinical significance or danger in newborn jaundice is the possibility of kernicterus. Kernicterus is a cerebral palsy–like phenomenon caused by the deposition of bilirubin in certain areas of the brain, in particular the basal ganglions. Involvement of other areas of the brain can cause varying degrees of deafness, mental deficiency, and other disorders. Kernicterus is a result of the diffusion of free indirect bilirubin across the blood-brain barrier in newborns and can result from a variety of causes, such as infection and prematurity. In fact, kernicterus in premature infants can occur without markedly elevated levels of serum bilirubin.[10]

Since indirect bilirubin is carried from the spleen to the liver by a carrier protein, it is unavailable for diffusion out of the circulation. If the level of bilirubin produced exceeds the carrying capacity of the serum proteins, however, some of the lipid-soluble bilirubin will be free in the serum. It is this lipid-soluble, free, indirect bilirubin that can diffuse into the lipid-laden brain. Free bilirubin can become elevated in the serum if (1) production exceeds the protein-carrying capacity, (2) the protein-carrying capacity is decreased, or (3) excretion is so slow that bilirubin accumulates faster than excretion and carrying capacity is exceeded.

In the healthy full-term newborn with adequate serum proteins and no history of drug ingestion, the serum-carrying capacity for bilirubin is rarely exceeded until the serum *total bilirubin* exceeds *25 mg/dl* and the *indirect bilirubin* level exceeds *20 mg/ dl*. Indeed, so-called physiologic jaundice should be of little or no concern at all in the healthy full-term newborn until the indirect bilirubin is more than 15 mg/dl.

Since premature infants have lower serum protein levels and thus lower bilirubin-carrying capacity, they are susceptible to brain damage from kernicterus at much lower serum bilirubin levels. Certain drugs carried in the serum, especially albumin, may bind to protein more tightly than does the bilirubin. These drugs can therefore displace bilirubin from its binding sites on albumin and cause an accumulation of free indirect bilirubin. Such infants will develop kernicterus at lower serum total bilirubin levels, since such a high proportion of the total will be free bilirubin. The list of drugs that will displace bilirubin is long, but only a few are clinically important. The two of primary importance are the sulfa drugs and aspirin.

These drugs are now rarely given to infants but are frequently given to mothers and can cross the placenta. They should therefore be avoided in the pregnant woman, especially late in pregnancy and just before delivery. The use of prostaglandins and oxytocin in labor has also been implicated in neonatal jaundice.[4]

The direct concern about jaundice is that it will cause brain damage from kernicterus. Kernicterus can, however, be avoided by (1) a clear understanding of the physiology of the bilirubin process, (2) careful observation of jaundice and laboratory testing of bilirubin levels, (3) correction of pathologic states, and (4) simple interventions that will be discussed later in this chapter.

PATHOLOGIC JAUNDICE

A discussion of the pathologic causes of jaundice is beyond the scope of this chapter. Suffice it to say that they can be divided into a few large groups of diseases and will be discussed only briefly to help the nurse in differentiating them from "physiologic" jaundice. It is important to recognize pathologic jaundice to intervene early to prevent kernicterus.

Pathologic jaundice of the newborn can be classified in three large groups: (1) disease causing increased red cell hemolysis, (2) deficiency of carrier protein or binding sites, and (3) liver and metabolic disease. Some pathologic jaundice overlaps several categories. Sepsis, for example, may increase red cell destruction (hemolysis) and also decrease liver function.

In the first category are Rh hemolytic disease, ABO incompatibility, congenital spherocytosis, and other hemolytic processes. All these diseases increase bilirubin by increasing red cell breakdown. The most severe of the group is Rh disease, which can serve as a model. If Rh disease is severe, the fetus can be affected. In the affected newborn, there is usually some degree of anemia at birth; bilirubin begins to rise immediately after birth (indeed it may be elevated in the cord blood, although the placenta usually clears much of it), and it rises rapidly on the first day. This rapid rise on day one clearly differentiates hemolytic disease from physiologic jaundice, which begins on day two or three and peaks much later. Hemolytic disease must be diagnosed promptly and treated vigorously frequently by exchange transfusion, to avoid serious consequence or even death.

The second category, the decrease in binding sites for bilirubin on serum proteins, has already been discussed. The main concern here is that kernicterus can occur at lower than usual bilirubin levels. Development of a laboratory measure of free bilirubin levels helps to define the problem.

Certain conditions, such as prematurity, sepsis, hypoxia, and use of drugs, may result in a decreased production of serum proteins. Low protein levels mean decreased bilirubin-carrying capacity and thus a likelihood of kernicterus at lower bilirubin levels.

In the third category are the various enzyme-deficiency diseases, such as Crigler-Najjar syndrome, Rotor's syndrome, and others; liver damage from sepsis or hepatitis (including cytomegalovirus, toxoplasmosis, hepatitis virus, rubella, and syphilis); obstruction to bile flow (congenital biliary atresia); and metabolic problems such as galactosemia and hypothyroidism.

Characteristically most of these diseases (except sepsis and hepatitis) have a *late* onset of jaundice, often after the first week of life, and a persistent jaundice for several weeks. These causes of jaundice are rarely confused with physiologic jaundice but may be confused with "breastmilk jaundice."

BREASTMILK JAUNDICE

Breastmilk jaundice (BMJ) is a term used too loosely by many people. Often any baby being breastfed who becomes jaundiced is said to have BMJ. Most of these infants in fact have "physiologic" jaundice, and a few may have some form of pathologic jaundice. The term BMJ should be reserved for a very small number of jaundiced infants who are being breastfed who have the following characteristics:

1. Jaundice begins 5 to 7 days following birth, *after* breastmilk has come in.
2. Bilirubin rises rapidly and reaches its peak between the seventh and the tenth day.
3. Bilirubin remains elevated and jaundice remains more or less evident for several days or weeks, sometimes as long as 3 to 6 weeks.
4. Bilirubin levels drop rapidly with temporary interruption of breastfeeding and rise again with its resumption.
5. All pathologic causes of jaundice are ruled out.

BMJ is probably responsible for no more than 1 in 50 to 1 in 200[5,11] cases of jaundice in breastfed infants and is often erroneously diagnosed. The cause of BMJ is unknown but is probably some compound in the milk that either increases red cell hemolysis or liver excretion of bilirubin. If the neonate is mature, breastfeeding need not be discontinued.

INTERVENTIONS

"Physiologic" jaundice in the newborn is a common entity affecting perhaps as many as 40% of all infants. If serial serum bilirubin measurements were routinely taken, there would probably be some elevation of serum bilirubin in all babies. A condition affecting such a large number of infants can therefore be referred to as "physiologic" and in general can be considered nonpathologic. Indeed, if the condition had pathologic significance, mankind would probably not have reached its present state of evolutionary development. Interventions should be conservative, with careful observation of the infant, avoidance of separation of mother and infant, and institution of light therapy if bilirubin levels rise excessively.

Light therapy

Light therapy has been a major innovation for infants with "physiologic" jaundice but is being remarkably overdone at the present time. The use of light therapy originated in South America in the 1950's but did not reach significance in the United States until the late 1960's and early 1970's, when it was introduced and its use extolled by Lucey of the University of Vermont. Studies in a number of centers around the country have defined and refined the use of light therapy on a more scientific and rational basis.

The initial data indicating the efficacy of light therapy came from biochemical laboratories where bilirubin in serum or other diluting fluids left undisturbed in a lighted area of the laboratory was seen to lose its yellow color after a few hours. What happened was that light in the blue end of the spectrum was absorbed by the yellow pigment of the bilirubin and caused a reaction in which the bilirubin became colorless and water soluble. This is identical with the physiologic reaction that enables the bilirubin to be easily excreted into the urine.

Only blue light in the 460 to 480 nm wavelength range is effective in accomplishing this, and thus plain light or even sunlight, which contains a broad spectrum of light wavelengths, is somewhat less effective than fluorescent light, particularly that which emanates from new bulbs or bulbs especially formulated to emit light in the blue end of the spectrum.

There are some dangers to light therapy in that the blue light can cause damage to the cornea and possibly to the retina. The eyes of the baby should therefore be covered during light therapy. Additionally, the light may cause the reduction of bilirubin to biliverdin, the green pigment that can also be excreted by the liver. This green pigment, biliverdin, may then be excreted into the bile and into the stool and may result in liquid green stools in a number of infants. This should be explained to the parents. If these stools become excessive and the baby sweats from the heat of the light, dehydration may occur. Fluid balance must therefore be carefully watched during light therapy, and frequent breastfeedings should continue to prevent dehydration. There have been occasional sporadic reports of DNA modification,[9] riboflavin deficiency,[6] and growth retardation in animals exposed to prolonged and intensive light therapy; however, none of these dangers have been specifically found in human infants exposed to relatively short and less intensive light than that used in the experiments.

In general, light therapy is an effective means of treating jaundice in babies, but because of inherent known and unknown dangers, I recommend its use conservatively. As indicated previously *there is no scientific evidence that bilirubin levels less than 20 mg/dl in the first 3 days of life and less than 25 mg/dl after that are of any harmful effect in full-term infants who are healthy and not receiving drug therapy.* I have arbitrarily chosen a bilirubin value of 15 mg/dl at which to institute light therapy to prevent the serum bilirubin from reaching a level of 20 mg/dl. If the bilirubin level is rising extremely rapidly (more than 1 mg/hr) light therapy is occasionally begun at a lower serum bilirubin level. With a premature or sick infant light therapy is begun at a still lower bilirubin level. In the otherwise healthy full-term infant, however, there is no scientific justification for instituting light therapy at serum bilirubin levels below 15 mg/dl.

If, in spite of light therapy, the bilirubin continues to rise and reaches a level that exceeds 20 mg/dl of indirect bilirubin in the first 3 days of life of 25 mg/dl of indirect bilirubin in the first 3 days of life or 25 mg/dl thereafter, I institute exchange transfusion as the treatment of choice for the serum bilirubin levels. It should be pointed out that this rarely if ever occurs in "physiologic" jaundice, and indeed, if bilirubin values are found to exceed 15 mg/dl, there should be a diligent search for some pathologic cause of the jaundice.

Treatment of pathologic jaundice

The treatment of pathologic jaundice requires first of all the identification of the cause of the jaundice and its elimination. It is frequently said that the treatment of pathologic jaundice is usually exchange transfusion; however, it should be pointed out that exchange transfusion is less effective than identifying and treating the primary cause of the disease. In Rh or ABO incompatibility the management is similar to that of "physiologic" jaundice except that light therapy or exchange transfusion may be initiated earlier if the bilirubin levels rise rapidly. Indeed, in the presence of severe Rh disease, exchange transfusion at birth when serum bilirubin levels are still low may be the best way to remove the Rh antibody–coated red cells and thus prevent hemolysis and jaundice. If the bilirubin is found to be rising at a rate exceeding 1 mg/hr shortly after birth, the bilirubin will probably reach pathologic levels (exceeding 20 mg/dl) within a few hours and thus the early use of exchange transfusion is indicated. If the bilirubin rises slowly, institution of light therapy at bilirubin levels between 5 and 10 mg/dl may be indicated, with the institution of exchange transfusion if the bilirubin level approaches 20 mg/dl.

Treating breastmilk jaundice

The cause of breastmilk jaundice is at present unknown. However, it is thought to be perhaps a combination of "physiologic" jaundice and some factor that is transmitted in the breastmilk. In 1964, Arias and associates[2] reported high levels of a steroid pregnane-3(alpha), 20 (beta)-diol in breastmilk and felt that this metabolite was the cause of breastmilk jaundice. Others[7,8] have disputed this contention, although all agree that the basic cause of breastmilk jaundice is probably the exaggeration of the "physiologic" jaundice process by some compound or hormone transmitted to susceptible infants in the breastmilk of certain women. Whatever this compound may be, it appears to be nontoxic and nonharmful to the infant except for the production of jaundice.

Two theories about the development of BMJ have been proposed: (1) that the hormone compound in the milk may increase red cell hemolysis and (2) that it may depress the glucuronyl transferase of the liver. Whatever the mechanism, breastmilk jaundice is rare and can usually best be managed conservatively. Since BMJ usually does not appear until about the fifth day after birth, following a rise in the albumin-carrying capacity of the blood, bilirubin levels can safely be allowed to rise to higher levels than when an infant is younger. I assume here that the neonate in question is otherwise a normal, healthy infant and that all other causes of jaundice have been excluded. If that assumption is true, it can also be assumed that the baby's blood-brain barrier has matured sufficiently to withstand bilirubin levels up to 25 mg/dl. If the infant is still in the hospital when BMJ develops, light therapy may be introduced at bilirubin levels in excess of 15 mg/dl, but since the bilirubin does not usually peak until 7 to 10 days after birth, the baby will usually be home before the peak. Exchange transfusion is rarely if ever needed in the infant with BMJ.

Exposure of the baby to sunlight or light at home may help to keep the bilirubin levels low. If, however, the bilirubin level rises significantly, interruption of breastfeeding for 12 to 24 hours will result in a marked fall. When the mother resumes breastfeeding the serum bilirubin level will slowly rise, usually not quite to its earlier level. If the bilirubin does rise to this level again (3 to 5 days), breastfeeding may possibly again be interrupted for 12 to 24 hours. This cycle may be repeated until the bilirubin level stays down or begins to fall permanently.

Having cared for thousands of breastfed infants, I have seen a few hundred with breastmilk jaundice and have done exchange transfusions for breastmilk jaundice on only two occasions in 20 years of medical practice. Indeed, these two transfusions were done in my younger years when I had less experience!

It must be emphasized again that rarely, *if ever,* should breastfeeding be interrupted because of the presence of jaundice. This is the case even in infants with pathologic jaundice. If the infant is sick, the breastfeeding may need to be momentarily interrupted during an exchange transfusion or intensive treatment with intravenous fluids and drugs; however, the mother can maintain her milk supply by pumping and resume breastfeeding as soon as her infant's condition improves. Giving moral support along with a breast pump or instructions in hand pumping is important at this time.

SIMPLIFIED GUIDE TO THE CARE OF THE JAUNDICED NEWBORN
Normal healthy infant

If jaundice begins on the first day after birth, pathologic jaundice should be suspected. A maternal history taken previously should alert the pediatrician at the infant's birth to the possibility of hemolytic disease, and appropriate preparations should have been already made. If there is no preexisting history, the baby's blood type should be determined, and Rh and Coombs' tests should be immediately performed to rule out the presence of blood group incompatibility and hemolytic disease. An examination of the peripheral smear of the baby should be made to rule out such problems such as congenital spherocytosis. A careful physical examination should be performed on the infant for signs of other diseases such as sepsis or hepatitis. In an American Indian or an infant of Mediterranean extraction, a test for glucose 6-phosphate dehydrogenase (G6-PD) should be done. Tests for hypothyroidism, galactosemia, and other metabolic diseases should also be performed. Medical intervention then consists of the following appropriate treatment if any pathologic conditions are found: light therapy at bilirubin levels between 5 and 10 mg/dl if the rate of rise in the bilirubin is less than 0.5 mg/hr; exchange transfusion if the bilirubin level exceeds 20 mg/dl or the rate of rise exceeds 1 mg/hr in the presence of known hemolytic disease or if anemia is present. Appropriate supportive treatment for other existing diseases should be carried out. Breastfeeding should be continued if the infant is not too lethargic or ill to suckle. For example, the mother can breastfeed the infant between exchange transfusions or during light therapy. Bilirubin lights, as well as mothers and infants, are portable.

If the bilirubin level begins to rise on the second or third day and rises slowly, daily or twice or thrice daily bilirubin levels should be determined for the infant once jaundice is detected. The number and frequency of the bilirubin determinations should be done according to the rate of rise in the serum bilirubin level and the clinical signs of jaundice. The infant should be examined to rule out pathologic causes of jaundice, and the maternal history should be examined. A blood group typing, Rh test, and Coombs' test are performed to exclude possible hemolytic disease of the newborn. Assuming that all the pathologic causes of jaundice have been ruled out, the infant can be conservatively managed by continuing breastfeedings and by the institution of light therapy if the serum bilirubin exceeds 15 mg/dl. Exchange transfusions should be carried out if the serum bilirubin exceeds 20 mg/dl in the first 72 hours after birth or 25 mg/dl thereafter. Since dehydration will increase the serum bilirubin level, it should be avoided by having the infant suckle more frequently to stimulate the early, optimal flow of breastmilk. The institution of supplemental feedings or water supplements at this time is *not* appropriate, since this will decrease the infant's suckling and thus inhibit the mother's milk supply.

Giving water supplements for jaundice is frequently encouraged by medical and nursing personnel in many hospitals. It is erroneously thought that the use of water feedings will prevent dehydration and thus prevent physiologic jaundice. Indeed, there is *no* scientific evidence that the institution of water feedings at this point will in any way affect the physiologic rise in bilirubin, and it may, in fact, deter the establishment of breastfeeding. Supplements are therefore to be strongly discouraged in the management of physiologic jaundice, but frequent "on demand" suckling should be strongly encouraged to establish the milk flow and prevent dehydration.

Nurses and physicians should encourage rooming-in or frequently take the baby to the mother. If the infant needs light therapy, the mother may breastfeed often by going to the nursery and removing the baby. This will in no way harm the baby. An even better method is to place the incubator or crib with the light over it in the mother's room so that the mother can breastfeed the infant as often as she wishes. In milder cases light therapy can be carried out at home by exposing the infant to light from a window or taking him outside. Another self-care measure at home is to use a "grow light" (a light bulb commercially available to aid in the growing of house plants). Careful instructions on its use, including protecting the infant's eyes, must be given to the parents.

If jaundice begins after the third day, breastmilk jaundice should be suspected. The infant with breastmilk jaundice is most effectively cared for by conservative measures: encouraging frequent breastfeedings and thus hydration of the infant and monitoring the bilirubin level carefully on a daily basis. After the first 3 days of life, bilirubin levels can be allowed to rise to 25 mg/dl before intervention is necessary. At that time, exchange transfusion is rarely if ever indicated. Simply interrupting breastfeeding for 12 to 24 hours will be sufficient to allow lowering of the serum bilirubin level with a slow rise over the next 3 to 5 days, possibly followed by another short interruption. During an interruption, the mother can be encouraged to continue to pump her breasts to maintain her milk supply, breastfeeding again at the end of the interruption. This has worked successfully for my patients in several hundred cases. No permanent interruption of breastfeeding is necessary.

Sick infant

In the infant who is at full term but is found to be sick from one cause or another, different techniques must be followed. Illness may be due to many causes, such as congenital abnormalities, sepsis, or intrapartum asphyxia. In these illnesses, the blood-brain barrier may be more susceptible to the transport of bilirubin at lower serum bilirubin levels. There may be more hemolysis or a decrease in albumin-carrying capacity for bilirubin. Thus the bilirubin levels cannot safely be allowed to rise as high as in well infants of the same age. The bilirubin level at which intervention should be carried out is generally lowered by approximately 5 mg/dl; that is, light therapy is introduced at a level of approximately 10 mg/dl and exchange transfusion carried out at 15 mg/dl. If the infant is able to take anything by mouth, he can be breastfed. In those infants who cannot, the mother's milk can still be given to her baby through a nasogastric tube until she can breastfeed her infant.

Premature infant

The rules for premature care must be as strict as or stricter than those for the sick infant. The premature infant will generally have lower serum albumin levels and thus less bilirubin-carrying capacity and will also have a blood-brain barrier that is more susceptible to the diffusion of bilirubin into the brain. Therefore it is important that the infant be monitored carefully and bilirubin levels controlled at lower values. If the premature infant is simply of a low gestational age but otherwise healthy and has no respiratory distress, sepsis, or other illness, then treatment is much like that for the sick infant. If the infant is both premature and ill, intervention must be still more conservative, and light therapy may be instituted at 5 mg/dl and exchange transfusion at 10 mg/dl.

Breastmilk for ill and premature infants has multiple advantages. These infants, particularly the sick ones, may be unable to suckle because of their illness or because of a lack of strength. However, breastmilk can be pumped from the mother and stored or frozen for later use for the infant. As the infant improves, the breastmilk can be given by nasogastric tube. Again, jaundice should not be the precluding factor in determining whether these infants can receive human milk either directly from the breast or administered indirectly through a nasogastric tube. The jaundice should be managed appropriately to the child's condition without reference to the source of milk, which in all probability contributes little or nothing to the course of the jaundice and, indeed, is beneficial overall for the infant.

SUMMARY

Jaundice in the newborn, in most cases, is an exaggeration of a normal physiologic process that can be managed conservatively and is not a contraindication to breastfeeding. If we understand the normal physiologic process and intervene only when absolutely necessary, there is no contraindication to the neonate's consumption of human milk either by direct suckling at the breast or by tube feeding for those who may be too small or too young to suckle.

Breastfeeding should never be interrupted because of "physiologic" jaundice and should be rarely if ever interrupted even for pathologic jaundice. Even in the presence of jaundice that is brought about by the breastmilk itself, there is no reason to interrupt breastfeeding permanently. Breastfeedings should be strongly encouraged by *all* mothers and for *all* babies.

REFERENCES

1. Arias, I.M., and Gartner, L.M.: Jaundice in breastfed neonates, J.A.M.A. **218**:746, 1971.
2. Arias, I.M., et al.: Prolonged neonatal unconjugated hyperbilirubinemia associated with breastfeeding and a steroid in maternal milk that inhibits glucuronide formation in vitro, J. Clin. Invest. **43**:2037, 1964.
3. Brown, W.R., and Wong, H.B.: Ethnic group difference in plasma bilirubin levels of full-term Singapore newborns, Pediatrics **36**:745, 1965.
4. Calder, A.A., et al.: Increased bilirubin levels in neonates after introduction of labor by intravenous E_2 or oxytocin, Lancet **2**:1339, 1974.
5. Gartner, L.M.: Jaundice in the breastfed infant. In Lawrence, R., editor: Counseling the mother on breastfeeding, Report of the Eleventh Ross Roundtable on critical approaches to common pediatric problems, Columbus, Ohio, 1980, Ross Laboratories.
6. Gromisch, D.S., et al.: Light (phototherapy)-induced riboflavin deficiency in the neonate, J. Pediatr. **90**:118, 1977.
7. Hargreaves, T., and Piper, R.F.: Breast milk jaundice: effect of inhibitory breast milk and 3 alpha, 20 abeta-pregnanediol on glucuronyl transferase, Arch. Dis. Child. **46**:195, 1971.
8. Ramos, A., et al.: Pregnanediols and neonatal hyperbilirubinemia Am. J. Dis. Child. **111**:353, 1966.
9. Speck, W.T.: Intracellular DNA modifying potential of phototherapy, Pediatr. Res. **10**:432, 1976.
10. Tunkel, S.B., et al.: Lack of identifiable factors for kernicterus, Pediatrics **66**:502, 1980.
11. Winfield, C.R., and McFaul, R.: Clinical study of prolonged jaundice in breast- and bottle-fed babies, Arch. Dis. Child. **53**:506, 1978.

ADDITIONAL READINGS

Countryman, B.A.: Breastfeeding and jaundice, Franklin Park, Ill., 1978, La Leche League International.

Dahms, B.B., et al.: Breastfeeding and serum bilirubin levels during the first 4 days of life, J. Pediatr. **83**:1049, 1973.

Gartner, L.M., and Lee, K.S.: Jaundice in the breastfed infant: new concept of pathogenesis. In Frier, S., and Eidelman, A.I., editors: Human milk: its biological and social value, Amsterdam, 1980, Excerpta Medica.

Simkin, P., Simkin, M.D., and Edwards, M.: "Physiologic" jaundice of the newborn, Birth Fam. J. **6**:23, 1979.

11

Slow weight gain

KITTIE B. FRANTZ

The slow-gaining breastfeeding infant is a perplexing problem in pediatric nursing. To those of us who are convinced that human milk is the best food for infants and that the psychologic benefits are of the highest value in feeding infants throughout the first year, it is quite a distressing problem. Although our cultural beliefs place a special emphasis on a fat infant as a "healthy" infant, medical science tells us that obesity is not a sign of health.

The mother, father, relatives, doctors, and neighbors express concern about an infant who appears thin or malnourished and looks as if he is not thriving. The problem is obvious when an infant acts hungry, is irritable, and cries often. Other slow-gaining infants appear quite satisfied and do not seem uncomfortable. These problems are carefully examined in this chapter to provide some practical answers. Although problems sometimes arise with breastfeeding, they almost *always* have solutions that allow mothers to continue breastfeeding. All too often with slow-gaining breastfed infants, the health-care provider summarily recommends weaning. With a little effort, a proper diagnosis can be made and the poor weight gain corrected without interrupting the breastfeeding.

FAILURE TO THRIVE
Normal criteria of growth

Although our culture perceives a healthy infant as a fat infant (the "Gerber" look), the appropriate growth criteria for the normal newborn require only that the infant's birth weight be regained at least by the third week.[4] Infants who are breastfed usually regain birth weight sooner. Weight norms collected in the last century show that infants should double their birth weight at about 5 to 6 months and triple their birth weight by 1 year.[15] Some bottle-fed infants tend to gain more weight than their breastfed counterparts do in the first months.[11] Here, too, the "ideal" baby has been equated with what is really obesity instead of appropriate growth and development. A genetic factor appears to define normal growth for the individual infant. Some mothers of slow-gaining infants often discover that they too were slow in gaining weight as infants. It may be

Sections of this chapter are taken from Frantz, K.B., Fleiss, P.M., and Lawrence, R.A.: Management of the slow-gaining breastfed baby, Keeping Abreast J. **3**:287, 1978.

that some of the fat infants are going to be more susceptible to disease than are some of the thin infants. It is known that fat infants are likely to become fat children[5] and later fat adults with all the implications of potential diabetes, high blood pressure, and heart disease.

Other important criteria to consider in the question of failure to thrive (FTT) are the infant's length and head circumference. An infant should be one and a half times the birth length at 1 year. Head circumference will indicate much about brain growth. In the first year an infant's head will grow 7.6 cm (3 inches); and it will grow another 7.6 cm in the next 16 years of life. Thus a lean infant with appropriate growth in length and head circumference may be a very vigorous, developmentally normal, healthy infant having only minor feeding problems.

Growth charts

How is a normal but slow-gaining infant differentiated from one who is failing to thrive? Plotting the infant's growth on a growth chart can give a clear indication of the infant's progress using standard deviations or percentiles as a criterion. For example, if an infant's weight is below the 3rd percentile line on a growth chart, this is one of the criteria for FTT. Each child, however, has an individual potential of growth and a

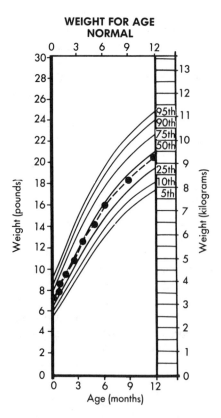

Fig. 11-1. Typical weight gain pattern of breastfeeding infant.

predictable growth curve (Fig. 11-1). Thus it is important to consider other factors when looking at the 3rd-percentile criterion of FTT. Familial weight and stature are also important. For instance, the weight and stature of a child with slight parents would be expected to fall well below the 50th percentile. Since percentiles are based on statistical data, 49 out of 100 children fall below the 50th percentile. Similarly 4 out of 100 children fall below the 5th percentile. Thus for some children, a slow weight gain is normal (Fig. 11-2). The same caution should be used in determining the predictable growth from his birth weight; for example, prematurity, low birth weight, or high birth weight should be evaluated.

The second FTT criterion is a drop of two percentile lines in a 56-day period for an infant under 5 months (Fig. 11-3) or a 3-month period for older infants.[3] If the infant was small, well developed, and on the 10th percentile at birth, dropping a little is not as significant as if he had dropped from the 75th to the 30th percentile. Plotting the weight gain on a predicted growth curve for a specific infant is really the best way to tell whether there is a deviation from the "normal" pattern.

An evaluation of nationwide growth curves shows that the Iowa growth curves are for much taller people, whereas the Boston growth curves are for shorter, slightly heavier babies. The Denver charts for the newborn give rates for smaller infants, but these

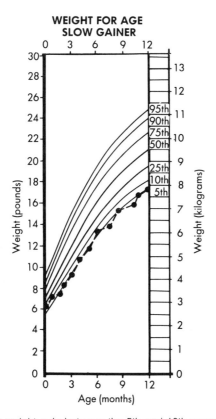

Fig. 11-2. Normal, steady weight gain between the 5th and 10th percentile in a healthy but small infant.

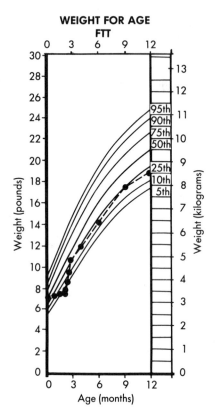

Fig. 11-3. Weight curve of breastfeeding infant who is failing to thrive with drop of two standard deviations within 2 months before correction of problem.

are based on infants born 1 mile above sea level who may be smaller than infants born at sea level.[6]

A typical FTT infant is described in the medical literature as having (1) a weight below the 3rd percentile, (2) a drop in length and head circumference growth, and (3) a fall of two standard deviations on a weight curve. As often described in the literature, this infant looks like a "little old man," acts lethargic, makes little eye contact, may resist being held, is developmentally delayed, may ruminate (regurgitate) after feeding, has unusual watchful expressions, is unable to be soothed or comforted, and is irritable.[2]

In contrast, many breastfed, slow-gaining infants are only growth-delayed in weight. They are usually alert and contented, make frequent eye contact, and smile readily. They love being held to the extent that they close their eyes at the breast and suckle poorly for long periods, only protesting when removed from the breast. They often breastfeed all day long in almost continuous feedings. They can be developmentally normal or even advanced, do not ruminate, and urinate normally because of their continual ingestion of foremilk, but they have infrequent stools because they do not suckle strongly enough to bring down the hindmilk or cream content.

What is the difference between FTT and healthy but slow-gaining infants? Why are they completely different with only a weight gain problem in common?

FACTORS CONTRIBUTING TO SLOW WEIGHT GAIN

A variety of factors can be responsible for a breastfed infant's growth not falling into his predicted curve. There may be problems with the infant, with the mother, with the breastfeeding technique, or any combination of these. For example, a sick infant is not always able to suckle well. Uusually when a breastfeeding infant fails to gain well, the first response is to discontinue breastfeeding and substitute formula-feeding. Only if the infant continues to do poorly is illness considered. Illness should be considered *first* before breastfeeding is stopped, or the diagnosis may be incorrect.

Infant problems

A glaring example is a mother who complained that her infant was not breastfeeding well and was getting little milk. She was told over the phone to stop breastfeeding and begin bottle-feeding. When examined later, the infant was found to have meningitis. Otitis media and urinary tract infections have been very common causes of poor suck-ling. Just like adults, infants sometimes lose their appetite when they are sick. Whether they are breastfeeding or bottle-feeding, they may make only a feeble attempt to suckle. A feeble attempt to suckle the breast yields less milk than from the bottle because milk flows more easily from a bottle.

Some infants with Down's syndrome have a weak suckle, whereas others suckle very well. The poor sucklers just need a little more encouragement, not a bottle. This is often true of neurologic disorders also. Mothers simply need more confidence that they are doing the right thing. Sometimes all that is needed to turn poor breastfeeding into successful breastfeeding is encouragement to the mother and an explanation about breastfeeding benefits.

Cystic fibrosis is associated with poor weight gain. One infant with cystic fibrosis who never had any other problems or illness in early infancy except poor weight gain was weaned from the breast at 18 months and began drinking cow's milk. His condition suddenly changed, and he developed all the other symptoms typical of an infant with cystic fibrosis. Breastfeeding this infant prevented the early development of the pulmo-nary symptoms of the disease. Although he was on the 3rd percentile from birth, he maintained a constant weight gain. Other conditions commonly associated with FTT are chronic regurgitation, intestinal malabsorption syndrome, chronic heart failure, idio-pathic hypercalcemia, Turner's syndrome, some chromosome disorders, renal insuffi-ciency, and some malignancies.

Hypothyroidism in the infant can also be a factor; however, recent studies indicate that human milk may contain some thyroid hormone to delay severe hypothyroidism.[14] Often initial symptoms of hypothyroidism are poor suckling, slow weight gain, and infrequent stools.

A rare problem is diencephalic syndrome (brain tumor). An example is the mother who was told she was not supplying enough calories to her infant. She was advised to switch to bottle-feeding when her child was 10 months old, and his weight fell two standard deviations. This information was confusing to the mother because the infant was an avid breastfeeder and ate more solid food than her eldest child did. The mother sought several opinions before the brain tumor was finally discovered when the child was 2 years of age.

Infants with jaundice sometimes do not suckle well because of lethargy in the first week, but this is no reason to stop breastfeeding. True breastmilk jaundice syndrome is caused either by steroids in the mother's milk or by other unknown factors that inhibit bilirubin reabsorption (see Chapter 10). It usually does not occur until the end of the first week or the beginning of the second week of life and rarely causes the lethargy found in hyperbilirubinemia of other cause. Premature infants may often be slower to gain weight because of weaker suckling and frequent pausing during the feeding to rest. Identification and treatment of the illness or problem while preserving breastfeeding should be the ultimate goal.

Maternal problems

Problems with the mother can include poor nutrition, poor health, family stress, effects of drugs, or a lack of being able to nurture. One mother who sought professional help because her infant was not gaining well had taken thyroid medication before and during her pregnancy. She stopped taking it, fearing that the drug would harm her infant. At 2 months of age, her infant had not regained his birth weight. What had happened? She had symptoms of hypothyroidism. Correcting the mother's thyroid medication dose will often result in the infant's again gaining weight. Thyroid-deficient mothers may not produce enough milk, and this lack of adequate milk can be one of the diagnostic signs of hypothyroidism in the mother.

Drugs taken by a woman, particularly birth control pills, can decrease her milk supply. Other drugs that are sometimes suspect are antihistamines in large regular doses, sedatives, and barbiturates. Some mothers can do without these drugs while breastfeeding or at least lower the dose if the physician agrees.

Extremely poor nutrition in the mother can somewhat decrease the quantity of milk but has little effect on its composition. Mothers who are *very* poor eaters over a long period of time may not produce quite enough milk. The result is an infant who has to breastfeed more frequently to make up for the differences in volume. Analysis of human milk shows few differences in the amount of protein in the breastmilk of well-nourished Swedish mothers and starving mothers in Pakistan and Afghanistan. Vitamins and minerals were slightly less in the malnourished mothers, but the milk of these mothers had more immune factors.[9] In the United States, breastfeeding mothers are usually given extra vitamins to make up for any deficiencies in their diets. In the case of poor nutrition, proper counseling about diet should be done with referral to government food subsidy programs (WIC) for women who qualify.

Some clinicians feel that stress and emotional upsets may cause problems. If a mother is under a great deal of tension or if she has ambivalent feelings about breastfeeding, she may have problems "letting down" enough milk for her infant. A poor let-down does not reward the infant, so he may develop a lazy suckle, which fails to extract enough milk or stimulate an adequate milk supply. Some stress can be alleviated, but if that is not possible, other suggestions can be made. A glass of wine, soft music, and a comfortable chair may help improve the let-down during a feeding. At least one clinician has found that "grooming" the infant (stroking, singing to the infant) relaxes the mother, enhancing her maternal feelings and thus her let-down.[16] I have found, however, after working with 300 poorly gaining breastfed infants in the last 6-year period, that poor weight gain associated with poor milk ejection is rare.

Difficulties in the mother-infant interaction and a lack of attachment likewise must be considered. This has been termed environmental FTT and refers to the emotionally deprived infant who fails to gain weight because he has not established trust in a single caretaker and has given up hope. This infant is usually developmentally as well as growth delayed. This FTT is usually seen in bottle-feeding infants who participate in some sort of self-feeding (such as bottle propping) with very little positive interaction between the mother and the infant.

Environmental FTT has also been seen in the breastfeeding mother but rarely. This probably occurs more often in the emotionally deprived mother who was forced into breastfeeding by a well-meaning relative or allergist. It can also be seen in the infant who was placed in a nonnurturing child care setting while his nurturing mother went back to work.

Improper breastfeeding techniques

Although a sick infant or sick mother may be a factor in slow gaining for infants, by far the most common factor I see in clinical practice is improper breastfeeding techniques. Even though infants have been breastfed for thousands of years, some women, in our culture especially, need help to breastfeed successfully.

Scheduling and limited sucking time. One problem of technique is breastfeeding on a 4-hour schedule. Mothers start off observing this feeding schedule in the hospital or are wrongly advised to follow it at home. Infants who are fed formula feed on a 3- to 4-hour schedule, and breastfeeding mothers are often given advice appropriate for bottle-feeding. The lower protein and different types of fat plus the higher amount of lactalbumin in human milk are more easily and rapidly assimilated, making breastfeeding almost a continuous feeding situation. Newborns may breastfeed every 2 or 3 hours or even more often. Premature infants need to breastfeed even more often because of a smaller stomach capacity and a slightly weaker suckle. *Limiting the time and frequency of suckling to a 4-hour schedule is inadequate for breastfed infants to gain sufficient weight.*

Cow's milk also has about three times more tryptophan, a soporific agent, than does human milk. Thus infants fed cow's milk or cow's milk–based formula may sleep more than do breastfed infants.[3] This could be a disadvantage for the bottle-fed infant in that as the result of more frequent feedings the breastfed infant is held more often, cuddled more, and interacted with more frequently. To the mother who does not like being on call 24 hours a day, frequent breastfeeding may seem a disadvantage. When explanations are given, however, most mothers seem to relax and accept this schedule.

In addition to restricted scheduling of feedings, consumer literature often wrongly advises limiting the amount of suckling time to prevent sore nipples. If the proper breastfeeding techniques are followed and the infant is not allowed to "chew the nipple," it is not necessary to limit suckling time, especially after hospital discharge. When mothers do limit breastfeeding to 3 or 5 minutes on each breast, the infant cannot breastfeed long enough to stimulate the milk let-down and thus obtain adequate milk to gain weight after the third or fourth day of life. Hall[8] points out that since cream content is much higher toward the end of the feeding, restriction of suckling time could rob the infant of necessary calories. Most free pamphlets given to mothers about breastfeeding give inaccurate advice, and mothers are led to believe that this is the right thing to do. No wonder they cannot understand why their infants are still crying and losing weight when they have faithfully breastfed 5 to 10 minutes on each side every 4 hours as they thought they should.

When a mother restricts breastfeeding time and then supplements her infant who is still obviously hungry, she begins, unwittingly, the process of weaning. The breasts receive less and less stimulation, and the milk supply continues to decrease until the infant ultimately rejects the breast in favor of the faster flowing bottle. For years the medical profession believed that infants obtain 80% to 90% of the milk from the breast in the first 5 minutes, but this assumption is no longer accepted.[8] The milk is let down several times during a feeding, and the volume of milk received depends on the length of the feeding and the strength of the infant's suckling. Even in a normally suckling infant, 5 minutes is not adequate. Women should switch breasts *several times during the feeding* to assure a let-down and breastfeed very often so the infant has an opportunity to obtain adequate milk. More important than even the frequency or duration of the feedings is the strength of the suckle in facilitating the let-downs and obtaining an adequate amount of milk and fat content for the infant.

Supplemental bottles. Supplemental feedings with bottles may increase the weight gain, but they often ruin the chance of successful breastfeeding. The use of supplemental bottles causes the infant to go longer periods between feedings, thus reducing the amount of breast stimulation. Also, the sucking action in feeding from an artificial nipple is quite different from suckling the maternal nipple. In breastfeeding, the infant's jaws compress the areola behind the nipple, which has been drawn far back into the infant's mouth by a forward-backward tongue motion and some suction. This jaw compression forces the milk toward the nipple. The posterior tongue pushes the nipple up against the palate, which further pushes the milk out of the nipple and down the pharynx. The infant's lips purse downward with the jaw action. This is a threefold "chewing" action that can be easily observed in the normal breastfeeding infant.

When sucking an artificial nipple, however, the action of tongue, lips, and jaw is very different. Since liquid flows easily from the bottle nipple, infants frequently position the tongue at the tip of the rubber nipple, thrusting forward and slightly upward to slow down the flow to keep from gagging. The jaws do not need to compress the nipple to extract the liquid, so there is little chewing movement of the jaw. When the infant tries to suckle the breast in the same way, he fails to extract the milk from the breast effectively or to stimulate the milk let-down. This is called "nipple confusion" and often results in a frustrated infant who begins to prefer the bottle. Removing the bottle supplement and stimulating a stronger suckle at the breast may be all that is needed.

Improper positioning. An improper breastfeeding position can create suckling problems. If the infant is not held closely enough, the infant's jaws grasp and manipulate only the nipple instead of compressing and manipulating the areolar portion of the breast. When this happens, the infant may not be able to stimulate a good let-down of the milk, and the mother will surely develop a protracted case of sore nipples. Also, nipple suckling does not allow adequate extraction of milk from the sinuses under the areola by compression. Babies who suckle the breast with a nipple shield over the areola also cannot effectively compress the sinuses under the areola to obtain sufficient milk.

Breastfeeding from only one breast at a feeding. Mothers should breastfeed from both breasts, but sometimes hospital routines recommend breastfeeding on only one breast per feeding. The mother's discomfort from an episiotomy or cesarean birth may make it hard for her to turn over to reposition the infant. Eventually the mother becomes accustomed to breastfeeding with only one breast per feeding and may not be stimulating an adequate supply of milk or providing enough milk for the infant. Of course, some mothers can breastfeed from just one breast and never have problems, but it should be kept in mind that infants who are *not* gaining weight adequately may begin to gain weight when both breasts are used at each feeding.

Both breasts have a let-down response at the same time. Even though one breast is being suckled, the pooling of let-down milk in the unused breast may also increase the likelihood of breast infection for the mother.[1]

True, mothers have breastfed successfully in the most absurd situations, positions, and surroundings, yet their infants thrive; however, when an infant fails to thrive, consideration must be given to *all* possible factors to help solve the problem. At the same time, support should be given for continued breastfeeding.

Negative "flutter" suckling. Most slow-gaining breastfed infants I have seen do what I call "flutter suckling." This nonnutritive suckling action is a more rapid suckle in which the infant does not draw the nipple well into the mouth. Instead, there is a licking of the nipple, followed by a very rapid uneven gumming or chewing motion of the jaws so that the areola is not well compressed, and the nipple is not drawn back into the mouth for the posterior tongue to do its job. Some infants tongue thrust more outwardly instead of drawing the breast inward. They may thrust their jaws downward instead of bringing them upward to compress the breast. The infant often falls off the breast easily if the mother moves her arm. Milk is only available to the infant when it leaks out, when milk let-down occurs, or when he momentarily suckles well.

Any time an infant is not gaining well, it is important to observe breastfeeding to determine how the infant suckles and whether the mother is using poor techniques. Practical ways of handling this include telling the mother, "I've just examined your infant and he's pretty upset. Why don't you feed him to calm him down"; or "Why don't you sit down and let him breastfeed and I'll watch what your *baby* is doing. He might be doing something wrong." Remember that the mother comes in feeling that *she* has done something horribly wrong if her infant is a slow gainer. Discussing immunizations or other things can be accomplished as the mother and infant are being observed, to put her more at ease.

As an example of FTT because of a suckling problem, the infant in Fig. 11-4 dropped two standard deviations in weight without a corresponding drop in height or head circumference. Fig. 11-5 shows the same infant after his flutter suckling problem was corrected.

Inhibited or unstable let-down. Occasionally mothers do have problems with an inhibited or unstable milk let-down reflex. If a mother is tense, it can momentarily affect the release of prolactin and oxytocin and thus inhibit the milk let-down reflex. At the same time, it is disturbing how much literature suggests that all mothers must be totally relaxed to breastfeed successfully. During World War II, however, the incidence of breastfeeding in France increased from 20% to 97%. That was certainly a period that fostered tremendous tension, yet women breastfed successfully because there was nothing else to feed their infants. It is absurd to generalize that unless a mother is a relaxed person, she cannot breastfeed.

When a severely stressful situation inhibits the let-down, supportive assistance can

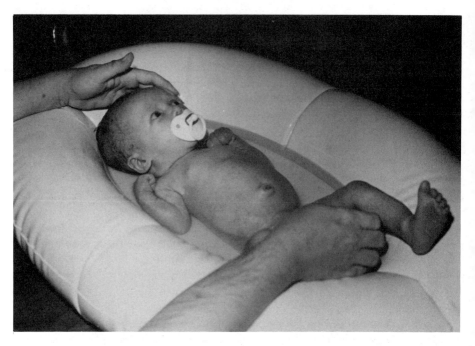

Fig. 11-4. A 2-month-old breastfed infant with failure to gain adequate weight.

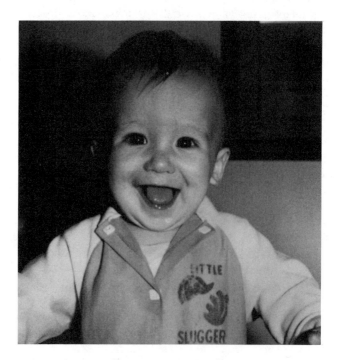

Fig. 11-5. Same infant still breastfeeding at 7 months and gaining satisfactorily after correction of suckling problem. No supplements given and solids begun at 6 months.

usually help. This can be the "booze and snooze" method recommended by Pryor[13]: a little wine, a glass of beer, a nap, soft music, a back rub, or a warm bath before feeding time. Often encouragement and praise are helpful. Sometimes all that is needed is getting the family or the husband to be supportive. Some situations, such as wife battering, cannot be corrected by the medical health-care provider alone. Referral to a psychologist, social worker, or family counseling service is a valuable adjunct to pediatric nursing care. Although chlorpromazine (Thorazine) has been used for insufficient let-down, I have found that it tranquilizes mothers so much that they are unable to function adequately, and I do not recommend its use.

Other factors that interfere with milk let-down include hormonal problems, fatigue, excessive amounts of coffee or soft drinks high in caffeine, smoking, and some drugs. Although many mothers may not be affected at all by them, they are important to consider when dealing with a slow-gaining infant. At times, it may be helpful to administer oxytocin in the form of a nasal spray (Syntocinon). It is usually sprayed into the nostril about 1 minute before breastfeeding to elicit a milk let-down. Mothers who dislike spraying it in the nose can spray it in the throat (pharynx) instead with the same effectiveness. However, it has a rebound effect (reverses the action) when used for more than a few days, so it is not something a mother could use throughout the course of breastfeeding. It is expensive, but it can be helpful, some believe, in initially proving to a mother that she has the ability to let down her milk. Its use should be followed by teaching the mother other ways to facilitate a natural let-down reflex.

On the other hand, suggesting oxytocin or discussing the let-down with a mother can create so much apprehension that she then has further trouble letting down. Minimizing the importance of the let-down while trying to build her confidence may be all that is needed; problems with the let-down reflex are not often the primary cause of the slow weight gain.

THE SLOW-GAINING INFANT SPECIAL HISTORY

So many factors are involved in evaluating the slow-gaining breastfeeding infant that Fleiss and I developed the "Slow-Gaining Special History" form (see box on pp. 222-223). This is a helpful history-taking tool in gathering all information needed to make a good assessment of the situation.

Some of the questions may deal with sensitive issues. I have found that the body language used during the interview is important. Standing with the history sheet in hand is not conducive to getting the kinds of answers needed. It helps to sit next to the mother after inviting her to sit down and breastfeed the infant. Ask questions and discuss them in a "chatting" way, face-to-face in a relaxed manner. Questions can be worded so they are not threatening to the mother. Remember that the mother may not only be very worried but may also have her mother-in-law, aunt, and everyone else telling her she is going to kill her infant if she does not begin bottle-feeding him. Being friendly and kind to the mother while asking questions will relax her, and she will respond freely to the questions. Such a relaxed atmosphere while taking the history has often resulted in mothers' confiding things they would not normally say on a first visit.

Taking the maternal history

In taking the special history, each question is explained to the mother. For example, when discussing smoking, point out that some mothers smoke and breastfeed with no

NO.____ DATE:_____

SLOW-GAINING INFANT SPECIAL HISTORY

Mother

Name_____

1. Do you smoke?_____ Which brand?_____ How many per day?_____
2. Any thyroid problems at any time in your life?_____
   Are thyroid medications being taken now?_____ What kind?_____
   Dose?_____ Last time you had your blood tested for thyroid level?_____
3. Coffee?_____ How many cups per day?_____ Caffeinated sodas?
   (Colas)_____
   How many caffeinated sodas per day?_____
4. Are you taking any medications?_____ Birth control pills?_____
   Prescription?_____ Nonprescription?_____ Which vitamins?_____
5. Do you have a busy life-style?_____ If so, why? (Name activities)_____
   _____
6. Alcohol consumption?_____ How much per day?_____ Week?_____
   Month?_____
7. When baby breastfeeds, do you feel: Tingling_____ Burning_____
   Filling_____
   Feeling_____ Leaking on other side_____ Nothing_____
   Other_____
8. Marriage relationship: Good_____ Average_____ Poor_____
   Are you seeing a counselor?_____ Other children?_____ Ages_____
   Breastfed?_____ How long?_____
9. Quiet environment for nursing?_____ If not, why? (Describe) Example:
   Loud music, freeway noise, dogs barking?_____
   _____
10. Do you have any blood pressure problems?_____
11. Are you in good health?_____ (Describe problem)_____
    _____
12. Do you eat regular meals?_____ How do you rate the kind of food you eat?
    Good_____ Poor_____ Excellent_____ Brief diet history_____
    _____
13. Any source of anxiety or tension?_____ Describe_____
    _____
14. How many children in your family while growing up?_____
    What number were you?_____
15. How would you describe your mother when you were little? Busy_____
    Warm_____ Troubled_____ Great housekeeper_____
    Other_____ Distant_____ Nurturing_____
16. What advice has she given you about spoiling the baby?_____
    _____

Baby

Name_____ Date of birth_____
1. How often is the baby fed in the daytime?_____
2. Breastmilk only?_____ Other?_____
   Do you feed from each breast at each feeding?_____
   How long on each breast?_____
3. How long does the baby take to finish a feeding?_____
   Does the baby pause a lot during feeding?_____

SLOW-GAINING INFANT SPECIAL HISTORY—cont'd

4. Who initiates end of feeding? You_____ Baby_____
5. How do you rate his suckling? Poor_____ Weak_____ Strong_____
   Average_____ Don't know_____
6. Number of wet diapers per day?_____ Are paper diapers used?_____
7. Number of stools per day?_____ Per week?_____ Consistency?___
   Color_____
8. Burping easy?_____ Technique used?_____ When burped?_
   Does he spit up?_____ Vomit?_____ How often?_____
9. Activity of baby: Active_____ Placid_____ Average_____
   Developmental progress: Average_____ Advanced_____ Slow_____
10. Is a pacifier used?_____ What kind?____ How much usage?_____
    Does he suck his thumb or fingers?_____
11. Night sleep pattern: Time put to bed_____ Is this on a regular basis?___
    List awake times:_____
12. Baby healthy?_____ Any problems since birth?_____ If so, what?_
    Jaundice?_____ How high was the bilirubin?_____
    Had any medications?_____ If so, what?_____
13. Ever had a urinalysis?_____ When?_____ Any other tests
    (Especially those for slow weight gain?)_____
    If so, what?_____
    Where?_____

Birth history

1. How long were you in labor?_____
2. Were medications given during labor or delivery?_____ If so, what?_____
3. First time the baby was put to breast was_____ hours/minutes after birth.
   Did the baby take to it easily?_____
4. Was it a difficult birth?_____ If so, describe problem:_____
   _____
5. Home birth?_____ Hospital with rooming-in?_____ Hospital with
   baby only in the nursery?_____ Were you separated from the baby for
   any length of time?_____ If so, why?_____ And how long?_____
6. Any medications taken during pregnancy?_____ If so, what?_____
7. Any medications taken after birth?_____ If so, what?_____

problems, yet other mothers may not do well. Ask the mother who smokes heavily to reduce her smoking to less than 10 cigarettes a day. A suggestion to eliminate the cigarettes she really does not need (such as the ones smoked while talking on the phone or having a cup of coffee) evokes a receptive response from most mothers. Many have found it quite easy to cut down this way. If the mother must smoke, she should do it in a room away from the infant. This may cut down "side stream" smoke as an irritant to the infant. Of course, the question arises, "What about marijuana?" Whether mothers smoke marijuana, tobacco, or other substances, none are proven good or harmless around other people, especially infants.

Thyroid problems. When asked about thyroid problems, some mothers reveal that they had problems during adolescence but not since. Since pregnancy can change thyroid levels, such mothers need to be checked again. A low thyroid level can decrease milk production. It is important to know whether a mother is on thyroid medication, as well as the dose, type, and last date she was tested. Perhaps a mother has been on the same dose for 5 years and has had two pregnancies since without any further thyroid assessment.

Caffeinated beverages. Beverages such as coffee, chocolate, tea, cola, and some noncola soft drinks (sodas) may inhibit lactation because of caffeine, especially if used in large amounts. Limiting the caffeine may improve lactation in some mothers. Other mothers can consume large amounts of caffeine and never have a problem with their infants' weight gain.

Medicines. To many mothers, oral contraceptives and nonprescription drugs such as cold remedies (antihistamines and diuretics), headache remedies, sedatives, and vitamins are not considered "medicines." Some mothers may insist they use none of these medications until they are asked, "What do you do if you have a headache?" or "What if you can't sleep at night?" The answer to this question reveals what they really do use. Improper use of vitamins can also create problems. It is known that excessive vitamin B_6 (pyridoxine) blocks lactation by depressing the release of prolactin from the pituitary gland.[7] Oral contraceptives, antihistamines, and diuretics have all been implicated in decreased lactation. Other drugs may create problems by making an infant overly sleepy or irritable (see Chapter 6). Several other useful references on drugs and breastfeeding are also available. If at all possible, the mother's medications should be stopped, or those drugs that have been shown to decrease lactation should be changed.

Alcohol. Most mothers also deny much alcohol consumption. Ask how much is used each day, each week, and each month. Generally, they will say use is occasional. If a mother is abusing alcohol, it creates problems. She will not be breastfeeding often enough, and the infant may be so sleepy that he sleeps through feedings. This mother needs special help for alcoholism. Obviously she was abusing alcohol during her pregnancy, and the infant may have the evident characteristics of fetal alcohol syndrome—one of which is a poor weight gain for organic reasons.

Nutrition. The evaluation period can be a good time to talk to a mother about nutrition. Find out what foods she likes. This will give a glimpse of any cultural or ethnic foods she is inclined to use. Then recommend foods, especially those high in protein, from a list of foods familiar to her cultural or ethnic background that can be convenient, yet very nutritious. It is as important to know how a mother rates her diet as it is to know what she eats. This information will reveal her knowledge about good nutrition. Take a brief diet history. Some mothers with poor nutrition do not realize it and need good advice.

It is important for mothers of slow-gaining infants to eat regular, well-balanced meals. A woman may try to skip breakfast if she is alone, if the husband skips breakfast, or if they have no other children. If she gets busy with the infant or his siblings, she may also forget to eat lunch.

Inadequate nutrition creates maternal fatigue. As a result, the mother may let the infant sleep too long between feedings or use a pacifier excessively. The quality of the milk may not be seriously affected, but the quantity may diminish. If the only meal a mother has each day is dinner, one solution is to have her keep nutritious foods on hand to eat during the day, such as nuts, seeds, raw vegetables, fruit, cheese, or fruit juice. She can snack while she is breastfeeding the infant.

General health. It is important to know whether the mother is in good health. This is not to imply that an unhealthy woman cannot breastfeed, but she may need assistance in correcting problems that contribute to her not feeling well. This and fatigue can slow down milk production or inhibit milk let-down. For example, if the mother has had high blood pressure problems but has stopped medications during pregnancy, she may need to be reevaluated.

Milk let-down. Assess the milk let-down reflex by asking what sensations the mother feels when breastfeeding. Before asking this, however, explain that some women do not feel the let-down and that that is *normal*. Some mothers are familiar with literature descriptions of the reflex, and they worry about it when they do not experience it. Their worry then further inhibits the let-down. Mothers are very relieved to know it is all right to not feel it. When asked whether she can hear the infant swallow when breastfeeding, a mother may say the infant chokes and swallows well, but she feels that there is no let-down. She can be taught that this is a sign of let-down. Leaking milk on one side while breastfeeding on the other or feeling a tingling, filling, burning sensation can also be pointed out to mothers as a sign of milk let-down. Besides providing information, such discussion also encourages the mothers.

Stress. Unusual stress in the mother's environment can have a direct relationship to breastfeeding. One mother was having trouble breastfeeding her third infant. It was discovered that barking dogs that disturbed her every time she sat down to feed the infant were the cause. Another mother was married to a jazz musician and really could not stand her husband's practicing on the drums all the time. She had him practice somewhere else and had no trouble afterward. Of course, there are always mothers with several children noisily playing in the room all the time they breastfeed and it does not disturb them. However, keep in mind that this chapter deals with the mother whose infant is not doing well, so each possible factor should be considered.

Almost always, mothers deny having a busy life-style. By joking about it the nurse finds out more. Ask something like, "Haven't you had anything that's cluttering up your life?" and exaggerate as if she has a horrendous schedule, such as being chairman of the PTA, plus several other organizations and running a 15-child car pool twice a day. Mothers will usually giggle or laugh at this approach and begin mentioning specific activities they are involved in. Many mothers do not consider themselves busy, so questions must be specific.

One mother was out every day as a Jehovah's Witness missionary with the infant in a stroller. She didn't understand why he wasn't gaining because he slept so beautifully in the stroller as she went from door to door. She was breastfeeding "on demand" and felt that was all she needed to do. After conferring with her church, she was able to leave her service for a while to stay home and breastfeed more often to correct the weight gain problem.

It is important to ask about the marital relationship. Often, if there is a marital problem such as an unsupportive husband, infidelity, wife beating, or other conflict, it reflects on the breastfeeding. In working with a mother whose infant was gaining fine, treatment was interrupted when she moved to Tucson, and the infant then lost a great deal of weight. When she came back to Los Angeles, the infant began gaining again. When asked what happened, she admitted she had left her husband. When she returned to him and worked with a marriage counselor, the infant's weight improved. Some women may be able to breastfeed well in spite of such problems, but it could be a major factor in a slow-gaining infant for other women.

Past experience with breastfeeding. Asking about the past breastfeeding history with other children can give important clues about what is happening with this slow-gaining infant. If the mother has breastfed other infants very successfully, then the breast is "proven," and other factors such as her health or some factor related to the infant may be more likely. If she reports having had problems breastfeeding other infants, the factor may be related more to her physically or emotionally, or it may be a matter of technique. Also, part of a mother's "busy" life-style may relate to the care of other children and their activities, so fatigue may be a factor this time.

Problems in nurturing. A woman's mothering skills are a learned behavior from the way she herself was mothered by her own mother. Ask about her early childhood and her relationship with her mother. The family structure may also give clues as to the type of mothering she received as a child. Sometimes a busy mother with numerous children finds it easy to delegate the care of the youngest child to an older sibling. Find out what advice her mother has given to her concerning the care of her baby. It may reveal that her own mothering had not been nurturing.

One mother of a slow-gaining infant presented a perplexing history. Her answers to all the questions about how often the infant breastfed gave no clues to the problem, and when observed, the infant suckled well. The examiner later ran into the mother at a conference where the breastfeeding was observed to be in fact infrequent and the feedings short. When the mother was confronted with the observation, she denied it but agreed to keep a log of feedings for a week. The mother was surprised to learn that indeed the feedings were short and infrequent. She then revealed that she was so neglected as an infant that she was diagnosed as retarded at the age of 9 months. Through infant stimulation done by her aunt, the woman made a full recovery. This young mother said she had a "creepy" feeling every time she breastfed and really felt that the feedings lasted "like an eternity." Discovering the problem enabled the mother to deal with her feelings and learn new mothering skills, which resulted in an immediate weight gain for the infant.

A home visit may be in order if nonnurturing mothering is suspected. Peculiar behavior between mother and child may be obvious while the history is being taken: lack of eye contact between mother and infant, lack of talking to or caressing the infant, derogatory comments to the infant such as "you little brat, are you wet again?" or jerky forceful movements as the mother handles the child.

When a nonnurturing mother's physical and emotional needs are met, she is better able to meet the needs of her infant. One mother said after receiving help, "I guess I was jealous of the baby. I never got any love from my mother, so deep down inside I just *couldn't* give it to my baby." Part of this mother's therapy was to sing to the infant and stroke her while breastfeeding. The infant stroked back and began to break away and smile and coo while feeding, which was the love returned that the mother so desperately needed.

Taking the infant history

Feeding frequency. Often, when I have asked mothers how often they feed the infant, they respond in surprise, "Well, on demand, of course!" If a mother has come knowing she will receive support in her breastfeeding, she is especially surprised by the question because she feels she is doing what the breastfeeding books recommend— breastfeeding "on demand." It is surprising, however, what "on demand" means to mothers. A mother might say, "Oh, he's such a good infant, he breastfeeds every 6 hours and doesn't give me any trouble at all!" And even after explaining to her that he needs to breastfeed more often, she replies, "But I'm breastfeeding him on demand!" Another mother may complain about her infant wanting to breastfeed every 2 hours and she has been holding him off to every 4 hours, resulting in his weight loss. That is when a detailed explanation becomes necessary about the differing consistency of fat and proteins in human milk and cow's milk or formula, which accounts for the rapid absorption of the human milk and need for frequent breastfeeding (every 1 to 3 hours for young infants, whereas those 6 to 7 months or older may go 4 to 5 hours).

However, if a mother says the infant is fed continuously, and she cannot ever put him down because he cries, that is often a clue that the infant is doing some ineffective suckling. This baby must breastfeed almost constantly because he cannot obtain enough milk in a shorter amount of time. This is especially likely when the infant is not gaining weight and is doing nonnutritive flutter suckling. This infant may also often breastfeed with his eyes closed, pausing frequently.

Supplements. Ask whether the infant is being fed breastmilk only or whether he is getting other foods. When solids are administered too early, the milk supply may diminish, especially if solids are fed to the infant just before breastfeeding. Solid food given to an infant whose digestive system is not ready to assimilate it may stay in his stomach longer and cause him to not be hungry for 4 hours. Some mothers will be supplementing because they were advised to do so by a doctor. If the infant is still not gaining, even with a prescribed supplement, it can be a clue that something may be wrong with the infant.

While the infant is being evaluated for the cause of the slow weight gain or even loss, breastmilk can be supplemented without the use of a bottle. The Lact-Aid Nursing Trainer (see Chapter 13) adds extra milk while breastfeeding and often improves the suckle.

Pausing. It is normal for infants to pause during breastfeeding. Excessive pausing by an infant is common for premature infants who tire easily. Other infants may be weak from inadequate calories and need to pause for rest. Infants with a neuromuscular dysfunction have to pause to rest after building up too much muscle tone. If excessive pausing occurs toward the end of the feeding, it can indicate that the infant is only breastfeeding well for about 5 minutes and spending the rest of the time at leisure. In such a situation, the infant may need to be switched from one breast to the other more often to stimulate new milk let-down and renew interest in stronger suckling.

Swallowing. Most mothers do not know what swallowing sounds like and cannot tell you if their infants swallow or not. Other mothers of slow gainers frequently describe swallowing as *only* in the first 5 minutes of the feeding. These babies often breastfeed with their eyes closed throughout the feeding. This can be a clue that the rest of the feeding is nonnutritive flutter suckling that obtains little or no milk. By listening to normally gaining infants, the nurse can learn this sound and imitate it for the mother. When swallowing stops or slows down, the mother should be instructed to take the infant off the breast, burp him to awaken him a bit, and put him on the other breast. If this "switch nursing" is done frequently during the feeding, it may be enough to encourage regular swallowing that results in a good weight gain.

Terminating the feeding. Who terminates the feeding? Is it the mother or the infant? If the mother feeds the infant until he falls asleep or stops breastfeeding himself, it is probably adequate. But an infant can also prematurely fall asleep after only 5 minutes of breastfeeding, so the mother thinks he is done. This is not adequate breastfeeding time. If the mother terminates the breastfeeding, it may not be adequate. One mother said, "I breastfed him for 10 minutes on each side and then I put him down. I can't understand why he cried again and was not satisfied." Some infants swallow air with the milk and feel full and sleepy. When the suckling slows down, an infant should be burped to create more room in the stomach and renew interest in feeding. This may need to be repeated several times along with switching back and forth from breast to breast.

Suckling. Asking the first-time mother how she rates her infant's suckling may be unfair, since she has nothing to compare it with. If this is her second, third, or fourth infant, she may say that the infant suckles much differently from her other infants, or that he just does not suckle right. Sometimes a mother will say that a friend breastfed *this* infant and could hardly feel him suckling. These comments could be clues that the infant has a poor suckle. Most mothers of slow gainers report that the infants do breastfeed the strongest at night. This could be due to a more relaxed mother, a baby who has a better muscle tone from sleeping, or an easier side-lying position for the infant. Many mothers will say the infant was suckling very well and then suddenly at 2 to 3 weeks of age his pattern changed and he seemed not to suckle as strongly. In the first 2 to 3 weeks, infants have a "reflex suck" that tends to be stronger and more automatic than the suckle. Most mothers produce more milk than they need in the first few weeks. Through discussion and observation, the nurse can rather easily discover whether the infant is doing nonnutritive flutter suckling—sucking on his tongue, or pausing excessively. Infants tend to suckle a finger stronger than a breast, so testing the strength of the suck with a finger may be invalid, but this finger assessment could give a good idea of how the baby uses his tongue. You should feel the tongue slide in and out on the underside of your finger horizontally. If you feel the tongue moving up and down vertically in the mouth intermittently *or* an *outward* horizontal thrust, you might suspect a nonnutritive, inefficient suckling pattern.

To tell whether an infant is sucking his tongue, observe his cheeks carefully. If he sucks his tongue, the fat padded area will be drawn in deeply with every suck. Pull down the lower lip. If only the infant's gum can be seen and the tongue is not visible between the gum and the breast, the tongue has been sucked up to the roof (hard palate) of the infant's mouth. The tongue sucker often makes a "clicking noise" when he suckles the breast.

Persistent poor suckling, even with a Lact-Aid Nursing Trainer, and persistent primitive neuromuscular movements of the infant's body (tonic labyrinthine reflex), or a prolonged need to use the Lact-Aid Nursing Trainer over more than a 4-month period may suggest a neurologic dysfunction. Since the tongue, jaws, and lips are operated by muscles, which are innervated, it seems quite logical that a neurologic dysfunction would first manifest itself in a feeding problem. Referral to a physical therapist who has had specialized training* in assessing and treating feeding problems based on the research

*Neuro-Developmental Treatment Association, Inc., P.O. Box 14613, Chicago, Ill. 60614.

of Morris, Bobath, and Meuller[17] can improve the efficiency of the infant's suckling. Most often, however, the problem is only transitory and due to an immature central nervous system. As the infant matures, the feeding problem disappears (3 to 9 months).

Occasionally I have seen infants who actually push against the mother with their hands almost as if they are trying to pull away while they breastfeed. They keep losing the breast, are easily distracted, and get very fussy at the breast. They do minimal suckling. Such infants want a fast milk let-down and refuse to wait for it. A Lact-Aid Nursing Trainer has been used with these infants to keep their interest long enough to build up the supply and enhance the milk let-down. This pushing away may also be a manifestation of the increased muscle tone and hyperextension of the head and extremities seen in the neuromuscular disorder, which responds so well to physical therapy. The Lact-Aid Nursing Trainer has also been helpful in correcting nonnutritive flutter suckling and excessive pausing. Observation of suckling and the infant's body position while feeding is essential, and as more experience is acquired, faulty suckling and positioning become easy to detect and correct.

Elimination. The number of wet diapers the infant has each day can be revealing. Six to eight very wet diapers a day is considered a sign of adequate fluid intake in a breastfed infant. The infant who has only one or two wet diapers, whose diapers are just barely wet, or who is not gaining well obviously is not getting enough fluid intake. Paper diapers absorb more and do not feel as wet as cloth diapers, so it is important to know which is being used. The number of stools a day may not be as important as changes in stools. For example, a normal breastfed newborn infant can have a stool with every diaper change. A young infant who generally has frequent stools but suddenly has very few that have the same color and consistency as before may not be receiving enough milk. On the other hand, going without a stool for several days, sometimes as long as 2 weeks, is common around the third month, corresponding to a growth spurt. This should *not* be confused with an infrequent stool in the unsupplemented breastfed newborn under 2 months, which may indicate poor milk intake.

Color and consistency are important. If a mother says her infant has stools like hard pellets but says she is only breastfeeding, it is not likely to be true. Stools of breastfed infants can be liquid, thick like toothpaste, pleasant smelling, yellowish or greenish in color, and have tiny curds or strings of normal mucus, but they are not hard. Stools of formula-fed infants are brownish yellow, thick, sometimes hard, and have a bad odor. One mother told me she was totally breastfeeding, yet her infant's stool was brown, was like hard pellets, and smelled terrible. When I confronted the mother with the possibility that something was wrong with the infant and suggested further tests, the grandmother admitted to having given him a bottle each afternoon and night because she did not think the infant was doing very well. The formula had made the infant constipated, uncomfortable, and full, making him a problem breastfeeder.

Burping. Much of the literature and word-of-mouth advice indicates that breastfed infants never need to be burped. Although it is needed less often than with bottle-feeding, some infants do swallow air and burping is necessary. Otherwise they feel full and fall asleep before finishing a feeding. After a while this can reduce the milk supply. Assist mothers of the slow-gaining infant in learning how to burp their infants during a feeding so they may be encouraged to take more milk and suckle more strongly. Excessive crying or hyperextension of the head in infants with a neuromuscular disorder also may lead to air swallowing, so burping just before feeding may be helpful.

Activity and development. Ask mothers to rate their infants as active, placid, or average. Their answers are very revealing. Some will describe the low-weight infant as extremely active. This may be the infant who flips himself over in the crib at 1 month old, arches his back or head, and is practically on his hands and knees. This activity is burning up all the calories he gets and may also be a sign of an increased muscle tone found so often in a neuromuscular disorder. If the mother says she cannot wake the infant, this may indicate that the infant is too placid or possibly sick. If a mother has nothing to compare her infant with, she may think he is just average, but most mothers will suggest active or placid.

Asking the mother how she rates his development may give you a clue as to how she views him. Couple this with your assessment of his development to see whether you agree. If she says he is slow and you rate him as advanced, it may be that she has no knowledge of normal developmental milestones. Explaining his accomplishments to her can raise her esteem of the child, which will have a positive effect on their relationship.

Pacifiers. It is important to know whether pacifiers are used and what type they are because they can change suckling patterns just like the bottle nipple does. Suggest more frequent breastfeeding rather than use of the pacificer to help correct suckling problems and build up the milk supply. Some infants resort to sucking their thumb or fingers a great deal at the third or fourth month, especially during teething. This activity can greatly shorten the feeding, thereby causing a sudden onset of poor weight gain.

Sleep patterns. Night sleeping patterns are especially revealing. Sleeping through the night can be considered any 6-hour stretch and usually does not occur until 8 to 12 weeks of life.[12] A young infant put to bed at 7 PM who wakes up at 7 AM has gone too long between feedings. Suggest that the mother wake the infant and breastfeed before she goes to bed, and in extreme slow gain problems, suggest that she also wake him in the middle of the night to breastfeed. A mother seeking help for her slow-gaining infant will cooperate by doing anything asked of her to help her continue breastfeeding. Sometimes this additional breastfeeding is enough to make the difference.

Health of the infant. Were there any problems since birth? If the infant had jaundice, how high was the bilirubin? Did the infant ever suckle well? Did the suckling then deteriorate when the infant became lethargic with jaundice? Did the infant have sepsis or return to the hospital for a problem? These are all clues as to what could have effected a change in the infant's suckling patterns. It is very helpful to point out to mothers that poor suckling may be the infant's fault. Mothers have a heavy burden of guilt, and blaming the infant helps them relax immediately. Try joking to the infant, saying, "See, it's your fault, and we've got to do something about it so Mommy can enjoy breastfeeding you!" The mother will usually laugh and say she never realized it could have been the infant. She probably has thought it was her, not the baby, and perhaps everyone has been telling her she was doing something wrong.

A urinalysis should be routine protocol when dealing with a slow-gaining infant. Many urinary tract infections have been detected when the only symptoms were the poor suckling and weight gain. These low-grade infections can change suckling patterns and make infants lethargic.

Sometimes a mother is told that her infant's slow gain is solely because of breastfeeding. One infant had breastfed and gained well until, at 10 months, he stopped gaining. The physician insisted that he be weaned from the breast immediately, since the infant was too old and did not need to breastfeed any longer. The infant was also eating solids in addition to breastfeeding, but by 1 year he had dropped by two standard deviations. After she consulted a second physician, a urinalysis was suggested, which revealed a urinary tract infection. The original physician treated the infant with ampicillin but still insisted on weaning the infant. When the mother consulted the second physician again, it was suggested that the mother request an intravenous pyelogram (IVP), since it is unusual for males under age 4 to have urinary tract infections. The test revealed gross congenital urologic anomalies, which were then repaired surgically, but the infant had already lost partial function of one kidney because of reflux. Had this mother followed the advice to wean and accepted "inadequate milk" as the diagnosis, the infant's condition would not have been detected as soon, and kidney damage would have been much more extensive than it was. This is an important lesson on why it is unwise to blame breastfeeding immediately for slow gaining problems, especially if an infant has been doing well but suddenly stops gaining.

Ask if any other tests have been done for slow weight gain, since mothers have sometimes had a previous evaluation before coming in to your institution for another opinion. Repeating previously done tests is unnecessary and expensive. Make it clear to the mother that if she does have a problem with breastfeeding, no matter what the problem is, it can be worked out. All too often, when an infant fails to gain weight, and before consulting anyone for help, a mother will switch from breastfeeding to the bottle because of pressure from a family member.

Taking the birth history

Sometimes slow gaining is attributable to a sick infant or mother, or to breastfeeding technique, but at times, knowledge of the birth history can reveal other factors that may be involved.

Labor and delivery. If a mother was in labor for 3 days and became exhausted, perhaps the infant was also, thus establishing a poor suckling pattern. Perhaps because of being too tired, suckling was weak and the infant learned improper suckling behavior.

For a time it was felt that the first bottle given to the infant imprinted improper sucking patterns. This can still be a factor for some infants; however, it has been noted that in a few home births when no bottles were given, some infants developed a poor suckle. Some may have learned breastfeeding improperly after a very long labor. Others may have had a neuromuscularly affected poor suckle from the beginning.

It is known that medications given during labor and delivery can result in a very lethargic infant, who when put to breast establishes an incorrect suckling pattern. The longer the infant waits after birth to be put to breast, the more likelihood there is of developing improper suckling patterns. For the infant who has been in intensive care for a long time and fed by bottle, the transition to the breast can be very difficult. The infant tries to suckle the breast the same way he sucks the bottle nipple. Asking the mother whether the infant started out suckling well and when the suckling deteriorated can reveal that the infant may not have been doing well physically. If the infant never breastfed well, it may be that suckling never got off to a good proper start.

Bonding behaviors recorded by many delivery nurses could be a useful clue. Klaus and Kennell[10] have well documented the effects of poor bonding at the time of delivery.

Until recently some emergency cesarean births allowed no bonding time, which may have caused poor attachment.

Even if a mother has had rooming-in, find out the breastfeeding advice she was given. The mother may have been limiting feedings to every 4 hours, and just 3 to 5 minutes per breast, or one breast per feeding, according to the advice she received, her own observations, or instructions in a pamphlet given to her. Rooming-in ideally should provide an opportunity for staff to educate the mother and get her off to a good start breastfeeding while supporting frequent feedings.

Medications during pregnancy. In discussing medications in pregnancy, also look for the drug abuser, the mother who may be using heroin or other street drugs. Using the word "medication" is more polite than saying "drugs." Make it clear as you ask the question by saying, "because some medications will pass through the placenta or sometimes the breast and affect the infant," and "We just want to make sure this isn't the problem." Most mothers are genuinely concerned and may say something like, "Well, I've been chipping during my pregnancy but now I don't breastfeed the infant after I've used." (Chipping is street language for using heroin occasionally.) A mother may admit she uses diazepam (Valium) several times a day because a psychiatrist prescribed it for marital problems. Even if mothers fail to volunteer the information in the discussion, they will certainly think about it, and perhaps try to avoid drugs on their own later.

A mother who has taken phenobarbital for preeclampsia during pregnancy may find that her infant just does not suckle well at all in the first few days after the birth. Her obstetrician and pediatrician need to work together to solve problems brought about by maternal medications.

The use of the "Slow-Gaining Special History" form has been extremely helpful in working with mothers whose infants have trouble gaining weight. Originally, the form was one page. It has been expanded to its present length as more work was done in lactation. Others who have used it in the past have found it helpful in managing assessment and interventions for slow-gaining breastfed infants.

SUMMARY

Although breastfeeding is a physiologic and normal process, problems such as slow weight gain occasionally occur. In assessing the mother and infant with a slow weight gain, remember that they are two individuals, not just one. Thus the nurse must assess the mother as well as the infant. An important key to assessing them is to actually observe the mother and infant together, particularly during breastfeeding. Speaking positively to and about the infant may greatly improve the mother's feelings about the infant who is causing her so much worry. An example would be, "Look how adoringly he looks at you!" or "I love how she smiles, don't you?"

Perhaps the biggest mistake in working with mothers and infants is assuming that mothers know more about breastfeeding than they really do. Most health-care providers fail to give mothers sufficient information and encouragement. Mothers practice improper techniques, and infants then may develop ineffective suckling patterns.

It is essential to carefully analyze breastfeeding technique to discover any underlying problems in the mother or infant, or both. The infant who does well, then fails; the infant who never has done well; and the newborn who just cannot seem to suckle well all present different problems and different methods of management that are summarized in Table 11-1. In working to correct the mother's breastfeeding technique, arrange for close follow-up. A suggested protocol appears with Table 11-2. Suggesting "switch nursing" when the infant's suckle slows and swallowing stops is often all that is needed if technique has been the major problem. Then, if problems persist, often the Lact-Aid

TABLE 11·1

Summary of problems and interventions with slow weight gain when organic causes have been ruled out

Factor	Antecedent conditions	Nursing action
Simple mismanagement of breastfeeding	Mother removes baby before he finishes feeding to (newborns need 30 to 60-min feeds). Long intervals between feedings (4 hr or more). Mother tries to promote sleeping more than 6 hr at night before 8-12 wk. Mother gives more water than breastmilk in fear of jaundice.	Weight gain improves with proper counseling of mother.
Lazy suckler	Infant breastfeeds with eyes closed. Infant suckles and swallows audibly only during let-down—the rest of the feeding is done with a nonnutritive suckle. Infant breastfeeds frequently (every 1 hr or continuously) to make up for decreased volume obtained during feeding. Infant fusses furiously when put down. Infant sleeps 8 to 14-hr stretch at night from first month.	Weight gain improves by stimulation of productive suckling (switch breasts and awaken infant when swallows cease, awaken infant at least every 4 hr at night).
Sudden onset at 3-5 mo	Breastfeeds with eyes open. Sucks fingers all the time so not breastfeeding as often. Shortened feedings lately due to excessive finger sucking. Teething. May or may not sleep long periods at night. Early or heavy introduction of solid food (reduces interest in breastfeeding).	Weight gain improves by breastfeeding whenever fingers go into mouth, enticing longer feeds in a quiet room, removing fingers and substituting breast if a baby quits in mid-feeding or slows down on solid foods.
Emotionally deprived infant	Rare in breastfed infant Mother gives history of feeding that is contradictory. History of poorly mothered mother or of child abuse/neglect. History of recent mother/infant separation (for example, mother working and non-nurturing daycare environment). Mother encourages pacification in nonfeeding ways (swing, pacifier).	Weight gain improves by baby being stroked and cooed to during longer, more frequent feedings.

Continued.

TABLE 11-1—cont'd

Summary of problems and interventions with slow weight gain when organic causes have been ruled out

Factor	Antecedent conditions	Nursing action
Immature central nervous system or neuromuscular disorder	Poor suckling because of poor muscle coordination of mouth and body positioning (hypotonia, hypertonia). Breastfeeds with eyes closed. Fusses when put down. Breastfeeds continuously and when put on a 2-hour schedule, weight drops. May or may not sleep long periods at night. Suckles more strongly at night if breastfeeding then. May give history of difficulty attaching to breast at birth, prolonged sore nipples, or mastitis in early months indicating improper suckle. May suckle well with first let-down only but not with subsequent let-downs. Attempts at stimulating better suckling produce a 28-56 gm (1-2 oz)/wk weight gain but usually will not gain that well.	Use of Lact-Aid Nursing Trainer improves weight gain, suckling, and therefore mother's milk supply, but when Lact-Aid Nursing Trainer removed, poor suckling resumes immediately. Suckling improves by neurodevelopmental physical therapy over a 3- to 4-mo period.

TABLE 11-2

Protocol for intervention with slow-gaining breastfed infant when no organic cause is apparent

Assessment	Intervention
First assessment	Take history and suggest to parents some changes as per history findings. Review baby and mother assessment findings. Observe feeding—suggest switching breasts when swallows slow down. Obtain urinalysis.
Second assessment (4-7 days later)	Check weight to see if suggested changes worked. If so, check weight two or more times to establish continued pattern of correction. If no gain, (greater than 57 gm [2 oz]/week), discuss Lact-Aid Nursing Trainer with family. Observe feeding to see if suckling improved. Observe infant's posturing for abnormal hyperextension of head/or extremities while feeding. Suggest referral to neurodevelopmentally trained physical therapist if poor posturing or tongue and jaw thrusting noted.

Nursing Trainer will be useful as a means of providing supplement and correcting suckling problems. The Lact-Aid Nursing Trainer should not be used as a substitute for education and support but only as a useful tool when it is really needed.

Always keep in mind that each mother and infant dyad is unique. Sometimes nothing is discovered to account for a slow weight gain, and it just may be that some infants gain slowly for a while and then grow more rapidly, so in the long run it balances out. In these situations, close follow-up just to be sure nothing is wrong is all that can be done. Weight should be considered as just one criterion of growth and development. More important is preserving and enhancing the special bond that comes with breastfeeding for both the mother's and infant's emotional health while any medical or psychologic problems are discovered and treated.

REFERENCES

1. Applebaum, R.: The modern management of successful breastfeeding, Pediatr. Clin. North Am. **17:**212, 1970.
2. Fischhoff, J., Whitten, C., and Pettit, M.: A psychiatric study of mothers of infants with growth failure secondary to maternal deprivation, J. Pediatr. **79:**209, 1971.
3. Foman, S.: Infant nutrition, Philadelphia, 1974, W.B. Saunders Co.
4. Frantz, K.B., Fleiss, P.M., and Lawrence, R.A.: Management of the slow-gaining Breastfed Baby, Keeping Abreast J. **3:**287, 1978.
5. Garn, S., and Clark, D.: Trends in fatness and the origins of obesity, Pediatrics **57:**443, 1976.
6. Gifford, S., and Lieberman, B.I.: Evaluation of growth charts, Issues Compr. Pediatr. Nurs. **4**(2):1, 1980.
7. Greentree, L.B.: More dangers of vitamin B_6 in nursing mothers, N. Engl. Med. **300:**141, 1979.
8. Hall, B.: Changing composition of human milk and early development of appetite control, Lancet **1:**779, 1975.
9. Hambraeus, L., et al.: Nutritional aspects of breastmilk and cow's milk formulas. In Hambraeus, L., and Hannson, L.A., editors: Food and Immunology Symposium No. 2, Uppsala 1975, Swedish Nutritional Foundation.
10. Klaus, M.H., and Kennell, J.H.: Maternal-infant bonding: the impact of early separation or loss on family development, St. Louis, 1976, The C.V. Mosby Co.
11. Lawrence, R.: Breastfeeding: a guide for the medical profession, St. Louis, 1980, The C.V. Mosby Co.
12. Moore, T., and Ucko, L.E.: Night waking in early infancy. I. Arch. Dis. Child. **32:**33, 1957.
13. Pryor, K.: Nursing your baby, New York, 1973, Harper & Row, Publishers, Inc.
14. Sach, J., Amado, O., and Lunenfeld, B.: Thyroxin concentration in human milk, J. Clin. Endocrinol. Metab. **45:**171, 1977.
15. Vaughan, V., McKay, R., and Nelson, W.: Textbook of pediatrics, Philadelphia, 1975, W.B. Saunders Co.
16. Weichart, C.: Lactational reflex recovery in breastfeeding failure, Pediatrics **63:**799, 1979.
17. Wilson, J.W.: Oral-motor function and dysfunction in children, Proceedings of May 1977 Symposium, Division of Physical Therapy, Department of Medical Allied Health Professions, School of Medicine, The University of North Carolina, Chapel Hill, N.C., 1977.

ADDITIONAL READINGS

American Academy of Pediatrics: Breastfeeding: a commentary in celebration of the International Year of The Child, Pediatrics **62:**591, 1978.
Barnard, M., and Wolf, L.: Psychosocial failure to thrive, Nurs. Clin. North Am. **8:**557, 1973.
Bosma, J.: Human oral function in oral sensation and perception, Springfield, Ill., 1967, Charles C Thomas, Publisher.
Davies, D., and Evans, T.: Failure to thrive at the breast (letter), Lancet **2:**1194, 1976.
de Swiet, M., Fayers, P.L., and Cooper, L.: Effect of feeding habit on weight in infancy, Lancet **3:**892, 1977.
Eppink, H.: Experiment to determine a basis for nursing decisions in regard to initiation of breastfeeding, Nurs. Res. **18:**292, 1969.
Fleiss, P.: Says infant's failure to thrive no reason to halt breastfeeding, Pediatr. News, June 1977.
Forsum, E., and Lonnerdal, B.: Effect of protein intake on protein and nitrogen composition of breastmilk, Am. J. Clin. Nutr. **33:**1809, 1980.
Gilmore, H., and Thomas, R.: Critical malnutrition in breastfed infants, Am. J. Dis. Child. **132:**885, 1978.
Glaser, H., et al.: Physical and psychological development of children with early failure to thrive, J. Pediatr. **73:**690, 1968.

Glaser, H., et al.: Happy to starve, Arch. Dis. Child. **52:**974, 1977.

Hufton, I., et al.: Nonorganic failure to thrive: a long term follow-up, Pediatrics **59:**73, 1977.

Ingram, T.: Clinical significance of the infantile feeding reflexes, Dev. Med. Child Neurol. **4:**159, 1962.

Jelliffe, D.: Doulas, confidence and the science of lactation (editorial), J. Pediatr. **84:**462, 1974.

Koel, B.: Failure to thrive and fatal injury as a continuum, Am. J. Dis. Child. **118:**565, 1969.

Leonard, M., et al.: Failure to thrive in infants, Am. J. Dis. Child. **111:**600, 1966.

Lozoff, B., et al.: The mother-newborn relationship: limits of adaptability, J. Pediatr. **91:**1, 1977.

Mueller, H.: Facilitating feeding and pre-speech. In Pearson, P.H., and Williams, C.E., editors: Physical therapy services in the developmental disabilities, Springfield, Ill., 1972, Charles C Thomas, Publisher.

Newman, C., and Alpaugh, M.: Birthweight doubling time: a fresh look, Pediatrics **57:**469, 1976.

Salariya, E., et al.: Duration of breastfeeding after early initiation and frequent feeding, Lancet **2:**1141, 1978.

Shaheen, E., et al.: Failure to thrive: a retrospective profile, Clin. Pediatr. **7:**255, 1968.

Shapiro, V., Fraiberg, S., and Adelson, E.: Infant-parent psychotherapy on behalf of a child in a critical nutritional state, In The pyschoanalytic study of the child, vol. 31, New Haven, Conn., 1976, Yale University Press.

12

Breastfeeding support in the high-risk nursery and at home

PAULA MEIER
JAN RIORDAN

The mother who chooses to breastfeed her high-risk baby experiences many concerns and needs that distinguish her from the woman who breastfeeds a healthy infant. Although individuals can do much to assist these mothers in establishing and maintaining lactation, their special concerns and needs are most effectively addressed by an organized breastfeeding support program.

A breastfeeding support program for mothers of high-risk babies should be based on principles of normal lactation that have been adapted to the needs of women and their premature or sick newborn infants. Nurses, parents, and interested consumers can be instrumental in the development and implementation of such a program.

HISTORICAL DIMENSIONS

Although many professionals regard breastfeeding the high-risk infant as a transient and revolutionary trend, the literature contains references that refute this assumption. Budin[30] in 1870 reported his policy of encouraging breastfeeding among mothers of premature infants. His rationale was psychologically based: he felt that such a policy facilitated mothers' maintaining interest in their babies. In the 1930's Lundeen,[41] a neonatal nurse, argued that premature babies should be fed their mothers' milk, at least until they reached a weight of 4 pounds. Her suggestions for facilitating lactation without the aid of mechanical breast pumps included manual expression and the nursing of a healthy infant at one breast while collecting milk from the other. A similar procedure was used to put small premature infants to the breast: one breast was stimulated by a healthy baby to elicit the let-down reflex; the premature infant, whose suck was much weaker, was breastfed at the other breast.

In the 1940's and 1950's neonatalogy began to evolve into a scientific and academic specialty.[14] This development interested physicians, who had previously considered newborn care to be within the realm of traditional "woman's work," preferring instead to treat more challenging disorders and illnesses. Doctors subsequently replaced nurses in the primary care of premature and healthy newborn infants. As this professional transition occurred, many of the long accepted principles of premature care were subjected to clinical investigation. The frequent use of mothers' milk for nutrition of the premature infant was one such principle. As physicians became interested in nutritional research, the first acceptable alternatives to breastfeeding appeared, thus facilitating the move away from mothers' milk as the optimal source of nutrition for premature babies. The trend in artificial feeding of these infants persisted into the early 1970's.

The conversion of premature "stations" to regional Neonatal Intensive Care Units (NICU's) in the late 1960's and early 1970's effected a major change in the types of infants cared for in these facilities. One such group of babies consisted of the very small premature infants, previously considered incapable of survival. Although these infants did not die from prematurity, as they had in the past, many developed complications from the combined effect of their immaturity and their treatments. Necrotizing enterocolitis (NEC), an often fatal syndrome resulting from bowel hypoperfusion, was one of these complications. In the mid-1970's researchers began to hypothesize that the immunologic properties unique to human milk might protect the infant considered susceptible to the development of NEC.[6,49] Exploration of this relationship generated a new wave of interest in the use of mothers' milk for premature infant nutrition.

HUMAN MILK FOR PREMATURE INFANTS

Although studies concerning the immunologic composition of human milk have identified many antiinfective properties,[28,49,56] the macrophage has been delineated as the source of protection against NEC.[49] Since these and other live cells are destroyed with processing of any type,* debate was instantly generated concerning the advisability of feeding banked milk to preterm babies. Pitt[49] approaches the issue as one of risk vs. benefit. She describes the potential for contamination in collection and storage of expressed milk, which, if processed, might be of minimal immunologic benefit in providing protection from NEC.

This renewed interest in the use of human milk for premature infant feeding generated another series of investigations—those that contrasted the composition of human milk with growth requirements for the low birth weight baby. Researchers† published studies and commentaries suggesting the inadequacy of mothers' milk with respect to protein, sodium, and calcium, since requirements for these nutrients by the growing premature baby exceed those for the full-term infant. Suboptimal growth rates have been reported among premature infants fed pooled, expressed human milk.[15,16]

Räihä et al.,[50] however, compared rates of growth among four groups of appropriate-for-gestational age (AGA) premature infants fed three types of formula, each with varying amounts of protein, and pooled, banked human milk. They found no statistically significant differences in mean rates of weight gain among the four groups and suggested that high-protein feeding of premature infants might be not only unnecessary but also detrimental to subsequent growth and development. The basic issue underlying these discussions is whether prematurely born infants should be expected to continue to grow at intrauterine rates. This question remains unanswered but has been extensively reviewed by Heird.[26] It must be emphasized that the studies on which these thoughts

*References 13, 18, 22, 32, 36, 47, 49, 57.
†References 15, 16, 20, 21, 26.

and conclusions have been based were performed on samples of expressed milk from mothers breastfeeding *full-term*, not *preterm*, infants.

Although Atkinson, Bryan, and Anderson[4] are often cited as the first researchers to report data suggesting differences in composition between milk produced by mothers delivering at full term and those delivering prematurely, this issue was recognized as early as 1969. At that time Stevens[54] published data on the milk protein concentration of 10 mothers delivering premature, low birth weight infants. He noted the potential for absolute differences, in addition to rates of change with progressive lactation. Stevens' method was not well controlled by today's standards, but he did generate the original question of interest.

Atkinson, Bryan, and Anderson[4] published subsequent data (1978) reporting that the total nitrogen concentration of milk was higher among their sample of mothers of premature infants than among the women delivering at full term. Although the nitrogen concentration for both groups decreased over the first month of lactation, the absolute values remained significantly higher in the group of mothers delivering prematurely. Atkinson, Bryan, and Anderson also noted no significant differences in the volumes of milk produced by the two groups of women, concluding that premature delivery does not affect ability to lactate.

Reactions to this report were quite varied. Foman and Ziegler[19] responded that greater controls over study design were needed. They also specified that additional data describing relative concentrations in carbohydrates and fat in "premature" milk should precede alteration of established feeding practices based on the research findings. The study by Atkinson, Bryan, and Anderson, however, stimulated further research that tested the general hypothesis that composition of milk produced by mothers delivering at full term differs from that produced by women delivering prematurely.

Subsequent studies have further refined the nature of the differences between preterm and full-term human milk. Atkinson, Anderson, and Bryan[3] compared the relative nitrogen composition in the two types of milk, reporting that protein nitrogen was higher in premature milk throughout the first 4 weeks of lactation. This difference is consistent with the protein requirements of premature infants.

Schanler and Oh[51] also reported differences between milk produced by mothers of premature babies and that produced by mothers of full-term infants. They noted higher concentrations of total nitrogen, sodium, and calcium in the former group but found that differences between the two groups decreased over the first month of lactation.

Similar findings by Gross et al.[24] included greater amounts of protein, sodium, and chloride but lesser amounts of lactose in pre-term milk. They, too, found that differences between the two groups decreased over the first month of lactation and that at the end of that time composition of the milk was not significantly different. These researchers also analyzed milk from the two groups of women for relative amounts of fat, energy, potassium, calcium, phosphorus, and magnesium. The samples did not significantly differ with respect to these components. This study did not, however, use samples of milk representative of complete 24-hour collections. This factor may have influenced the data.

Other research has been directed toward identifying differences in mineral content between premature and full-term milk.[5,9,33,34] The results from these investigations are inconclusive, although the researchers agree that premature milk is more suited to the needs of the premature infant than is full-term milk.

A more recent area of research distinguishing the two types of milk concerns energy and lipid components. Since the energy value of milk is directly related to lipid content, this topic is particularly relevant when considering the dietary needs of the premature baby. Clandinin et al.[12] have published recent data concerning fatty acid accretion in the development of the spinal cord in fetuses and infants. They note that the developmental changes in accretion of fatty acids parallels the processes of myelination and increasing neuromotor activity. They suggest that their data are "indicative of minimal fatty acid requirements for synthesis of spinal cord tissues in the normally growing human fetus and neonate" (p. 5) and that they can provide a basis for computation of dietary requirements.

Absorption of dietary lipids is, however, more problematic for the premature baby than for the full-term infant; steatorrhea is higher among the former group. Human milk fat and unsaturated fatty acids are most easily absorbed. The absolute amounts and the relative composition of human milk fat differs from that of cow's milk. This factor and the presence of lipase in human milk[28] probably influence the more effective digestion and absorption of human milk fat by premature infants. Williamson et al.,[57] however, caution that this lipase activity may be decreased with heat processing of human milk.

Guerrini et al.[25] found an inverse relationship between gestational age and fat content in human milk. Anderson, Atkinson, and Bryan[1] reported that premature milk was consistently higher (20% to 30%) in lipid and energy content in their sample of women. Such differences are consistent with the higher energy needs of small premature infants. Spencer and Hull[53] propose that other factors markedly influence the lipid content of expressed milk; their data appropriately address the need for lipid "quality control." The investigators studied the lipid content of 274 samples of expressed milk that was used for premature infant feeding and noted a wide range in lipid content depending on a number of variables: the time of day the milk was expressed, whether it was foremilk or hindmilk, and its method of administration to infants. They emphasize the importance of routine surveillance of lipid content in milk fed to premature babies to ensure minimal acceptable standards. It is apparent from the preceding research concerning the specific nature of premature milk that more data are needed for conclusive recommendations on this subject. A major variable requiring investigation is the extent (if any) to which composition of milk varies with the degree of prematurity of the infant, since most comparison groups in the literature have been divided only into "mature" and "premature." This is especially important, since the nutritional requirements of the very low birth weight infant differ considerably from those of the larger premature baby. The American Academy of Pediatrics (AAP) Committee on Nutrition, however, has published a report[13] summarizing the literature and issuing a conclusion concerning the use of human milk for premature feeding:

> At this time the Committee considers it optimal for mothers of low birth weight newborn infants to collect milk for feeding their own infants fresh milk (p. 856).

This statement is consistent with professional attempts to develop nursery programs that support breastfeeding of high-risk infants.

Reports in the literature that provide practical assistance in the areas of program development or specific techniques for supporting lactation in mothers of premature infants are not nearly as abundant. Choi[11] has described the principles of milk expression and parent support with respect to nursing the premature infant. Henderson and Newton[27] and Stewart and Gainer[55] have published practical suggestions for counseling breastfeeding mothers who are separated from their infants; their reports, however, do not address program development or many of the specific needs of mothers of premature babies. Meier[43,45] has described the development and implementation of such a program, emphasizing the need to initiate feedings at the breast in premature infants not according to weight but to the ability to suck safely and effectively. Pearce and Buchanan[48] published data comparing weight gain in small premature infants who were nursed at the breast with that of a comparable group of babies fed expressed mothers' milk with a bottle. Infants in their experimental group began feeding at the breast at a mean weight of 1324 gm (about 2.8 lb). The authors found no significant difference in weight gain between the two groups of premature infants. They concluded that professional emphasis should be directed toward providing support to facilitate mothers' feeding their premature infants at the breast rather than exclusively toward techniques of processing and storing expressed milk.

COPING WITH THE BIRTH OF A HIGH-RISK INFANT

To provide effective breastfeeding support, the nurse must understand parental reactions to the birth of a premature or sick infant. Caplan[8] was the first author to describe the birth of a premature infant as a crisis for the mother, delineating the overlapping phases in a manner consistent with Lindemann's classic work.[39] Kaplan and Mason[29] later described "psychological tasks" associated with learning the maternal role when infants are prematurely born. Numerous authors* have subsequently proposed models describing maternal or parental reactions to the birth of premature or ill newborn infants. There is general agreement that certain characteristic behaviors are quite common among parents confronting this situation. The nurse who provides breastfeeding assistance must be aware of these behaviors to appreciate their effect on the breastfeeding process.

Initial parental reactions to the birth of a high-risk infant usually include shock, disbelief, and an emotional "numbness" when told of their infant's problems. During this period parents ask questions that reflect denial or an inability to fully comprehend the situation with which they are confronted. Patience during this time is essential to effective intervention. Parents need to hear the same information repeated at regular intervals, since they are often unable to accept and understand it without such repetition.

As time passes, parents develop the ability to understand that their infant is seriously ill. Consequent reactions include manifestations of anger, guilt, and depression. Their questions are usually directed toward establishing a cause or reason for their infants' problems. As this phase progresses, parents often express feelings of helplessness, loss of control, and isolation. Many have physical symptoms such as insomnia, anorexia, or extreme fatigue. Effective intervention at this time must permit parents to express and work through these feelings and reactions. It is also essential that they realize that these are normal responses to their situation. Intervention should not focus on "cheering them up" or attempting to dispel these feelings through lengthy, factual discussions. Finally,

---

*References 7, 10, 31, 38, 42, 52.

the nurse should recognize ways in which parents can exercise control over the situation they are confronted with, effectively reinforcing these efforts. It is during this time that initiation of parental caretaking functions is helpful. Breastfeeding is one such activity.

THE DECISION TO BREASTFEED THE SPECIAL-CARE INFANT

The decision to breastfeed a premature or sick newborn infant is considerably more complex than the comparable one to breastfeed a healthy infant. Although innumerable factors affect this decision, the common ones can be isolated into two categories. The first grouping of factors consists of those related to the parents' level of knowledge about breastfeeding the premature infant. They include the practical concerns about milk expression, storage, adequacy of supply, and the rationale for using mothers' milk in premature nutrition. These are information-related issues that few women have been exposed to before the birth of a high-risk infant. Fortunately, they can be anticipated, and answers to these questions are readily available.

The second clustering of factors includes parental reactions to the birth of a high-risk infant. Unlike the mother who chooses to breastfeed a healthy baby, the mother of the premature or sick newborn infant must cope with feelings of loss while attempting to attach to her infant. The very complex task of integrating the processes of loss and attachment inevitably influences the decision to breastfeed. The decision to breastfeed commonly includes two types of rationale by the mother, which reflect her attempt to cope with feelings surrounding her infant's illness. A mother may decide to breastfeed because she feels she is giving her baby something that no one else can; this is a healthy attempt to establish control over feelings of helplessness. Another woman might feel that she is "compensating" for having been responsible for her baby's problem. One mother stated, "I felt the need to apologize to my baby," reflecting a healthy coping mechanism to deal with feelings of guilt. For those mothers who had planned to breastfeed throughout pregnancy, such as manifestations may be less apparent.

Some women experiencing anticipatory grief are unable to invest the emotional commitment that milk expression requires. They quite justifiably fear tangible attempts to "attach" to a baby whose survival is threatened, since this maximizes their vulnerability. Such mothers usually decide not to breastfeed or to delay milk expression until their babies' conditions are more stable. Although the decision to breastfeed the high-risk baby must remain with the parents, it is the responsibility of the health professional to ensure that the decision is an *informed* one. This entails informing them of relevant information concerning the specificity of "premature" milk and the immunologic benefits of human milk for the special-care baby. Only by receiving such important information can parents make a truly informed decision.

A written supplement that addresses these and other important issues relevant to the decision to breastfeed should be made available to parents, since the nature of the crisis usually precludes their complete retention and understanding of oral communication. An example of such a publication is *Breastfeeding Your "Special Care" Baby,*[44] a consumer-oriented booklet developed at Michael Reese Hospital, Chicago, and included at the end of this chapter. The section entitled "Should You Nurse?" summarizes common parental concerns. Written material has the additional advantage of introducing mothers outside the institutional support system to the idea of breastfeeding a special-care infant;

this is particularly helpful if health-care providers are unable or unwilling to share relevant information with them.

Some parents, for any of a number of reasons, are still ambivalent and indecisive after obtaining relevant information. In such instances it is usually advisable to encourage the mother to initiate milk expression, emphasizing that it can be temporary and that the mother can decide to stop at any time. The nurse should also mention that the mother's milk is of greatest benefit to the infant during the first few weeks after birth. It can be carefully explained that it is easier to terminate milk expression after 2 weeks than it is to initiate lactation at that time. This approach necessitates that the nurse communicate in a caring, noncoercive manner with the parents and that she ultimately support the parents' decision even when it sharply conflicts with her own.

THE INITIAL BREASTFEEDING CONFERENCE

Once parents have made the decision to breastfeed their special-care baby, the nurse should schedule a conference with them to develop an initial plan. This session, which usually takes about an hour, should take place in a private room, preferably away from the patient care area. The two purposes of the initial breastfeeding conference are to assess the mother's support systems for breastfeeding her premature or sick baby and to develop with her an initial plan for milk expression. This mother is considered a *breastfeeding* mother whether her milk is given to her infant directly from her breast or, temporarily, by other means. Although it is tempting to include innumerable facts and suggestions during this conference, the nurse must remember that the mother is confronting a crisis and will be unable to remember information that is not immediately useful to her. For this reason, the content discussed during the initial breastfeeding conference should generally be restricted to the following five areas: identifying a support system, reviewing the lactation process, acquiring a suitable breast pump, establishing a milk expression and storage plan, and explaining the feeding plan. Each of these content areas will be developed in detail, and a practical intervention strategy will be emphasized. In addition, each section includes background information and supportive rationale to facilitate understanding of the specific content.

Identifying a support system

Since mothers who breastfeed premature infants describe a lack of professional and peer support of their decision as a major problem, it is essential that the nurse help the mother identify potential people who can fulfill this need. Questions such as "Have any of your family members or close friends breastfed their babies?" will usually elicit maternal perceptions of support within her immediate environment. If a mother does identify such a friend or relative, the nurse can further inquire whether any of these women has ever used a breast pump for milk expression.

If there are no apparent sources of support for breastfeeding, the mother should be referred to another woman who can provide reinforcement for her decision and basic assistance with common breastfeeding questions. Ideally, the nursery staff should maintain a list of several mothers who have expressed milk for their special-care babies. These women should preferably represent a wide geographic and cultural group that reflects the entire population served by the individual nursery. In addition to providing breastfeeding support, these women, who have had a similar experience, can assist new mothers in coping with the crisis of a complicated birth. They can also identify with those emotional factors affecting the breastfeeding process. Parent organizations (self-care groups) of special-care infants exist in several metropolitan areas; others are now developing. La Leche League International is another referral source; most local chapters know of members who have had experience with long-term milk expression. The important principle, however, is that each mother should leave the initial breastfeeding conference aware of the necessity of attaining effective support and with definitive plans for doing so.

Reviewing the lactation process

This area should be restricted to essential topics during the initial breastfeeding conference. Of particular importance is helping the mother distinguish between milk production and milk ejection. Although this information is relevant to all breastfeeding mothers, it is crucial when milk expression must be substituted for the infant's feeding at the breast. Many of the problems of mothers who breastfeed premature or sick babies are related to a temporary unresponsiveness of the let-down reflex. Teaching mothers how to recognize the sensations associated with milk ejection is important in helping them with breastfeeding problems should they occur. A mother's positive or negative response to "Are you currently having a let-down reflex?" is necessary in assessing a temporary breastfeeding problem. This topic should also be supplemented with written information comparable with the section "How Lactation Works" in *Breastfeeding Your "Special Care" Baby*[44] at the end of this chapter.

Acquiring a suitable breast pump

Selecting a suitable breast pump is an essential component of the initial breastfeeding conference, since milk expression should begin as soon as possible after birth. In giving the mother this information for the first time, however, the nurse should be aware of normal maternal reactions to the thought of milk expression by mechanical means. Few women even know that breast pumps exist; most consumer-oriented literature concerning breastfeeding addresses only the needs of the healthy mother and infant. Initial reactions of women to milk expression by pump range from mild disappointment to unquestionable revulsion. One mother's first comments compared the pump to a "milking machine for cows." The nurse should be aware of the fact that using a breast pump is one more reminder of the loss associated with a complicated postpartum experience. These feelings compound those resulting from the crisis surrounding the infant's condition.

Breast pumps that can be suitably used by mothers of special-care babies must meet certain criteria. First, they should be convenient, efficient, and comfortable to use, since milk expression is often prolonged over several weeks or even months. Second, the ability to adequately clean and sterilize all parts that come into contact with expressed milk is essential. Liebhaber et al.[37] and Pitt[49] have reported the increased potential for milk contamination with expression by a breast pump. Donowitz and Wenzel[17] have described an incident in which expressed milk became contaminated with *Klebsiella*. Subsequently the breast pump was found to be grossly contaminated with the organism. It is therefore essential that all the collecting equipment be thoroughly scrubbed or sterilized (see instructions in *Breastfeeding Your "Special Care" Baby*) and that the pump itself be properly serviced and maintained. The small plastic pumps with the suction-creating ball but no separate collection device (often referred to as bicycle horns) should not be used for milk expression, since the interior of the ball device cannot be adequately sterilized. Third, it is preferable that the collecting container be constructed of hard plastic, rather than glass, since leukocytes have been reported to adhere to the latter surface.[47] Finally, the pump should not present an unreasonable expense to the parent, since third party reimbursement for breast pump purchase or rental is not universal. The cost is, however, tax deductible as a legitimate medical expense.

Breast pumps can be divided into two broad categories: electric and manually operated ones. Both have certain advantages and disadvantages for the mother of the premature infant. Although the nurse does not need to discuss each of these with the mother, she should be aware of the various available products. For that reason specific breast pumps will be described in this section; emphasis will be on suitability of the pump for use with the mother of the special-care baby.

The Egnell and the Medela electric pumps are excellent machines for prolonged milk expression. These devices are extremely comfortable and convenient to use; the mother simply determines the desired level of negative pressure (from "low" to "normal") and then turns on the machine (Fig. 12-1). The pumps operate by internal mechanisms that produce a gentle, cyclic suction, simulating a breastfeeding infant. The collecting devices disassemble for thorough cleaning and sterilization. The flanges (nipple shields), those parts of the collecting devices that fit over the breast, are manufactured in different sizes. During the initial breastfeeding conference, the nurse should evaluate which size is correct for the individual mother. It must be sufficiently large to permit the "back and forth" movement of the nipple, a motion essential to proper conditioning of the letdown reflex in the mother who will use the pump for a prolonged time. It must not, however, be so large that the outer rim of the shield does not form a tight seal around the breast. An excessively large shield will allow air to enter between the rim and the breast during the negative pressure phase of the pumping cycle and interfere with optimal emptying of the breasts. Pumping is more comfortable if the inside of the flange is moistened with sterile water before starting, thus reducing irritation to the areola and nipple.

Comfort and ease of operating the Egnell and Medela pumps make them the machines of choice for the mother who must initiate and maintain lactation without her infant feeding the breast. Each special-care nursery should own an electric pump for mothers to use while visiting their babies. The Egnell Company recommends that each area of an institution with breastfeeding patients have its own pump for purposes of infection control. It is also recommended[23] that an electric pump used by a mother having a radioactive scan be removed from general use for several days, the length of time depending on the specific radioactive agent. Nurseries that serve a large breastfeeding population should therefore have at least two pumps, in the event that one malfunctions or must be removed from service.

The Egnell and Medela pumps, considerably more expensive than manually operated models, preclude individual purchase for home use. They are, however, available for rental from a variety of outlets (drug stores, hospital supply stores, and private homes) throughout the United States. The companies will supply a listing of local outlets on request. Another alternative for special-care nurseries is to establish their own unit-based

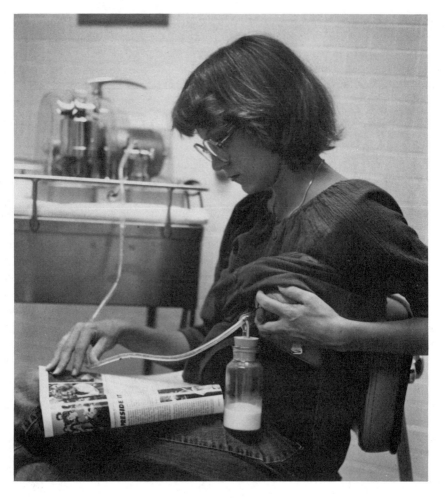

Fig. 12-1. Electric pump is comfortable, convenient, and efficient to use. (Courtesy Michael Reese Hospital and Medical Center, Chicago, Ill.)

outlet for pump rental. The companies can provide details necessary for the implementation of such a project.

Manually operated pumps include a number of acceptable products; two are particularly suited to the needs of mothers of high-risk infants. The Kaneson (Marshall) pump (Fig. 12-2) consists of inner and outer hard plastic cylinders that disassemble for easy cleaning. The flange, which is attached to the inner cylinder, fits over the breast; a plastic ring is inserted to adapt the device to the size of the mother's nipples. Suction is created by the mother's alternately extending and releasing the outer cylinder in a forward/backward motion while holding the flange securely over the breast. Several rapid movements in sequence provide the nipple stimulation necessary for eliciting the let-down reflex. Once the reflex is triggered, the mother can gently massage the breast with the hand holding the shield in place, while continuing to gently extend (not releas-

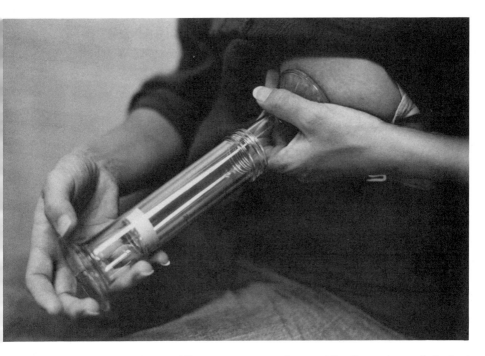

Fig. 12-2. One hand holds flange of Kaneson pump onto breast while other moves cylinder back and forth. (Courtesy Michael Reese Hospital and Medical Center, Chicago, Ill.)

ing) the outer cylinder. This constant negative pressure sufficiently empties the breast once milk ejection has begun. Leaning slightly forward while pumping prevents milk from flowing back to the opening. Ease of operation and plastic, nonbreakable construction are advantages of the Kaneson pump. A disadvantage is that the pump is easily tipped over, spilling the expressed milk. To avoid this, the nurse should instruct the mother to place the cover on the pump as soon as milk expression is completed.

The Loyd-B-Pump (Lopuco, Inc.) is the other manually operated device that facilitates milk expression for the mother of the special-care infant. The pump consists of two components: the pump body, which creates the negative pressure, and the glass collecting device. To use the Loyd-B-Pump, the mother grasps the "triggerlike" part of the pump body in one hand and holds the flange of the collecting unit firmly over the breast with the other (Fig. 12-3). The milk ejection reflex is elicited by alternately creating suction with the pump body and releasing it with the valve adjacent to the collection device. This series of movements is repeated until milk begins to flow freely with the let-down, and then a gentle negative pressure is created and maintained with the pump body. The hand holding the shield in place can be used to massage the breast, facilitating complete emptying.

Although the Loyd-B-Pump is comfortable to use, it has two major disadvantages. The collecting device is constructed of glass, which may promote leukocyte adherence[47] and is susceptible to breakage. Although the collection bottle is easily replaced (it is a standard 4-ounce baby food jar), the flange must be obtained from the company. The second negative factor is the degree of manipulation required to operate the pump. Since

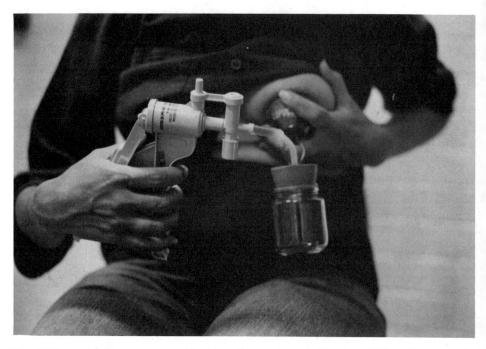

Fig. 12-3. Loyd-B-Pump is operated by triggerlike mechanism. (Courtesy Michael Reese Hospital and Medical Center, Chicago, Ill.)

suction and release phases are controlled by different parts of the pump, a reasonable amount of practice is required to use it effectively and efficiently. Although this is usually a minor problem for mothers with healthy infants, it can present a major psychologic obstacle for those coping with crisis and loss. These are, in perspective, minor limitations of the product and certainly should not preclude its use by mothers of special-care babies.

The Kaneson and Loyd-B-Pumps are comparably priced and can be secured in a variety of ways. They are available for purchase from the respective companies (listed at the end of this chapter) or designated local outlets. Ideally the institution should supply either the Marshall or Loyd-B-Pump to all mothers who require prolonged or temporary assistance with milk expression. These devices can be purchased in bulk and stocked by the hospital pharmacy or central supply department. When needed, they can be ordered and charged to the mother's or infant's account; such a procedure usually complies with criteria for third party reimbursement.

Each maternal situation is individual; a pump suitable for one mother might not be for another. Factors such as expense, availability, and projected duration of milk expression should influence the nurse's recommendation. Although the electric pump is usually the machine of choice, it may not be accessible to the mother. By discussing alternatives with her, the nurse can develop an individualized plan based on maternal needs and resources. An option is for the mother to use the electric pump frequently during her visits to the nursery, supplementing her milk expression at home with a manually operated device. Each nursery should establish and maintain relations with the major breast pump companies, the local La Leche League chapter, and nursery mothers who have used the various products. By effectively using these resources, the health-care professional can provide optimal assistance in the selection of a breast pump suited to the individual needs of mothers of special-care babies.

Establishing a plan for collecting and storing milk

Probably no topic in neonatal nutrition has been the subject of more controversy than methods of collecting and storing expressed human milk. Since there are no definitive answers to some of the questions involved, a number of health-care professionals have chosen not to support a nursery-based breastfeeding support program. Certain guidelines based on the available literature, however, can be developed to provide a framework for specific procedures and protocols.

Once milk expression has been discussed, mothers usually ask about the frequency of pumping. Quite simply stated, milk expression should be consistent with an uncomplicated breastfeeding experience with minor modifications. The mother expressing milk, like the mother breastfeeding a healthy infant, should begin as soon as possible after delivery. Since milk expression is initially difficult on demand, the nurse should advise the mother to use the pump every 3 hours during the waking hours and once during the night, if possible. Often, a full night's sleep for the fatigued mother is more advantageous than the extra stimulation of her milk supply. Such decisions must be highly individualized. Recommendations concerning the duration of pumping should be based on comparable reasoning: approximately 5 minutes per breast initially, progressing to 10 or 15 minutes per breast over the first 3 or 4 days.

Appropriate milk processing and storage are more complicated issues, and the potential untoward effects are more serious. The nurse must therefore adequately address proper hygiene and strict attention to storage protocols during the initial breastfeeding conference. The approach for sharing this information should generate caution, not fear, within the parents. Basic rationale for these procedures and protocols must be included, since this knowledge facilitates parent compliance.

Before initiating discussion of milk storage, the nurse should review with the mother proper aseptic technique while collecting milk. She should wash her hands immediately before manipulating the breasts or using the equipment. Although some professionals advocate extensive nipple cleansing, the necessity for such a practice is not documented, nor is it advisable. The collecting device, including all pump parts that could theoretically contact milk, needs to be sterilized twice a day, either in boiling water or in a dishwasher, and scrubbed with soap and hot water before each use. The mother should also be cautioned not to cough or sneeze while handling the equipment.

Expressed mother's milk can be processed and stored in a number of ways[32]; there is no consensus[13] in the literature at the current time on a single optimal method.[13] Although heat processing destroys undesirable pathogens, it adversely affects the protective immunologic components in human milk.[18,22,36,47] Williamson et al.[57] found that heat treatment also appeared to alter fat absorption in preterm infants fed human milk and postulated that milk lipase might be inactivated with this process.

Freezing is an acceptable alternative to heat processing of expressed milk.[13] Storage of milk by freezing preserves many desirable immunologic properites,[36] although milk leukocytes are inactivated by this process[36,47] (Table 12-1). Freezing does not, however,

TABLE 12-1 _____

Effect of pasteurization and freezing on breastmilk

Method	Lysozymes	Leukocytes	IgA	Lactoferrin
Heat treatment (62.5° C [144.5° F] for 30 min)	Slightly or not altered	Destroyed	Slightly or not altered	Reduced by two thirds
Freezing	Slightly or not altered	Destroyed	Not altered	Slightly or not altered

destroy bacteria,[13,32] as does heat processing, so scrupulous attention to aseptic technique when handling milk or equipment is mandatory.

In addition to the immunologic advantages associated with freezing in contrast to heat processing, there are several practical considerations. First, the freezing method is usually readily available; most families have at least a small freezer compartment, and most institutions can acquire a small freezer with minimal difficulty. Second, freezing milk, rather than processing it with heat, is considerably less expensive, since no specialized equipment is required. Third, freezing is a less complicated method that is easily accomplished without the assistance of a trained technician; this is untrue of heat processing. These practical issues should be considered when deciding on institutional protocol for milk processing and storage.

A frequently asked question is how long expressed milk can remain frozen and still be considered adequate for infant consumption. Although there are no reliable data addressing this issue, reputable sources describe isolated samples of milk that have been frozen for up to several years. On biochemical and bacteriologic examination, this milk was found to be entirely appropriate for infant feeding. This is not to suggest that these figures be used as guidelines. In the absence of contradictory data, however, there is no reason that frozen milk cannot be stored for at least the several weeks of a baby's hospitalization. Anecdotal reports suggest, however, that if milk is to be frozen for several weeks, it should be stored in a hard plastic or glass container. Although inconclusively documented, frozen milk stored in soft plastic containers for several weeks has been noted to acquire the odor of the plastic.

There remains also the distinction between milk storage in a freezer compartment and storage in a deep freezer[32]; the latter ensures an unfluctuating temperature, whereas the former does not. Although no specific guidelines exist, it is reasonable to generalize that the length of time milk is frozen in a refrigerator-freezer should be minimal before transfer to a deep-freezing unit. Hypothetical estimates on limits of this time are generally 1 to 2 weeks. Based on substantiated and anecdotal data, the following guidelines are recommended:

Guidelines for storing breastmilk

Fresh breastmilk: Use within 30 minutes or refrigerate.

Refrigerated breastmilk: Use within 24 hours in 4° C (40° F) refrigerator.

Frozen breastmilk: Keep 1 to 2 weeks in a refrigerator-freezer unit, longer if in an 18° C (0° F) freezer that is a separate compartment from the refrigerator. Keep in hard plastic containers.

Thawing breastmilk: Thaw under running water, first cold and gradually warmer until the milk has liquified. Do not refreeze.

When at all possible, infants should be fed fresh milk that has not been processed by any method.[13] This ensures optimal nutritional and immunologic benefit to the premature infant. Although there is a deficiency of supporting evidence in the literature, most experts agree that human milk is bacteriologically acceptable for feeding for 24 hours after expression, providing it has been refrigerated.[16]

During the initial breastfeeding conference, the nurse can very generally discuss the differences between fresh and processed milk. Mothers can then plan to freeze all milk except for that which is most recently expressed. The fresh milk may be used at any time within a 24-hour period, preferably alternated with feedings of frozen milk. Parents who understand the immunologic advantages of fresh milk can fully participate in their infant's nutritional plan. Allowing parents to share the responsibility for such a plan helps to meet their natural needs for control over their situation, thereby channeling these feelings in a constructive manner.

Expressed milk can be stored in any of a variety of sterile containers. The small graduated infant nursers provided by commercial formula companies are especially suitable. These presterilized bottles are plastic, which eliminates the problem of potential breakage and maximizes preservation of leukocytes.[47] (Leukocyte survival is important only when fresh milk is stored, since processing in any form inactivates live cells.) They are also small, which facilitates storage, and the durable construction prevents accidental puncture or leakage associated with the use of sterile plastic bags. There is seldom a charge for these products, so they can be distributed to mothers as needed. The collecting bottles should *always* be labeled with the date and the baby's name.

Transporting expressed milk to the special-care nursery requires maintaining the same conditions under which milk has been stored (fresh or frozen). For this purpose small cold storage chests and refreezable ice packs are handy. When it is impossible for relatives or friends to transport milk to the nursery on a regular basis, several options should be considered. First, the nurse can attempt to locate a hospital employee who lives near the family and can bring expressed milk to the nursery between parent visits. If this is impossible, resources in the institution's ''Patient Services'' or ''Volunteer'' Departments should be explored. If the hospital is nonsupportive in this respect, local parenting and breastfeeding support organizations should be approached. In arranging for milk transport, the nurse should recognize and use the universal humanistic appeal of a project designed to benefit premature or ill newborn infants.

When expressed milk reaches the special-care nursery, it must be immediately frozen or refrigerated. Labeling separate shelves or areas for each baby's milk serves two major functions. It organizes the milk within the freezer or refrigerator, and it communicates to the parents that the mother's expressed milk is desired. The milk represents an emotional investment of the mother—a visible sign of her relationship with her baby. Careless storage or handling practices, resulting in discarding of milk, are extremely frustrating and often demoralizing for the mother. Treatment of expressed milk by the professional staff should reflect respect for these maternal feelings and the effort involved.

Expressed milk must be warmed to at least room temperature before it is used for infant feeding. Heating refrigerated milk should be a gradual process; approximately half an hour should be allotted. If commercial infant feeders are used, they can be placed within a paper cup filled with lukewarm water. If milk is frozen, thawing by the same method will take an hour. Milk should *never* be placed in very hot water to effect more rapid warming. Such a procedure potentially affects milk in a manner similar to heat processing, altering desirable nutritional and antiinfective characteristics.

It is essential that written protocols be developed for milk collection and storage to ensure uniform compliance with aseptic technique. These materials should reflect documented research rather than individual opinion and sentiment. They should also be practical, demonstrating awareness and use of available resources. Information relevant to collection and storage should also be written for parents to supplement discussion during the initial breastfeeding conference. This can be a very complex topic, especially for parents who already feel somewhat helpless and confused; written materials can be reviewed at a time when comprehension is better.

Explaining the feeding plan

Parents are often unable to place their infant's nutritional plan within the framework of an overall management regimen. They may have little or no understanding of when and how their baby will receive expressed milk or on what basis such decisions are made. For this reason the nurse should conclude the initial breastfeeding conference by describing a tentative feeding plan for the infant, delineating those factors that will directly influence it. The following is an example of such an approach:

> Since your baby's respiratory problem is consuming so much of his energy, it is best that he not be fed for the next few days. He will get the nourishment he needs during that time from the intravenous feedings. As he continues to need less assistance with his breathing, we will gradually begin to feed him the milk you express. To do this we will pass a tiny tube through his nose into his stomach; we will then feed him your milk through that tube. Once he grows and takes a few feedings from a bottle he will be ready to begin to feed at the breast. Judging by his weight and his condition, that will be about 3 weeks from now.

The nurse should emphasize that the time periods are only *guidelines* and can vary with the infant's condition. Such an individual evaluation, however, is extremely advantageous in facilitating parental integration of the nutritional plan and the baby's overall condition.

COMMON PROBLEMS DURING MILK EXPRESSION

The time between the initial breastfeeding conference and the premature infant's feeding at the breast is characterized by certain predictable problems. Mothers should be aware of the potential occurrence of these problems and of where they can receive assistance. Early identification and intervention are essential for optimal resolution.

The most frequent problem mothers have in expressing their milk is inhibition of the let-down reflex. Since this mechanism is greatly affected by emotional and psychologic factors, a suboptimal response among mothers of sick newborn infants is not unusual. For instance, the stimuli that normally enhance the let-down reflex—touching, smelling, hearing, and seeing her infant—are absent. As one mother described this experience, "there's nothing about a machine that makes me feel motherly." Instead of the usual sensations, the let-down "stimulus" is the sound of an electric pump.

This problem can be recognized by careful assessment. The mother usually notes difficulty producing an adequate volume of milk and describes sensations inconsistent with those accompanying the milk-ejection reflex. The nurse should assure the mother that this problem is normal and temporary and acknowledge the mother's expression of feelings of frustration, disappointment, and depression. Several ways to increase the milk flow have been discussed by mothers who participated in the breastfeeding support program at Michael Reese Hospital and Medical Center in Chicago[43]:

1. Encourage the mother to sit or lie down, take a few cleansing breaths, and relax for at least 5 minutes before beginning milk expression.
2. Suggest that she put a picture of the baby beside the breast pump where it is easily seen.
3. Advise the mother to massage the breast she will first empty for 1 minute before applying the pump.
4. Suggest that she then use the pump for about half the time allotted to that breast, interrupting milk expression to massage the breast again.
5. Instruct the mother to pump again until the milk spray lessens, then switch to the other breast, repeating the above procedures until both breasts have emptied (usually about 15 minutes per breast).

Pumping is time consuming, boring, and tiring. Talking with a friend, reading, or watching television will often relieve tedium and even facilitate the milk flow. Milk expression at home is sometimes more tolerable with family support and involvement. One mother's young daughter "pumped" along with her mother, placing the extra breast pump flange over her breast. Fathers, too, have been known to assist by manipulating the manual pumps when mothers become fatigued.

In the nursery the let-down reflex can be facilitated by encouraging the mother to hold her infant (condition permitting) while expressing milk. The psychologic benefit of doing so cannot be overstated. A special room in the hospital near the nursery should be set aside for mothers to express milk. A private area with a comfortable homelike atmosphere and furnishings is optimal. Such a location need not be large, and the lack of an allotted physical space should not be a deterrent. At Michael Reese Hospital, one of two seldom used isolation rooms was converted into a breastfeeding area. It was subsequently furnished with a comfortable reclining chair, some plants, and a homemade quilt, which served as a wall decoration. A sign stating "Mother Breastfeeding" was ordered; when attached to the outside door it ensured privacy. This conversion took place without additional expense and conveyed to parents that breastfeeding is a valued and supported behavior in the special-care nursery.

Another common problem among mothers of special-care babies during milk expression is the decrease in milk volume following worsening of their infants' conditions. This situation is almost universal among mothers of very small premature infants, since these babies' clinical course is characterized by series of "ups and downs." In assessing this problem the nurse must attempt to identify when the mother first noticed the decrease in volume. Occasionally a woman will recognize the relationship between the change in the infant's condition and the onset of the problem. Most of the time, however, the nurse will need to explain this to the mother. Understanding the causal relationship of the two events must precede a mother's attempts to resolve the problem. Although the temporary decrease in supply is usually a result of emotional interference with the milk-ejection reflex, the previously mentioned techniques are often inadequate.

The mother is experiencing a very real crisis, of which the breastfeeding problem is only one manifestation.

Nursing intervention in this very common situation consists of acknowledging the mother's feelings of loss and assuring her that this is her body's reaction to a very upsetting situation. The nurse should emphasize that this is a *normal* response and that it is temporary. The mother should be reassured that whatever volume of milk is expressed is sufficient to maintain lactation and (if appropriate) reminded that the amount of stored milk is sufficient to meet the baby's requirements during this time. The nurse should also stress the fact that her milk flow will increase after the crisis resolves. Probably of most benefit, however, is the initiation of a parent-to-parent referral to provide needed encouragement and support. A mother who has experienced the same situation in the same nursery is an invaluable resource during this time. Finally, the nurse should not emphasize the volume of milk in her subsequent interaction with the mother. A follow-up question such as "How are things going with you today?" is less threatening than "Were you able to express more milk than yesterday?" Chronically stressed as she is, unintentional remarks by the hospital staff can be devastating to and exaggerated by the mother. One young mother, tearful after a physician's comment that she was not expressing enough milk, was prepared to stop trying. She persisted, however, after reassurances from a hospital nurse, and eventually completely breastfed her infant for a year. It is instructive to note that she remembered the physician's remarks years later.

One other problem is sufficiently common during the period of milk expression to indicate its mention in this section. This is the failure of the infant (usually premature) to adequately gain weight when fed his mother's milk via nasogastric or nasojejunal tube. Although the ideal rate of growth for prematurely born infants has not been documented,[21,26] most neonatologists feel that weight gain should proceed at a rate comparable with intrauterine figures. This goal can be achieved by manipulating concentration and relative caloric composition with commercial formulas. Weight gain from these products has become accepted as the "standard" with which other sources (including expressed mother's milk) are compared.

The mother who feels that her milk is inadequate in meeting her baby's needs may understandably become depressed and threatened. Her reaction is characterized by ambivalence: wanting to breastfeed but feeling that perhaps commercial formula is better for her baby. Such an attitude is often conveyed by health-care professionals. These mothers are referred to as "self-centered," for not thinking of their babies' needs but only of their own desire to breastfeed. The nurse must remember that mothers in this situation feel very vulnerable and require a tremendous amount of reassurance and support.

Contrary to what many neonatologists prescribe, the first solution for this problem should not be formula. There are a variety of reasons for a slow rate of growth on expressed mother's milk. Since the caloric value of milk is directly related to the fat content, ascertaining this measure should be the first step in the process. Lucas et al.[40] have described a simple method to determine fat content of mother's milk that is inexpensive and practical. Lemons et al.[35] replicated the technique with similar findings. Termed the "creamatocrit," this method requires that two hematocrit tubes be filled with samples of the mother's milk. They are sealed and centrifuged similar to the comparable hematocrit technique. The creamatocrit is the percentage of fat in the tube. Using the linear regression charts in either article, the nurse can estimate fat and caloric content of the milk sample.

If the fat content is below average, the nurse should continue her assessment of the problem. Diurnal variation in fat content of milk produced by mothers delivering at full term has been described,[28] and it has been reconfirmed in a recent study.[53] Fat content is known to increase near the end of a feeding, after the milk-ejection reflex has occurred.[28,53] By testing the creamatocrit of each sample of milk expressed within a 24-hour period, the nurse can assess whether there is a wide variability in fat content. If so, the milk could be pooled to provide a consistent fat intake.

Another reason why infants occasionally fail to gain weight on feedings of mother's milk is mechanical problems of administering feedings by nasogastric or nasojejunal tube.[53] The fat portion of the milk can adhere to the lumen of the tube and not reach the infant. This can be overcome by adequately flushing the tube with water following a bolus feeding. If the milk is being administered with an infusion pump, the position of the syringe or other device holding the feeding is very important. Since the fat layer will settle to the top of the milk, the syringe should be stabilized in an inverted position. Fat, which is on the top, is infused before the rest of the milk; it would otherwise be lost in the infusion tubings. These techniques, although quite simple and effective, are often overlooked in the assessments conducted by health-care professionals. This is unfortunate, since in the absence of contradictory data most physicians will elect to convert feedings from mother's milk to commercial formulas.

PUTTING THE PREMATURE INFANT TO BREAST

The criteria for initiating feeding at the breast for the premature infant are extremely varied and usually reflect opinion rather than empirical data. Most, however, recommend an arbitrary weight that must be achieved before breastfeeding is begun. Only two reports[43,48] in the literature address a policy of premature infants' feeding at the breast on the basis of only sucking and swallowing ability. In both instances the infants began to breastfeed weighing slightly under 3 pounds. No untoward effects were noted.

The following techniques were developed and implemented at the Michael Reese Hospital Special Care Nursery over a 3-year period. Instrumental to the development and refinement of these techniques were the nursery mothers, who patiently learned with the professional staff. This mutual sharing of knowledge and experience became the foundation for the entire breastfeeding program but was especially important in developing the techniques for breastfeeding the small premature infant.

When the nurse, parents, and physician agree that an infant is ready to feed at the breast, a brief interview should be held with the parents. The purpose of this conference is to clarify their expectations concerning initial breastfeedings. Mothers often expect that their babies will breastfeed either unrealistically well or poorly; expression of these feelings is helpful in planning for the experiences. Clarify with the parents that the first several sessions should be regarded as ''getting acquainted'' periods. A reasonable goal for these first experiences is simply to assist the infant in grasping the nipple in a manner conducive to breastfeeding. It should also be emphasized that the volume of milk ingested is not of concern; the infant at first will almost always require at least a partial

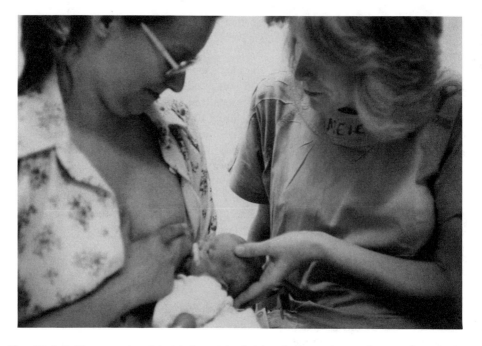

Fig. 12-4. Putting premature infant to breast for first few times requires assistance of another person to immobilize infant's head. (Infant weighed 3 pounds.) (Courtesy Michael Reese Hospital and Medical Center, Chicago, Ill.)

supplement with expressed milk by feeding tube. It is important that the mother realize that her baby will not remain hungry if he ingests only a small volume at the breast.

Putting the small premature infant to breast should occur only under rigidly controlled circumstances. The infant must be warmly dressed and wrapped in blankets. There should be no evidence of apnea or bradycardia with feeding. Finally, a nurse should remain with the mother and infant at all times during the first several breastfeeding sessions. Sitting, rather than standing, next to the mother conveys the nurse's intent to assist and guide the process—not to direct it.

The mother should be comfortably seated, preferably in a reclining easy chair. She begins by massaging her breast and elongating the nipple. This facilitates the infant's grasping the nipple by maximally increasing its length and decreasing its diameter. The mother then cradles her baby in one arm and guides her breast with the opposite hand. The nurse then grasps the infant's head securely in her hand, moving the infant to a nearly upright position. With her hand in this position, she guides the baby's mouth onto the nipple (Fig. 12-4). Occasionally infants require more assistance; if so, the nurse can use the other hand to help the baby open his mouth more widely or to move the tongue to the floor of the mouth (Fig. 12-5).

Once the infant grasps the nipple, the nurse should exert a gentle but constant pressure on the back of the infant's head (Fig. 12-6). This facilitates the infant's sucking and increases the area of the areola drawn into the mouth. It also stabilizes the head,

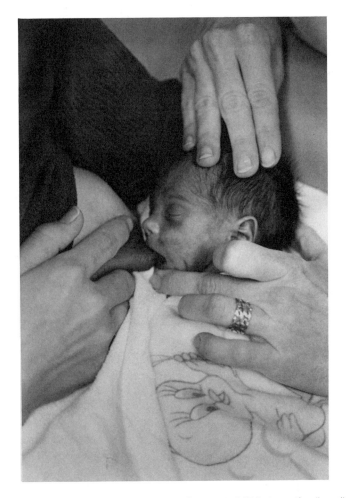

Fig. 12-5. Some premature infants require more assistance to initiate breastfeeding. (Infant weighed 2 pounds 13 ounces.) (Courtesy Michael Reese Hospital and Medical Center, Chicago, Ill.)

preventing the baby from pulling away, which quickly exhausts the small premature infant. This position should be maintained throughout the time the baby grasps the nipple.

When the baby has been positioned at the breast, the nurse should quickly assess maternal behavior. A mother is justifiably nervous during this initial experience and usually needs to be reminded to relax her face, neck, shoulders, and arms. Taking a few slow, deep breaths also facilitates milk ejection.

Babies' abilities to breastfeed during these first sessions vary quite widely. Some infants behave as if they had always been breastfed; others require several attempts to adequately grasp the nipple. Most small premature infants will feed only at one breast before burping and falling asleep. There is no reason, however, if an infant is not too fatigued, that the second breast cannot be offered.

As mothers become more skilled at and comfortable with breastfeeding, the nurse

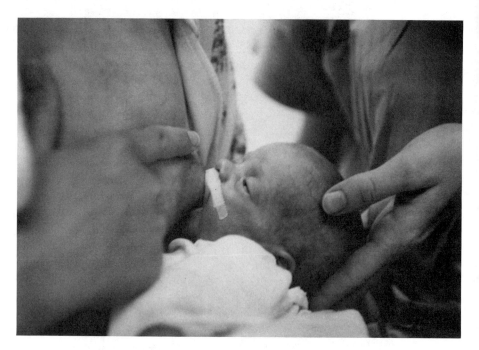

Fig. 12-6. Constant pressure exerted on back of premature infant's head enables him to suck more effectively. (Courtesy Michael Reese Hospital and Medical Center, Chicago, Ill.)

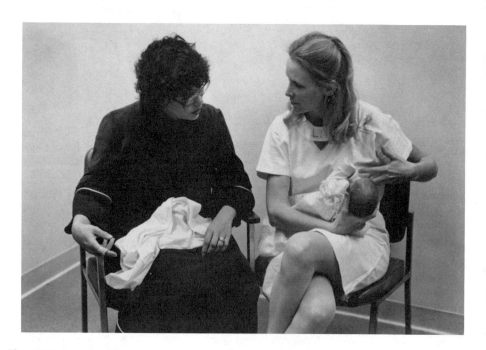

Fig. 12-7. The "transitional" position incorporates opposite arm supporting premature infant's tiny body. Other hand manipulates breast into baby's mouth. (Courtesy Michael Reese Hospital and Medical Center, Chicago, Ill.)

can move from the role of assistant to observer. The usual positions for feeding a large, healthy infant, however, require adaptation for the small premature infant. Cradling the tiny baby in the arm is unsatisfactory, since the infant tends to collapse into "a little ball." The recommended transition position for mothers just beginning to independently breastfeed small premature infants is shown in Fig. 12-7. The baby is held in the arm opposite the breast at which he will feed. The arm extends the length of the infant's back and neck, and the mother's hand grasps the baby's head to stabilize its position in relation to the breast. The other hand is used to elongate the nipple and compress the breast just proximal to the areola. The mother then moves the infant to a semisitting or an upright position, guiding him onto the breast. The hand that supports the infant's head continues to exert a gentle pressure to facilitate and maximize the baby's sucking efforts (Fig. 12-8). This position allows the mother unrestricted visibility of the infant

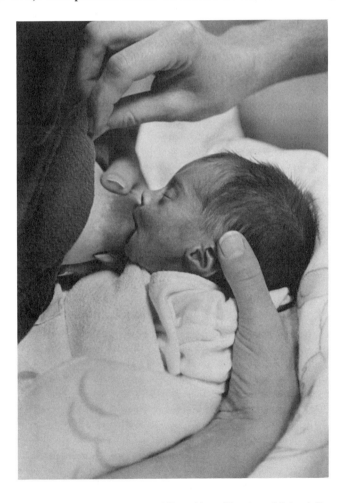

Fig. 12-8. Infant breastfeeding in "transitional" position. (Courtesy Michael Reese Hospital and Medical Center, Chicago, Ill.)

in addition to giving her complete control over his movements while at the breast. Mothers have found it universally effective.

For some reason, most physicians and some nurses are quite uncomfortable with the lack of exactness of milk intake when the premature infant breastfeeds. Mothers, too, are often concerned about adequacy of volume. Although weighing an infant before and after feeding (with the same clothing and diaper) is a fairly reliable indicator of intake, it is seldom necessary or advisable. When at all possible, mothers should breastfeed their premature infants on a semidemand basis, at intervals of 2 to 4 hours between feedings. Adequacy of intake should be based on several criteria. First, the nurse, while observing the mother and infant, should note the occurrence of the let-down reflex and the infant's subsequent sucking behavior. Second, the mother can be asked to estimate the volume the infant ingested. Nearly all women who have expressed milk for several weeks can distinguish between a full and empty breast and can fairly reliably estimate intake on how the breast feels before and after the feeding. If the mother is in doubt she can use the breast pump after the feeding to estimate the difference between that volume and the amount she usually expresses. Third, the infant can be observed for symptoms of satiety and adequacy of hydration. Finally, the infant can be weighed daily. These measures, although not entirely exact, should certainly be adequate for the healthy, growing premature infant.

Delay in initiation of nursing at the breast for the mother and her premature infant usually complicates the eventual transition from rubber nipple to breast when a certain arbitrary criterion (such as 5 pounds, or discharge) is achieved. The soft premature nipples supplied by the commercial formula companies require very little effort but an entirely different sucking mechanism, as described on p. 26.

Prolonged sucking on a soft rubber nipple results in the premature infant's reluctance to open his mouth sufficiently wide to grasp the mother's nipple and areola. This results in extreme frustration for both mother and infant. Our experience is that this problem can be prevented by early and frequent breastfeedings. Since few mothers, however, can remain available to breastfeed at all times, expressed milk should be fed in the least confusing manner. The NUK brand nipple has been proposed for supplementation of the breastfeeding premature infant[45]; when properly used, it gently forces the infant to open his mouth more widely, a movement that simulates feeding at the breast.

PREPARING FOR DISCHARGE

As discharge of the special-care baby approaches, parents confront a second crisis. Commonly expressed fears such as "I feel so helpless" are reminiscent of initial reactions to the birth of their infant. Impending discharge is characterized by simultaneous, but disparate, feelings of joy and apprehension, which can be overwhelming for the parents who still see their baby having special needs. For these reasons, planning for home care of the infant should be initiated as soon as possible after the baby's condition begins to stabilize.

Involving parents in infant care is a challenge to the health-care professional. Careful assessment of parent and infant needs and readiness for caretaking is a primary component. Ideally, parents should have unrestricted visiting opportunities, including a family care unit where they may stay overnight with their infants in preparation for discharge. In a protective, supportive environment such as this, parents have the opportunity to recognize and respond to infant needs, experimenting with and developing competent caretaking skills. This arrangement is especially worthwhile for the mother who is breastfeeding.

Neonatal staff members often wrongly assume that if a designated facility does not exist for such a program, it cannot be implemented. Such units, although philosophically appealing, are usually not funded by major health care institutions, because they do not generate income like the addition of surgical or other specialty beds. Despite this unfortunate situation, the implementation of progressive discharge programs for parents of high-risk babies is possible. Although designated physical space may be unavailable, portable cots or reclining chairs can usually be secured. Use of any available space—such as offices, conference rooms, or treatment rooms vacant during the evening and nighttime hours—should be considered. Such circumstances, although not ideal, are an improvement over the status quo and may lead parents to write letters about the deficiency in the physical environment.

Few mothers, however, regardless of support, are totally breastfeeding at the time of their infants' discharge. Factors such as geographic location, other children, and accessibility to transportation influence this situation. For these reasons, it is highly desirable that the breastfeeding premature infant be discharged to the parents as soon as medically indicated. There is really no justification for separating a mother and her healthy 1800-gm (3 lb 15 oz) infant for 7 to 10 days while the baby gains enough weight to reach a "mystical" 2000-gm (4 lb 6 oz) discharge weight. Early and comprehensive discharge planning combined with optimal follow-up support make home, rather than hospital, care an acceptable alternative for the breastfeeding premature infant who needs only to gain weight.

THE TRANSITION AND HOME CARE
Self-care support system

A major problem of breastfeeding mothers, especially those with premature babies, is the variation in quality and quantity of breastfeeding support after discharge. The community physician, health department professional, or extended family member, although often well intentioned, has usually had only minimal, if any, experience with the breastfeeding premature infant. The information provided by these people may sharply conflict with that which the mother received in the hospital. Parents should be aware of the likelihood of such a situation, as well as an alternative plan, before the time of discharge. Referring the breastfeeding mother to a community- or hospital-based self-help support group supplements professional health care and makes a difference in the transition of the infant to breastfeeding. This should be done as early into the home care planning process as possible so that mothers have the opportunity to establish relationships before the crisis of impending discharge.

A few parent support organizations for special care infants already exist. Such groups as those in Wichita, Kansas, or the Delaware Valley in Pennsylvania, offer parents a number of services, including breastfeeding support. Each mother is assigned to a "graduate" mother who periodically visits with her, either on the phone or in person.

The local La Leche League chapter can be another support system; many local chapters currently have members whose children were born prematurely or who have worked closely with such women.

A mother's individual needs and geographic location will influence the source of postdischarge breastfeeding support. As an absolutely minimal criterion, however, *no* mother should be discharged without having established contact with some source of self-care breastfeeding support.

Bottle to breast

The most obvious advantage for the mother during the transition from bottle to breast at home is increased accessibility to the baby for feedings on demand. If bottle-feedings have been extensively used in the hospital, transferring from bottle-feedings to breastfeedings requires that the infant completely repattern sucking actions using separate and diverse oral muscle actions to draw out the milk. If the infant has been feeding at the breast at least several times weekly on a regular basis, this transition is unlikely to be prolonged or difficult. It is, however, frustrating for nearly all mothers, since premature babies often have a weaker sucking reflex and tire before consuming adequate amounts of milk. Most mothers find the transition from breast pump to baby as difficult as the comparable situation of going from baby to pump. It is appropriate therefore to encourage mothers to keep rental breast pumps for at least the first week or two after their babies' discharge. Supplemental pumping is usually mandatory if the milk supply is to be maintained.

Because of their rapid growth and inability to ingest large volumes of milk at a feeding, most premature infants will demand to be fed at least every 2 to 3 hours and even more frequently during the first few weeks at home. Since continuous nutrition is so important for these babies, supplemental feedings may be necessary for a limited time after discharge. These can consist of milk that the mother has expressed to empty her breasts or a commercial formula, as suggested by the physician. Specific, but reasonable, guidelines for time intervals and supplemental feedings, based on the baby's weight and general condition, should be given to the parents before discharge.

The mother who has breastfed her premature baby on a regular basis before discharge is at an extreme advantage. With few exceptions, discharge recommendations should restrict supplementary bottle feedings to 45 to 60 ml (1½ to 2 oz) *following every other* breastfeeding. She should be encouraged to gradually decrease the amount and frequency of supplements over the first 2 weeks, at which time the baby should be totally breastfed. These guidelines will, of course, vary with respect to maternal experience and self-confidence; they must not, however, be so vague as to provide the mother with no structure. Instructions concerning assessment of hydration (number of wet diapers, color of urine) and weight gain (by physician, visiting nurse, or a reliable home scale) should also be included in discharge planning. No anticipatory guidance, however, can substitute for continual follow-up and support during the infant's transition to total breastfeeding after partial supplementation by bottle. Parents feel very vulnerable during this time, since home care of their infant presents an overwhelming responsibility; well-intentioned friends and relatives reinforce these feelings with questions such as "How do you know for sure the baby is taking enough milk; he's so little. . . ."

Helping parents *objectively* assess this situation on a day-to-day basis is an invaluable contribution of nurses or parent self-help groups.

If the mother is in the early stages of the transition to breastfeeding following discharge from the hospital, she should begin feedings at home by relaxing in a private place, away from other household activity, and sitting comfortably in an easy chair or rocker, with pillows supporting her back and on her lap. The optimal time for feeding is when the baby awakens before, not after, he begins to cry from hunger. The position for breastfeeding the premature infant will depend on his size and developmental abilities. At discharge the head lag of most premature infants is pronounced, necessitating cradling of the head, in the manner previously described as the transition position for breastfeeding in the hospital. Massaging and stimulating the breast to facilitate let-down, so that a few drops of milk appear on the breast, signals his taste buds for feeding readiness. The infant can then be helped onto the nipple. If the mother has not had experience breastfeeding before discharge, she may find it helpful to have assistance using the techniques previously described for these initial feedings.

The next chapter describes the use of the Lact-Aid Nursing Trainer in relactation and adoptive breastfeeding. The Lact-Aid Nursing Trainer can also be effective in supplementing the premature infant during the transition to the breast. Because the milk flows easily into his mouth without vigorous effort, the infant tires less during feedings at the breast. It can supplement breastfeeding with a commercial formula or with the mother's previously expressed milk. Its use can then be discontinued as the strength of the baby's suck increases.

General self-care concerns

Unlike the mother whose infant is discharged when she is, the mother of the premature infant has at least had time to physically recuperate after childbirth. The constant 24-hour demands of a small baby for frequent feedings, however, can quickly exhaust any woman. Since premature infants will usually not predictably sleep at long intervals during the nighttime for several weeks (or even months), the mother must learn to adapt her schedule to her baby's sleeping pattern, napping when her infant does. Anticipatory guidance concerning this situation will be helpful, especially if the nurse is able to explore some acceptable housekeeping alternatives with the mother before discharge.

First, household help for at least the first week is absolutely essential for the mother with a breastfeeding premature infant. Grandparents or other family members are often willing to live in and run the household, caring for any older children. Taking her father's suggestion "All you need to do is feed your baby," a mother literally did just that and in 1 week's time her infant gained 16 ounces on her breastmilk alone. Babies' fathers should, of course, be encouraged to arrange vacation time or a "paternity leave" to assist mothers during this time.

Following the prolonged separation from their infants, many women crave time along with them after discharge. This is a totally normal expression of the maternal-infant bond and should be recognized as such. The nurse can, however, help new parents evaluate the rationality of a plan for total seclusion of the family after discharge. Focusing on the reality of household tasks and how these can be performed by others, leaving the family free to interact, is a worthwhile intervention. Often, however, the need for uninterrupted private time with an infant supercedes objective reasoning.

A question frequently asked of nurses concerns what special precautions exist for foods and medications. Generally, unless a mother is allergic to a specific food, or if she observes untoward effects such as excessive gas, irritability, or stool changes in her infant after she has eaten a certain food, no dietary restrictions are necessary. She should, however, include at least two servings each of fresh vegetables and fruits a day to maintain water-soluble vitamins in her milk. With few exceptions, these mothers should continue to take prenatal vitamins during lactation, especially those containing vitamin C, since the level of this vitamin decreases with stress.

A disproportionate number of premature infants are born to teenage mothers who are known to have compromised eating habits. This presents a special challenge, since increasing numbers of these mothers now choose to breastfeed. Special emphasis should be made in motivating these young women to eat a balanced diet and avoid empty-calorie sugared foods. A mother's awareness that her food patterns influence her infant's health provides an incentive to improve her nutritional habits.

Ingestion of drugs or exposure to environmental hazards presents special problems for the mother breastfeeding her premature baby. The infant's small size and underdeveloped metabolic processes make him more vulnerable to the effects of these agents than is a healthy, larger newborn.

When the breastfeeding mother of a premature infant must take pharmacologic agents, the risk/benefit ratio should be carefully evaluated by the pediatric care provider. Often the mother is told to pump and discard her milk during the course of the drug therapy. This imposes a hardship for the mother, who may decide to stop breastfeeding entirely. The nurse can serve as an advocate for this mother in seeking out possible alternatives. First, the nurse can investigate whether the drug is potentially toxic in the prescribed dose. Few drugs are *absolutely* contraindicated in the breastfeeding mother, a finding many pediatricians are unaware of. Second, the nurse can suggest an alternative, less toxic drug that might be equally as effective. More information concerning effects of drugs on the breastfeeding infant may be found in Chapter 6. Appropriate parental information about drugs and the breastfeeding premature is included in *Breastfeeding Your "Special Care" Baby*.[44]

Alcohol ingestion, cigarette smoking, and exposure to environmental pollutants affect the breastfeeding premature infant in a manner similar to pharmacologic agents. Since each of these substances is known to be excreted in mothers' milk, with a potential for untoward effects on the infant, they should be avoided by the breastfeeding mother.

The nurse is a vital resource to the mother who desires to breastfeed her premature or sick newborn infant. As primary care providers, nurses can offer these women assistance in the form of counseling, education, and practical aids, which often make the difference between success and failure with respect to their goals. Recognition of the unique properties of breastmilk, especially beneficial to the premature or ill infant, reinforces the importance of a planned program for breastfeeding support in the hospital and at home. Also important is understanding the reactions and needs of parents during this time of crisis and their relationship to the breastfeeding process. We hope the insights, suggestions, and resources are helpful to all who work with these very special families.

A GUIDE FOR PARENTS

BREASTFEEDING YOUR "SPECIAL CARE" BABY*

INTRODUCTION

Like most parents, you have probably thought a lot about what life would be like once your baby way born, and how you would care for your infant. The fact that your baby requires "special care" has undoubtedly been quite a shock for you. In these first few days you will probably feel very confused and frightened, and you may think you'll have to change all the plans you've made for your baby. Although some temporary limitations may be necessary, you can still do many of the things you had planned. If one of your plans was to breast-feed your baby, we would like to help you do so. With the help of the nursery staff and this booklet, chances are good that you can.

SHOULD YOU NURSE?

The decision to nurse may be somewhat more difficult for you than for the mother who has experienced an uncomplicated birth and post-partum period. You may have planned all along to breast-feed, or you may have just begun to consider it. If you intended to use the last few weeks of your pregnancy to choose whether to breast or bottle feed and your baby was born prematurely, you may not feel prepared to decide. Nearly all parents have questions concerning a method of feeding; however, since you and your child have very special needs, this decision may be especially difficult for you. Following are some commonly asked questions about breast-feeding "special care" babies. Perhaps the answers will help you make the choice that is best for you and your family.

Is breast milk better for my baby?

Most pediatric authorities agree that mother's milk is the ideal food for the full-term newborn infant. Although less is known about the feeding of human milk to premature babies, research suggests the following advantages:

1. Mother's milk seems to be more easily tolerated than formula by the premature baby's stomach and intestines. Formula is made up of slightly different substances than those found in mother's milk, which may make formula more difficult for the small, premature baby to digest.
2. Mother's milk contains extra defenses against infection; this is especially true of colostrum, the early milk which is present in your breasts at the time your baby is born. These defenses, called antibodies, protect your child against several types of infection which might be especially serious for a premature baby.
3. Breast-feeding allows you to experience a comfortable closeness to your baby. This might be especially important to you, since you may not be having the physical contact you expected to have with your baby at first. Some mothers tell us that nursing is like 'making up'' for all the experiences they could not enjoy while their babies were too little or too sick.

One other point should be emphasized: if you choose to breast-feed, you need not commit yourself for a definite period of time. If you decide after a week or two to quit nursing, your milk will already have given your baby some very valuable defenses against infection.

Will I be able to produce enough milk?

Nearly all mothers are concerned about whether they will be able to produce enough milk for their babies, particularly if their breasts are small or if they describe themselves as "the nervous type." This is seldom a problem; the body tends to produce as much milk as the baby takes from the breasts. Therefore, the more frequently an infant nurses, the more milk the body produces.

If your baby is unable to nurse at the breast for a while, you will have to "express" the milk (obtain it from your breasts) and store it so that your baby can take it from a bottle or a feeding tube. Because milk production depends on regular milk removal from the breasts, establishing and maintaining an adequate milk supply will require some extra effort on your part. You will have to use a breast pump several times a day, so it helps if you are motivated and sincerely want to nurse.

Your milk supply depends not only on milk production but on your body's ability to let the milk flow from the breast once it has been produced. Normally, a baby's sucking at the breast triggers a reflex which causes milk to be forced from the breast to the baby. This mechanism is called the "let-down" or "milk-ejection" reflex. Many physical and psychological factors can interfere with this reflex, including stress and anxiety. Thus, if you are worried about your baby's well-being, it may take longer for the let-down reflex to work effectively for you, and you may begin to feel that you "don't have enough milk." Although this problem is only temporary, it can be particularly frustrating at this very vulnerable time in your life. Later in this booklet we'll discuss some ways you can encourage the "let-down" reflex.

Can I breast-feed following a Cesarean delivery?

Some people think that mothers who give birth by Cesarean delivery, especially prematurely, are not able to nurse. This is not true. Milk production begins as soon as the placenta (after birth) is delivered following your baby's birth, no matter how the baby is delivered. The delivery of the placenta causes some major changes in your body's hormone balance, and these changes ultimately cause the breasts to produce milk. Regardless of how your baby was born, you can breast-feed if you choose to.

Two common breast-feeding problems that many women experience following a Cesarean delivery are the physical discomfort of having undergone major surgery, and the discouragement and improper advice from those around them. The combination of these two things can make you nervous and uncomfortable and interfere with your let-down reflex. Your breasts will produce milk but be unable to release it. But keep in mind that this problem is only temporary.

Can I breast-feed if I'm taking prescription medications?

The question of which medications you may safely take while you are breast-feeding is a complex one. Nearly all medications which find their way into your bloodstream will also be present in your breast milk. The amount of medication that reaches your milk and its potential effect on your baby, however, vary greatly with the specific medication and the dosage. It is therefore impossible to answer the above question with a "yes" or "no." Most drugs *can* be safely taken by a nursing mother, but your doctor should decide which ones. Be sure to tell the doctor or nurse taking care of your baby about all medications you are currently taking. If you are uncertain about the name of a particular capsule or tablet, bring the medication and the bottle it is in to the nursery when you visit, so that the staff can determine whether or not you can safely take it while you are breast-feeding.

How will breast-feeding affect the other areas of my life?
Most parents are curious about the advantages and disadvantages of breast-feeding relative to loss of personal freedom, the use of supplemental bottles, or a mother's return to work. If you have questions like these—or other questions we may not have answered—the resources listed at the end of this booklet should be helpful to you in making your final decision.

HOW LACTATION WORKS
You'll probably feel more comfortable with breast-feeding if you first understand how lactation occurs. In this section of the booklet, we explain the basic processes of milk production and ejection.

Milk production
During the last few months of pregnancy, hormones in the mother's blood signal her breasts to produce a thick yellowish fluid called colostrum. You may have noticed some drops of this fluid on your breast or clothing before your baby was born. Colostrum is the first food your baby receives, before the thinner, blue-white "true" milk comes in.

Once your baby is born and the placenta is delivered, certain hormone levels in your blood fall quite rapidly. This change in hormone levels signals the brain to secrete a new hormone, called prolactin. Prolactin enters the bloodstream and causes certain cells in your breasts to begin to make milk. As the milk is produced, your breasts enlarge and become firm and warm. This process is referred to as "engorgement" or as "the milk coming-in."

The change of hormones in the blood may take only a few hours or it may take several days, which explains why some women feel engorgement within a day after birth while others must wait three or four days. We know, however, that the more stimulation the breasts receive during this time, the sooner the true milk replaces the colostrum. This is true whether the stimulation is a baby's nursing or the regular use of a breast pump.

Many people erroneously believe that the newborn baby doesn't receive any nourishment until engorgement occurs. But colostrum has several components which make it a nourishing food for your baby until it is replaced by milk. Colostrum is rich in protein and other nutrients your baby needs in the first days of life. It also has a laxative effect, helping your baby pass his or her first stools. Most important, it contains a very high concentration of antibodies, or defenses against certain germs which can cause infection. These infections can produce symptoms in newborn babies such as severe diarrhea. The antibodies are very beneficial to babies who require special care. That is why we suggest that you try to express milk, even if it's only for a week or two. In this way, your baby will receive the unique protection your colostrum provides.

Milk ejection
Milk production is only the first half of the lactation process, and is usually not a problem for any woman who has an adequate diet and drinks plenty of fluids. The other component of lactation—"milk ejection" or "let-down"—is sometimes a problem because physical and emotional factors can interfere with it.

Milk ejection is a reflex which causes tiny muscle cells in your breasts to tighten, squeezing milk which has already been produced out onto your nipple. This occurs in response to nipple stimulation, either by the baby's sucking or from use of the breast pump. Sometimes lightly rubbing a dry washcloth over the nipples will also provide this stimulation.

The response to stimulation may take from several seconds to several minutes. You can recognize it by three signs: a tingling (pins-and-needles) sensation in both breasts; milk flowing more freely from breasts; and mild abdominal cramping as your uterine muscles tighten. The let-down reflex may take several days to function effectively for you; for many women the "tingling'' sensation is so slight that it goes unnoticed for even longer. There are several ways you can encourage this reflex to work for you. The following sequence is particularly helpful:

- Try to follow the pumping schedule outlined later in this booklet, so that your breasts begin to "anticipate" milk removal on a regular basis.
- Sit down and put your feet up for five minutes before beginning to express your milk. Relax your arms and back and take several slow, deep breaths. Concentrate on feeling the tension leave your body.
- Place a picture of your baby where you can see it while you're expressing your milk.
- Do a complete breast massage (described in the next section), and continue to concentrate on relaxing your arms and back.
- Begin to use the breast pump.

If you still experience difficulty after trying these suggestions, please ask your baby's nurse for further help.

EXPRESSING AND STORING YOUR MILK

Expressing and storing milk for your baby may seem complicated at first. You'll find, however, that with a little practice, you'll master the entire procedure with no difficulty. Specifically, this process consists of four major parts: developing a milk-expression schedule; collecting and storing milk; locating a suitable breast pump; and cleaning the breast pump equipment.

A milk-expression schedule

If left to his own instincts, the newborn baby would breast-feed immediately after birth and every two to three hours thereafter. If you wish to breast-feed but must be temporarily separated from your baby, we recommend that you express milk from your breasts in a similar pattern. Generally, you should begin to express your milk as soon as you are able after your baby's birth—certainly within the first six to twelve hours after you deliver. Just tell your maternity nurse or your baby's nurse that you wish to breast-feed, and ask her to show you how to use a breast pump.

After using the pump for the first time, you should continue to do so approximately every three hours during the day. It is important that you maintain this schedule during the first two weeks, while your milk supply is being established; after two weeks you can be more flexible. It is not necessary to continue this frequent pumping during the time you are sleeping, but if possible you should try to express your milk once during the night.

As you use the breast pump, try to remember to alternate the breast that you first remove milk from each time. As a rule, the breast you begin with is emptied more completely than the breast you end with. If you continually empty one breast before the other, your breasts will produce unequal amounts of milk. This principle is true throughout the time that you lactate.

Before you place the pump on your breast, you should massage that breast. This simple technique helps to move milk from the outer areas of the breast into the milk reservoirs behind the areola and nipple, where it is easily removed with the breast pump.

To massage your breasts, first wash your hands well, then place the fingers of one hand over the fingers of the other hand. Using firm but not uncomfortable pressure, guide your hands from the outer areas of your breast to just behind the areola. Work around each breast in a clockwise direction until you've massaged the entire breast surface, being careful not to touch the nipple with your hands. Don't rush: you should spend at least a full minute on each breast.

Now you can attach the breast pump to express your milk. After two or three minutes, remove the pump and massage your breast again. Then reattach the pump to complete emptying the first breast. Repeat this procedure for the other breast.

Nearly all mothers experience some nipple tenderness in the first weeks of breast-feeding; this discomfort may be slightly exaggerated in mothers using a breast pump. You can minimize the tenderness by using the breast pump for only a few minutes at first, then gradually increasing the time. We recommend the following schedule in most cases:

First day: about 5 minutes at each breast each time you use the pump
Second day: about 8 minutes at each breast each time you use the pump
Third day: about 10 minutes at each breast each time you use the pump
Thereafter: 10 to 15 minutes at each breast each time you use the pump

(Remember to complete breast massage before and midway through pumping each breast.)

Collecting and storing milk

In collecting and storing your milk, your careful attention to cleanliness cannot be overemphasized. Breast milk is sterile (free from germs) at the time it is expressed, but bacteria can easily grow if it is handled carelessly. First, and most important, wash your hands thoroughly with soap immediately before touching your breasts or any of the equipment you use to collect and store milk. Take care not to cough or sneeze around collected milk or equipment. Wash your breasts and nipples once or twice a day with a clean cloth and warm water. Following these instructions will help keep your milk as free from germs as possible for your baby.

As soon as you decide that you wish to breastfeed your baby, a nurse will discuss with you how to collect your milk so that it can be fed to your baby. Most hospitals provide mothers with small plastic containers for storing expressed milk. These containers are always sterile until you break the wrappings or seals which keep them free from bacteria. When you have collected your milk in the breast pump equipment, pour into each container approximately the amount that your baby takes with a feeding (the nurse will tell you how much the first time). Then cover the container with its top. Be careful not to touch the milk or the inside of the container and top.

Once your milk is collected, label it with your baby's name (first and last) and the date. Then either freeze or refrigerate it immediately. There are two principles to consider in determining whether to freeze or refrigerate your expressed milk. Milk which has been refrigerated but not frozen contains the most defenses against infection, and is therefore best for your baby. But milk which is not frozen must be fed to your baby within twenty-four hours after its removal from your breasts in order to guarantee its freshness. Your baby's nurse can tell you what time your baby is to receive milk, so that perhaps once a day you can plan to bring a bottle or two of unfrozen milk to the nursery. Be sure to tell the nurse you have fresh milk as soon as you arrive in the nursery, so that it can be refrigerated until it is given to your baby. You can freeze the other bottles of your milk and bring them to the hospital when you visit. Milk which you freeze will be stored in the nursery freezer and thawed immediately before being fed to your baby.

Mothers often ask if they can freeze milk from several pumpings in the same container. There is no reason why you cannot do this, as long as the milk is removed from the freezer only long enough to add the amount you've just expressed. If you do this, you will probably notice that the milk forms a new "layer" with each addition. This is because the color and consistency of your milk vary slightly with each pumping. This is quite normal, and the layers will mix once the milk is thawed for your baby.

Locating a breast pump

Although it is possible to express your milk without using a breast pump, it is usually difficult to do so for more than a few days. If your baby must stay in the hospital after you leave, try to obtain a breast pump to use in your home. Several types of breast pumps are used in hospital nurseries and maternity areas. Ask your nurse or doctor which ones your hospital uses so that you can look for the same kind to use at home (it's easier not to change types). You can either rent an electric breast pump or purchase a hand-operated model.

Electric breast pumps are easier to operate and slightly more efficient at emptying the breasts than are hand-operated pumps. They are, however, generally larger and heavier, and can eventually result in greater expense. The Egnell electric breast pump is an effective and comfortable machine that is available for rental from outlets throughout the country. The rental fee consists of a one-time charge for the accessory kit and daily rate which ranges from about $1.70 to $2.50. The nurse involved in your baby's care will help you locate the Egnell pump outlet nearest your home. You should call this number as soon as possible and reserve a pump for the day you go home. Have a friend or relative pick up your breast pump before you leave the hospital so you can continue your milk-expression schedule without delay. If for any reason a breast pump is not available to you from the outlet you call, tell the nurse so that she can help you locate one somewhere else. If you are unable to locate an Egnell pump within a reasonable distance from your home, the company can be contacted directly at its offices in Cary, Illinois. You'll find the address and phone number in the last section of this booklet.

An alternative to the electric pump is one of the manual (hand operated) ones, such as the Loyd-B-Pump (Lopuco, Inc.) or the Kaneson (Happy Family Products). These devices are small, comfortable to use, and allow your milk to be collected under sterile conditions. Some hospitals routinely dispense the pumps to breast-feeding mothers who are separated from their babies, so you should inquire about this possibility. The pumps may also be purchased directly from the companies that manufacture them: the Loyd-B-Pump costs about $35, and the Kaneson is available for about $15. The address and phone numbers of these companies are included in the last section of this booklet.

There are other types of acceptable electric and hand-operated pumps. The only pump which should not be used to express milk for your baby is the manual one operated by a suction-creating bulb at one end. Since this pump has no collecting jar, your milk easily enters the bulb apparatus, a part of the pump which cannot be adequately sterilized. This milk would not be suitable for your baby.

Your local La Leche League chapter can also give you information about breast pumps. These women will know where all types of pumps can be located in your area, and can help you decide whether an electric or manual pump will best meet your needs.

Care of the breast pump equipment

As we said earlier, it is important that your milk be as clean as possible for your baby, so proper care of the breast pump accessory kit is essential. The collecting jar and all attachments which come into contact with your milk must be sterilized according to the following procedure. First, wash the equipment well in warm, soapy water. You can use a bottle brush to reach all the edges of the collecting jar, and a Q-tip to remove any milk which may have accumulated in the narrow opening in the breast shield attachment. Then rinse well with clear water. Place the three pieces in a large pan (padded inside with a dishcloth) of water, and boil for twenty minutes. If you have a dishwasher, you may use it instead of boiling your equipment.

It is not necessary to sterilize your equipment more than twice during the same twenty-four-hour period. You should, however, rinse the attachments after each pumping, and then wash them with warm, soapy water immediately before using them again. Always make sure to rinse away all the soapy water with clear water.

FEEDING YOUR BABY

The manner in which your milk is fed to your baby will depend upon several factors: his or her weight, maturity, and ability to suck, and the presence of respiratory or other problems. In many hospitals, small premature babies receive their mother's milk through a tiny feeding tube which delivers the milk directly into their intestines. This type of feeding runs continuously, so that the babies never receive more milk than they can tolerate at one time. Since they don't have to use their strength to suck milk from a bottle or your breast, they can save their energy and use it to grow.

Larger premature babies usually receive their mother's milk through a tube which delivers it to their stomach. These babies also save their energy by not having to suck, but because they are bigger and stronger, they can tolerate larger amounts of milk at each feeding. These infants receive mother's milk every two or three hours, then rest between feedings.

Other babies, depending upon their condition, may nurse at the breast or receive mother's milk from a bottle. Sometimes these babies take part of the feedings from a bottle or at the breast, and part from one of the types of tiny feeding tubes previously mentioned. Although most infants take their first nipple feedings with a soft, red "premature" nipple, they should be changed to the "Nuk" nipple as soon as possible. The Nuk nipple is very similar to the shape of a mother's nipple in the infant's mouth. With consistent use of the Nuk nipple, your baby begins to develop the muscles and movements needed to nurse at the breast. This makes the transition from bottle to breast a bit easier for most mothers and babies. If your nursery does not have the Nuk nipples for nursing infants, ask if you can purchase several and bring them to the hospital. They can be sterilized just like other nursery equipment.

Many parents ask how big their babies must be in order to breast-feed. Weight is not usually a major factor in deciding when an infant is able to nurse. Once your baby has reached a stable condition and has been able to take several feedings from a nipple, you may begin to feed at the breast. A nurse will remain with you the first few times you nurse your baby. Fathers are also welcome to participate in this very special event. In general, the first few nursing sessions are for you and your baby to get acquainted, so try to remember that very few infants will take to the breast right away. Most need some coaxing and time to adjust. Some babies may need the temporary assistance of a specially designed nipple shield or a "lact-aid" device before they can make the final change from bottle to breast. Your nurse will discuss these possibilities with you if they seem necessary.

Once you are able to begin nursing, we encourage you to breast-feed your baby as often as possible. This will help you and your baby adjust to each other and make your transition from hospital to home easier. If your schedule permits you to "room-in" and nurse your baby "on demand," the hospital staff will do their best to adapt the nursery routines and facilities to meet your needs.

WHERE YOU'LL FIND HELP

Mothers of "special care" babies have told us that they feel the problems and frustrations they experience with breastfeeding are different from those of mothers who are nursing full-term infants. For this reason, a mother who has previously nursed an infant from your baby's nursery can be a great help if you have temporary difficulties. If you would like to speak with an experienced nursing mother, please tell your baby's nurse. Some nurseries have an organized breastfeeding referral system, operated by the staff, volunteers, or interested nursing mothers. If your hospital does not have such a system, you may be interested in helping them initiate one later.

If this is your first experience with breast-feeding, you will undoubtedly have many questions which are not answered in this booklet. The following organizations and publications may help you answer those questions.

For breast-feeding advice, support, and help with common problems:

La Leche League International. Headquarters in Franklin Park, Illinois; phone (312) 355-7730, or check with directory assistance for the local group nearest your home.
The Complete Book of Breast-feeding, by M.S. Eiger and S.W. Olds. Workman Publishers, New York, 1972.
Nursing Your Baby, by Karen Pryor. Harper and Row Publishers, New York, 1973.
My Baby is a Special Care Infant, A Parents Guide to Neonatal Intensive Care, by Jude Langhurst; 1452 Melrose, Wichita, Kansas 67212.

"Nursing a Preemie: A Mother's Personal Victory" by Christine Schaffer. This is a brief article in the *Keeping Abreast Journal,* Vol. 2 (April-June, 1977), pages 132-136. You can get it from Resources in Human Nurturing (see below).

For breast-feeding equipment:

Egnell Pump Company, Inc., 412 Park Ave., Cary, Illinois 60013; phone toll-free 800-323-8750. Call for information concerning electric breast pump rental program.

Happy Family Products, 12300 Venice Blvd., Los Angeles, California 90066, phone (213) 390-9649. Toll-free order (800) 228-2028. Contact for information about or purchase of the Kaneson breast pump.

Lopuco, Ltd. 1615 Old Annapolis Rd., Woodbine, Maryland 21797; phone (301) 489-4949. Call for information concerning local purchase or C.O.D. orders directly from company.

Resources in Human Nurturing, 3885 Forest St., P.O. Box 6861, Denver, Colorado 80206; phone (303) 388-4600. Call for information about, or to order, the Lact-Aid Device for special breast-feeding problems.

La Leche League International (see address and phone number above).

Medela, Inc., 457 Dartmoor Dr., P.O. Box 386, Crystal Lake, Illinois 60014; phone toll-free 800-435-8316. Contact for information concerning electric breast pump.

REFERENCES

1. Anderson, G.H., Atkinson, S.A., and Bryan, M.H.: energy and macronutrient content of human milk during early lactation from mothers giving birth prematurely and at term, Am. J. Clin. Nutr. **34:**258, 1981.

2. Anderson, G.H., Atkinson, S.A., and Bryan, M.H.: Human milk feedings in premature infants: protein and energy balances in the first two weeks of life, Fed. Proc. **40:**890, 1981.

3. Atkinson, S.A., Anderson, G.H., and Bryan, M.H.: Human milk: comparison of the nitrogen composition in milk from mothers of premature and full-term infants, Am. J. Clin. Nutr. **33:**811, 1980.

4. Atkinson, S.A., Bryan, M.H., and Anderson, G.H.: Human milk: differences in nitrogen concentration in milk from mothers of term and premature infants, J. Pediatr. **93:**67, 1978.

5. Atkinson, S.A., et al.: Macro-mineral content of milk obtained during early lactation from mothers or premature infants, Early Hum. Dev. **4:**5, 1980.

6. Barlow, B., et al.: An experimental study of acute NEC: the importance of breast milk, J. Pediatr. Surg. **9:**587, 1974.

7. Barnett, C., et al.: Neonatal separation: the maternal side of interactional deprivation, Pediatrics **45:**197, 1973.

8. Caplan, G.: Patterns of parental response to the crisis of premature birth, Psychiatry **23:**365, 1960.

9. Chan, G.M.: Preterm and term breast milk calcium and vitamin D (abstract), Pediatr. Res. **13:**396, 1979.

10. Choi, M.W.: A comparison of maternal psychological reactions to premature and full-size newborns, Matern. Child Nurs. J. **2:**1, 1973.

11. Choi, M.W.: Breast milk for infants who can't breastfeed, Am. J. Nurs. **78:**852, 1978.

12. Clandinin, M.T., et al.: Fatty acid accretion in the development of human spinal cord, Early Hum. Dev. **5:**1, 1981.

13. Committee on Nutrition of the American Academy of Pediatrics: Human milk banking, Pediatrics **65:**854, 1980.

14. Cone, T.E.: History of American pediatrics, Boston, 1979, Little, Brown & Co.

15. Davies, D.P.: Adequacy of expressed breast milk for early growth or preterm infants, Arch. Dis. Child. **52:**296, 1977.

16. Davies, D.P., and Evans, T.J.: Nutrition and early growth of preterm infants, Early Hum. Dev. **2:**383, 1978.

17. Donowitz, L.G., and Wenzel, R.P.: Nosocomial klebsiella bacteremia in a newborn intensive care unit caused by contaminated breast milk, Clin. Res. **27:**818A, 1980.

18. Evans, T.J., et al.: Effects of storage and heat on antimicrobial proteins in human milk, Arch. Dis. Child. **53:**239, 1978.

19. Fomon, S.J., and Ziegler, E.E.: Milk of the premature infant's mother: interpretation of data, J. Pediatr. **93:**164, 1978.

20. Fomon, S.J., et al.: Human milk and the small premature infant, Am. J. Dis. Child. **131:**463, 1977.

21. Forbes, G.B.: Is human milk the best food for low birth weight babies? Pediatr. Res. **12:**434, 1978.

22. Ford, J.E., et al.: Influence of heat treatment of human milk on some of its protective constituents, J. Pediatr. **90:**29, 1977.

23. Giacoia, G.P., and Catz, C.S.: Drugs and pollutants in breast milk, Clin. Perinatol. **6:**181, 1979.
24. Gross, S.J., et al.: Nutritional composition of milk produced by mothers delivering preterm, J. Pediatr. **96:**641, 1980.
25. Guerrini, P., et al.: Human milk: relationship of fat content with gestational age, Early Hum. Dev. **5:**187, 1981.
26. Heird, W.C.: Feeding the premature infant, Am. J. Dis. Child. **131:**468, 1977.
27. Henderson, K.J., and Newton, L.D.: Helping nursing mothers maintain lactation while separated from their infants, Matern. Child Nurs. J. **3:**352, 1978.
28. Jelliffe, D.B., and Jelliffe, E.P.: Human milk in the modern world, Oxford, 1978, Oxford University Press.
29. Kaplan, D., and Mason, E. Maternal reactions to premature birth viewed as an acute emotional disorder. In Parad, H., editor: Crisis intervention, New York, 1965, Family Service Association of America.
30. Klaus, M.H., and Kennell, J.H.: Mothers separated from their newborn infants, Pediatr. Clin. North Am. **17:**1016, 1970.
31. Klaus, M.H., and Kennell, J.H.: Maternal-infant bonding: the impact of early separation or loss on family development, St. Louis, 1976, The C.V. Mosby Co.
32. Lawrence, R.A.: Breastfeeding: a guide for the medical profession, St. Louis, 1980, The C.V. Mosby Co.
33. Lemons, J., et al.: Composition of preterm breast milk, Pediatr. Res. **13:**403, 1979.
34. Lemons, J., et al.: Differences in sodium and nitrogen contents between preterm and term milk, Pediatr. Res. **14:**504, 1980.
35. Lemons, J., et al.: Simple method for determining the caloric and fat content of human milk, Pediatrics **66:**626, 1980.
36. Liebhaber, M., et al.: Alterations of lymphocytes and of antibody content of human milk after processing, J. Pediatr. **91:**897, 1977.
37. Liebhaber, M., et al.: Comparison of bacterial contamination with two methods of human milk collection, J. Pediatr. **92:**236, 1978.
38. Liefer, A.D., et al.: Effects of mother-infant separation on maternal attachment behavior, Child Dev. **43:**1203, 1972.
39. Lindemann, E.: The symptomatology and management of acute grief. In Parad, H., editor: Crisis intervention, New York, 1965, Family Service Association of America.
40. Lucas, A., et al.: Creamatocrit: simple clinical technique for estimating fat concentration and energy value of human milk, Br. Med. J. **1:**1018, 1978.
41. Lundeen, E.: The role or the nurse in the care of the premature infant, reprinted from a presentation to the American Congress on Obstetrics and Gynecology, Cleveland, Ohio, September 11-15, 1939.
42. Mason, E.: A method of predicting crisis outcome for mothers of premature babies, Public Health Rep. **78:**1031, 1963.
43. Meier, P.: A program to support breastfeeding in the high risk nursery, Perinatology/Neonatology **4:**43, 1980.
44. Meier, P.: Breastfeeding your "special care" baby, Chicago, 1980, Michael Reese Hospital Publications.
45. Meier, P.: Nursery update, Perinatology/Neonatology **4:**51, 1980.
46. Narayanan, I., Prakash, K., and Guyral, V.: The value of human milk in the prevention of infection in the high risk, low birth weight infant, J. Pediatr. **99:**496, 1981.
47. Paxson, C.L., and Cress, C.C.: Survival of human milk leukocytes, J. Pediatr. **94:**61, 1979.
48. Pearce, J.L., and Buchanan, L.F.: Breast milk and breastfeeding in very low birthweight infants, Arch. Dis. Child. **54:**897, 1979.
49. Pitt, J.: Breast milk and the high risk baby: potential benefits and hazards, Hosp. Pract. **5:**81, 1979.
50. Räihä, N.C., et al.: Milk protein quantity and quality in low-birthweight infants. I. Metabolic responses and effects on growth, Pediatrics **57:**659, 1976.
51. Schanler, R., and Oh, W.: Composition of breast milk obtained from mothers of premature infants as compared to breast milk obtained from donors. J. Pediatr. **96:**679, 1980.
52. Seashore, M., et al.: The effects of denial of early maternal-infant interaction on maternal confidence, J. Pers. Soc. Psychol. **26:**369, 1973.
53. Spencer, S., and Hull, D.: Fat content of expressed breast milk: a case for quality control. Br. Med. J. **282:**99, 1981.
54. Stevens, L.H.: The first kilogram: the protein content of breast milk of mothers of babies of low birth weight, Med. J. Aust. **2:**555, 1969.
55. Stewart, D., and Gainer, C.: Supporting lactation when mothers and infants are separated, Nurs. Clin. North Am. **13:**47, 1978.
56. Welsh, J.K., and May, J.T.: Anti-infective properties of breast milk, J. Pediatr. **94:**1, 1979.

57. Williamson, S., et al.: Effect of heat treatment of human milk on absorption of nitrogen, fat, sodium, calcium, and phosphorus by preterm infants, Arch. Dis. Child. **53:**555, 1978.

ADDITIONAL READINGS

Brooke, O., et al.: Protein concentration in milk from mothers of preterm and term infants, Biochem. Soc. Trans. **9:**69, 1981.

Chance, G.W., et al.: Post-natal growth of infants 1.3 kg. at birth weight: effects of metabolic acidosis, of caloric intake, and of calcium, sodium, and phosphate supplementation, J. Pediatr. **91:**787, 1977.

Clandinin, M.T., et al.: Extrauterine fatty acid accretion in infant brain: implications for fatty acid requirements, Early Hum. Dev. **4:**131, 1980.

Clandinin, M.T., et al.: Intrauterine fatty acid accretion rates in human brain: implications for fatty acid requirements, Early Hum. Dev. **4:**121, 1980.

Clandinin, M.T., et al.: Fatty acid accretion in fetal and neonatal liver: implications for fatty acid requirements, Early Hum. Dev. **5:**7, 1981.

Countryman, S.: Breastfeeding your premature baby, Franklin Park, Ill., 1980, La Leche League International.

Crawford, M., Hassan, A., and Livers, J.: Essential fatty acid requirements in infancy, Am. J. Clin. Nutr. **31:**2181, 1978.

Gibson, R., and Kneebone, G.: Fatty acid composition of human colostrum and mature breast milk, Am. J. Clin. Nutr. **34:**252, 1981.

Lemons, J., et al.: Four methods of expressing human milk, Pediatr. Res. **15:**669, 1981.

Lucas, A., Gibbs, J., and Baum, J.: The biology of human drip breast milk, Early Hum. Dev. **2:**351, 1978.

Nutrition and the early growth of preterm infants, Early Hum. Dev. **3:**373, 1979.

Rowe, J. et al.: Nutritional hypophosphatemic rickets in a premature infant fed breast milk, N. Engl. J. Med. **300:**293, 1979.

Schaffer, C.: Nursing a preemie: a mother's personal victory, Keeping Abreast J. **2:**132, 1977.

Schultz, K., Soltesz, G., and Mestyan, J.: The metabolic consequences of human milk and formula feeding in premature infants, Acta Paediatr. Scand. **69:**647, 1980.

Tibbetts, E., and Caldwell, K.: Selecting the right breast pump, Matern. Child Nurs. J. **5:**262, 1980.

Tyson, J., et al.: Growth and metabolic response of infants less than 1500 grams fed frozen human milk or whey-dominant premature formula, Pediatr. Res. **14:**511, 1980.

Zimmerman, A., and Hambidge, K.: Low zinc in mothers' milk and zinc deficiency syndrome in breastfed premature infants, Clin. Res. **28:**603A, 1980.

13

Relactation and induced lactation

JIMMIE LYNNE AVERY

THE CONCEPT
Definition

Defined most simply, relactation is the process of restimulating lactation after it has previously occurred. It can occur days, weeks, months, or even years after prior lactation has ended. Its purpose is to enable women to resume breastfeeding after an untimely weaning or to initiate breastfeeding that has been delayed by neonatal or maternal illness or prematurity. Relactation is also a feasible option for the mother who initially bottle-feeds her infant but later has a change of heart or discovers that her infant cannot tolerate infant formula.

The word *relactation* is often broadly used to describe any situation in which relactation techniques are useful. More accurately, it refers only to the reestablishment of lactation in women who have previously experienced puerperal lactation. Induced lactation refers to the initiation of lactation in nulliparous women, usually to breastfeed foster or adopted infants.

Historical perspective

As a therapy for breastfeeding problems, relactation often seems a new and rather startling concept. Actually, it is an ancient art, rooted in wet-nursing, and in traditional societies it has commonly been used when the infant's survival is at stake.[11,12] In certain cultures an infant whose mother dies is given to another mother to breastfeed. If none are lactating, one or more women initiate lactation to meet the infant's nutritional needs. Within non-Western cultures where breastfeeding is the norm, relactation and induced lactation have been regarded simply as aspects of normal lactation.

Perhaps the main reason that reports of relactation/induced lactation first appeared in scientific literature is that until recently, authors were physicians and anthropologists from Western cultures in which bottle-feeding was rapidly becoming or was already the norm. In their eyes relactation was an extraordinary phenomenon indeed, so it was natural their reports before 1973 appeared primarily among discussions of aberrant behavior and abnormal lactation.[8,17]

To the modern woman who must build her family by adopting, induced lactation presents an alternative that has not been available since the arts and skills of wet-nursing passed out of fashion. Even though adoptive breastfeeding has roots in wet-nursing associated with infant survival, when reports of relactation by modern women appeared in the 1970's,[10,20] they provoked much controversy.

General public reaction was negative. Adoptive nursing was viewed as impossible, physiologically abnormal, and possibly perverse. Until fairly recently, there was no proof that human prolactin existed,[19] and abnormal lactation was considered only as a result of disease, disorders, and certain drugs.[8,17,21] Also, "bonding" and "psychologic parenthood" were not yet issues in the study of human development and adoption. Thus it was no wonder that both the physical and emotional health of women who attempted induced lactation was questioned.

Since then, breastfeeding has increased in the United States and other Western cultures, particularly among middle-class educated women. Worldwide efforts are directed to reversing a breastfeeding decline within traditional societies and among less affluent women in Western cultures. Human milk has come to be regarded almost as a new wonder drug in neonatal medicine. Likewise, bonding, parenting, and other nurturing issues are the topic of the day in maternal, child, and family health. Thus it seems appropriate that relactation has come full circle to be regarded as an aspect of "normal" lactation and a valuable therapy in meeting infant survival and bonding needs.

Now that relactation is a respectable topic for serious research, data on relactation/induced lactation can enhance basic understanding of breastfeeding. An awareness of relactation, its applications, and basic method is valuable for breastfeeding in special situations and can play an important role in developing breastfeeding support protocols and programs.

MODERN APPLICATIONS

Before the 1970's, the initial purpose of relactation among modern women was to initiate breastfeeding for infants who were unable to thrive when bottle-fed proprietary formula. Publicity about their experiences prompted other women to use similar methods to breastfeed adopted infants, and it became a tool for encouraging women to relactate when confronted with breastfeeding problems. Today, relactation forms the basis for managing breastfeeding in a wide variety of special situations that fall into the following four categories.

Delayed breastfeeding

Maternal or neonatal illness or premature birth have often prevented breastfeeding. Today, breastfeeding can be delayed until the condition of the infant or mother makes it practical. Likewise, the mother who initially bottle-feeds can later elect to breastfeed.

Untimely weaning

Breastfeeding problems, return to work, inaccurate advice, hospital separation of mother and infant, or maternal medications need not result in a permanent and untimely weaning. Breastfeeding can be resumed.

Breastfeeding adopted infants

Women who adopt infants can *nurture* their infants at the breast, even though it may not always be possible to totally *nourish* their infants via lactation.

Lactation enhancement/supplementation

Severely diminished lactation can occur from a variety of complex and interrelated factors. Although women do not relactate in the literal sense, the principles and management techniques are the same. In certain situations, lactation may not be enhanced, and thus supplementation is required. A mother in my practice, for example, had extensive mammary surgery that severed her milk ducts. She was able to enjoy a breastfeeding relationship with two infants by electing to supplement at the breast by means of a Lact-Aid Nursing Trainer.

PHYSIOLOGY

Invariably, the first question a mother will ask is, "How is relactation possible?" Mothers benefit most from a very simple explanation, rather than an in-depth treatise on physiology. The nurse should explain that little is known about the precise details, since only recently have scientists been seriously interested in it for research.[7] Most of our knowledge has come from observing women who attempted it, from asking them questions about their experiences, and then from noting the ways in which relactation appears similar or strikingly different from both "normal" puerperal lactation and "abnormal" nonpuerperal lactation.

Normal puerperal lactation

The normal course of puerperal lactation and breastfeeding was thoroughly discussed earlier in this book. In summary, the hormones of pregnancy, primarily estrogen, progesterone, and prolactin, along with adrenal cortical steroids, prepare the breasts for lactation by causing an increase in the size and number of alveoli and ducts. The high levels of estrogen and progesterone prevent prolactin from exerting its lactogenic effect on alveoli. At birth, the expulsion of the placenta sharply reduces the levels of estrogen and progesterone, thus permitting prolactin to initiate milk production. Suckling stimulation after delivery causes continuing prolactin secretion, which promotes milk production. Suckling also stimulates release of oxytocin, the hormone responsible for milk ejection. Regular and frequent suckling supports lactation. The composition of lacteal secretion changes over time from colostrum to transitional milk and then to mature milk. Amenorrhea and an interruption of the fertility cycle are prolonged during lactation when suckling is frequent.

Mammary involution

If breastfeeding does not occur or if weaning takes place, the lactational structures within the breasts return to a nearly prepregnancy state. This resorption of alveoli and ducts is known as "mammary involution." It is highly likely that lactational structures in nonpregnant women, postweaning women, and women whose lactation is severely diminished are similar. Women who have attempted relactation within 2 months after delivery have reported greater milk production than women who attempted it later.[1-4] Other women who attempted to breastfeed adopted infants after having breastfed a prior nonadopted infant reported the need to provide supplemental nutrition in greater quantity and for much longer than they had expected. They had assumed or been told incorrectly that their prior lactation experience ensured success in fully relactating for the subsequent adopted infant. Information about mammary involution is a key issue in developing realistic expectations by clients about the success or failure of their attempts.

Abnormal nonpuerperal lactation

Abnormal nonpuerperal lactation can occur in men and children as well as in women. It is usually a symptom of some physiologic, psychologic, neurologic, or hormonal disorder or disease. It may occur as a side effect of certain drugs, such as chlorpromazine, from chemicals, or from hyperstimulation of the breast or nipple.[8,17] Among women, amenorrhea may also be present at the same time. Abnormal lactation may be present with pituitary tumors, thyroid disorders, or even starvation.[9] Symptoms of abnormal lactation have serious implications for health and should never be underemphasized. However, in some instances no physiologic cause is found, and it is assumed that the reason for abnormal lactation is psychologic.

Lacteal secretions in abnormal lactation can be similar to colostrum, transitional milk, or mature milk in composition. For example, in galactorrhea associated with hypothyroidism, the secretion resembled colostrum.[13,15] In women with a pituitary tumor, composition was initially similar to colostrum but changed over time to resemble normal milk, possibly as an effect of the regular stimulation that occurred when samples were collected for analysis.[13,15,21]

Relactation/induced lactation

In relactation, mammary involution can be partial or complete, depending on the duration after delivery or the length of time since weaning occurred. In cases of induced lactation, mammary involution is not a factor; but lack of alveolar or ductal proliferation is, since there has been no prior pregnancy or lactation. Since there is no sharp decrease in estrogen or progesterone such as occurs at birth with the expulsion of the placenta, some other factor or factors are responsible for lactogenesis.

Hyperstimulation of the breasts and nipples by suckling and massage has been most effective in stimulating lactation. However, if stimulation alone were sufficient, many women would be lactating as a result of stimulation as part of sexual activities. Motivation and desire are additional factors. Experimentally, women have been given a variety of drugs that are known to increase prolactin secretion or to reduce prolactin-inhibiting factor (PIF).[16,19,21] Others have been given high doses of estrogen and progesterone to simulate pregnancy and thus prime the breasts for lactation, with the expectation that sudden withdrawal of hormones might simulate the drop that occurs immediately after delivery.[1-5,22]

Women who relactate or induce lactation have a variety of breast and nipple changes during preparation and the early phase of lactogenesis. Breasts may seem firmer and perhaps larger and nipples may become more protuberant and sometimes darker. Menstrual patterns may change. Some women will have greater intervals between menses and diminished flow, perhaps decreased to spotting. Others may miss menses for several months after relactation, as in normal amenorrhea associated with breastfeeding.

Lacteal secretions initially may be clear, gray, or bluish drops from one or more nipple pores. Over time, the appearance becomes indistinguishable from transitional or mature milk. Analysis confirms that the composition is similar to mature milk, since there is no colostral phase in relactation/induced lactation.[13,15,21] Many women find that their milk production seems to progress in plateaus relative to their menstrual cycling, being diminished or at a static level just preceding menstruation, and increasing within 2 to 3 days after menses occurs. Table 13-1 shows similarities and differences of normal puerperal lactation, abnormal nonpuerperal lactation, and relactation/induced lactation.

TABLE 13-1

Similarities and differences of normal puerperal lactation, abnormal non-puerperal lactation, and relactation/induced lactation

Normal puerperal lactation	Abnormal nonpuerperal lactation	Relactation and induced lactation
Occurs only in women.	May occur in women, men, and children.	Occurs only in women.
Onset of lactation occurs at parturition.	May occur at any time, including at parturition as in certain galactorrhea conditions; abnormality may not be evident until long after parturition unless it occurs in a woman who does not breastfeed.	Can occur at any time after delivery, regardless of number of months or years. Can occur in postmenopausal women. Can occur in nulliparous women.
May occur without intent to breastfeed.		Done with intent to breastfeed.
Puerperally induced.	A pathologic symptom of physiologic, neurologic, endocrine, or psychologic dysfunction or disease (pituitary tumor). A result of hyperstimulation of nipples or breasts, such as suckling, rubbing, scratching, injury, or surgery. A side effect of drugs, chemicals, or hormones.	Induced by motivation, desire, and hyperstimulation of nipples/breasts by suckling, massage, use of mechanical pumps. A desired effect of certain drugs.
Breast proliferation during pregnancy is stimulated by estrogens, progesterone, prolactin, and other hormones.		
High levels of estrogen and progesterone during pregnancy inhibit lactogenic effect of prolactin.	Alveolar/ductal proliferation may occur, likely because of influence of prolactin alone. As side effect of prior use of estrogen (oral contraceptives). In starvation, marijuana use in males, as a result of suppression of male hormone testosterone, thus allowing estrogen and prolactin to cause proliferation of lactational tissues.	Estrogen given to cause alveolar/ductal proliferation before relactation/induced lactation may create changes similar to early pregnancy, thus inhibiting lactogenic effect of prolactin. Cyclical rise in estrogen/progesterone creates an early pregnancy state in breasts, which may appear as fluctuation in milk production; that is, decrease premenstrually followed by increased lactation during secretory phase.

TABLE 13-1—cont'd

Similarities and differences of normal puerperal lactation, abnormal non-puerperal lactation, and relactation/induced lactation

Normal puerperal lactation	Abnormal nonpuerperal lactation	Relactation and induced lactation
Lactogenesis is associated with decrease in estrogen and progesterone at parturition, which allows prolactin to exert lactogenic effect.	Lactogenesis theoretically associated with increase in prolactin secretion or reduction in PIF.	Lactogenesis is theoretically associated with increase in prolactin secretion or reduction in PIF.
Is sustained over time by breastfeeding or regular expression manually or with a mechanical pump.	Must be diagnosed and any pathologic condition treated. Lactation suppressant medications are often administered.	Sustained over time by breastfeeding or regular manual or mechanical expression.
Amenorrhea may be present to some degree.	Amenorrhea may or may not be evident.	Amenorrhea may be present to some degree.
Composition changes over time from colostrum to transitional milk and then mature milk.	Composition of galactorrhea milk may resemble colostrum, transitional milk, or mature milk.	Composition may resemble transitional milk and mature milk, but no colostral phase has been found.
In absence of breastfeeding, mammary involution occurs.		Mammary involution may be present to a degree, or complete in women who attempt to relactate.
In 1979, 23% of U.S. infants breastfed to age of 5 months (figure includes supplemented breastfeeding).		75% of infants breastfed up to or past the age of 9 months; of those, 31% received supplement; of supplemented infants, half or more of nutrition was provided by lactation.

POSITIVE OUTCOME VS. SUCCESS

On learning that it is possible to relactate or to induce lactation, women immediately express concern about their potential for success. Their questions create an excellent opportunity for anticipatory guidance in making informed choices and in planning for positive outcomes.

Relactation/induced lactation is a practice well worth supporting. Infants, their mothers, and families can derive nurturant benefits that may be more important than any nutritional or immunologic considerations. Because supplementation may be an ongoing necessary adjunct to breastfeeding, it is clear that breastfeeding does not have to be an all-or-nothing proposition. So many variables affect the ultimate experience of each mother and infant that it is more appropriate to abandon thinking of induced lactation/relactation in terms of success and to instead focus on planning and managing for a positive outcome. When confronted with the issue of success, help mothers shift their focus by talking with them in terms of "outcome" experienced by other women in similar situations.

COLLECTIVE EXPERIENCES

Some significant amount of "hard data" is important in planning how to educate and assist women who might benefit from relactation/induced lactation. A serious problem exists in gathering data, however. Most reports consist of isolated case histories, with no common grounds for interpreting or describing the circumstances. The few studies that have been done consist of surveys that are self-selecting, in that women contacted can choose whether or not to participate. Much of the information discussed here was obtained from such a survey by Auerbach and myself[1-4] in 1977.

Survey methods

More than 1300 women were sent questionnaires, 60% of whom were from a list of names supplied by the manufacturer of the Lact-Aid Nursing Trainer. About a third were self-referring individuals who learned of the study through professional journals and other publications that announced the study in progress. The remainder were referred through human milk banks, hospitals, and other organizations.

About 100 were returned with incorrect addresses. Nearly 300 women indicated they did not attempt to relactate. Thus the adjusted number contacted was 920, of whom 606 (66%) did complete a lengthy 15-page questionnaire. Only 2% refused to participate, and 32% did not respond. the sample was obtained over a 9-month period, and the respondents were divided into four groups:

1. Untimely weaned—those cases in which weaning occurred sooner than expected or planned by the mother
2. Premature—birth of a premature infant
3. Hospital separated—subsequent separation of mother and full-term infant because of hospitalization
4. Adopted infants—self-explanatory

In an effort to obtain data about "unsuccessful" efforts, the need for a balanced view of the experience was stressed in cover letters to women contacted. Thus 28% of the women provided information about their experiences, even though they were unable to establish breastfeeding via relactation/induced lactation.

The discussion that follows cites not only data from this survey but also findings from clinical experience. In spite of the obvious flaws in doing a self-selecting survey, it was striking that patterns that appeared do closely parallel not only our clinical findings but also reports from others in the field who have frequent contact with women in similar situations. For example, we draw on client records and market data from worldwide distribution of Lact-Aid Nursing Trainer products to more than 10,000 clients worldwide since 1969.

Additional data were gained through the operation of a Denver-based relactation clinic over a 6-year period, 1971 to 1977. Over 2000 clients were counseled by three staff members. A lactation clinic in a large metropolitan area of Southern California reported handling about 1200 relactation clients annually, as of 1981. Information from staff indicated findings similar to our own and those of the survey.

Willingness of infants to suckle the breast

As shown in Fig. 13-1, many infants unwilling to suckle initially eventually accept the breast with patience and perserverance on the part of the mother. Thus conveyin

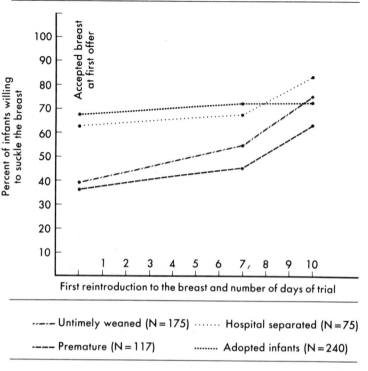

Fig. 13-1. Changes over time in infants' willingness to suckle the breast during relactation efforts. (Modified from Auerbach and Avery, 1979.)

to the mother that the initial feeding is in no way a pass-fail test relieves tension that the mother almost always feels during the introductory feedings. Of the adopted infants, almost 70% accepted the breast initially. Those who did not accept the breast at first showed less inclination to begin suckling after 10 days of effort than did the other groups.

Duration of breastfeeding after relactation

An encouraging number of infants breastfed for a long time after relactation/induced lactation. The length of breastfeeding in all four groups is given in Fig. 13-2. Approximately 75% of the untimely weaned infants continued to breastfeed past 1 year of age. About one third of the premature infants had weaned at 1 year, whereas only one fifth of the adopted infants had ceased breastfeeding when they reached their first birthday. Overall, of those infants who accepted the breast, 75% breastfed up to or beyond 9 months.

Volume of milk

This was difficult to measure, because there was no way to calculate milk volume. Volume could only be estimated by the amount of liquid supplements needed in addition to the mother's milk. Thus a decrease in the number of supplemented feedings or in the amount of the supplement indicated that the volume of milk produced by the

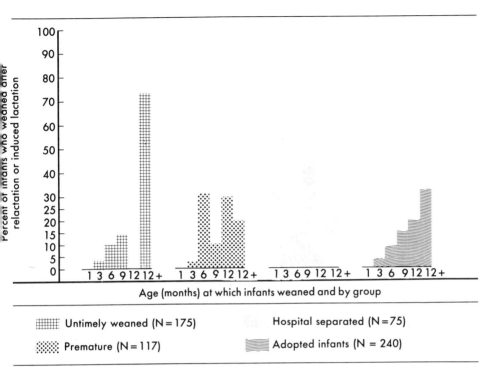

Fig. 13-2. Duration of breastfeeding after relactation or induced lactation. For all groups combined, nearly 75% of infants breastfeed up to or past the age of 9 months. (Modified from Auerbach and Avery, 1979.)

mother had increased. Fig. 13-3 shows the changes in supplementation of infants who were untimely weaned up to 12 months. The survey also showed that of the premature infants, 54% were supplemented at every feeding initially, but by 12 months of age, none were supplemented more than one to three times a day. Only 31% of all the infants still received supplemental formula at each breastfeeding. Of the infants who were being supplemented, most received half or more of their nutrition from their mother's milk.

Women in the survey who breastfed adopted infants, in general, needed to provide more supplement and for a longer time than women in the other categories. Those who had breastfed a previous child gave somewhat less supplement, because their breastfeeding style provided more opportunity for suckling than the more restricted style practiced by women inexperienced in breastfeeding. Some women were breastfeeding an older nonadopted child at the time they adopted an infant. Because they were already lactating, they expected their milk yield to increase sufficiently to totally nourish both children. Despite their optimism, the younger infants did not gain adequate weight without supplementation.

Certainly, more data are needed before we can gauge how widespread the relactation trend has become and more accurately assess outcomes. However, the remarkable achievement of the women surveyed must be recognized. Many of them had little or no helpful information at the beginning and were frequently exposed to hostility from oth-

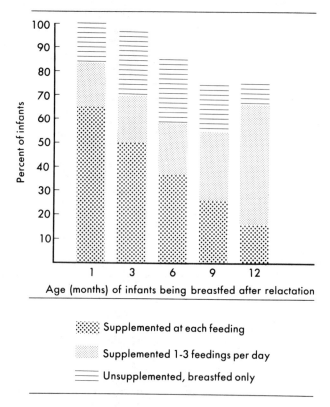

Fig. 13-3. Changes in supplementation (refers to supplemental liquid food [infant formula]) of untimely weaned infants after relactation. Infants who accepted the breast equal 75% of 175 infants studied in the group. (Modified from Auerbach and Avery, 1979.)

ers who questioned their motives. In spite of inadequate support and some outright misinformation, they prevailed magnificently. Those who did not "succeed" but chose to report a disappointing experience must also have their contribution recognized, since it lends a much needed balance to the whole picture.

CONTROVERSY ABOUT POTENTIAL MILK YIELD

Since the early 1970's, there has been much controversy about potential milk yield for women attempting relactation/induced lactation. A key factor seems to be lack of knowledge about mammary involution. In adoptive breastfeeding, women who have borne and breastfed children often wrongly assume it will be easy to stimulate a fully adequate milk supply for a subsequent adopted infant. For such women, the need to continue supplementation has wrongly been regarded as a failure not only by the mothers, but by others as well. This also applies to other relactation situations. Quite often, the inability to attain a fully adequate milk supply has been attributed to a lack of maternal motivation or to some deficiency in the quantity or quality of the infant's suckling.

Another controversy about milk yield relates to the method used for supplementation. For example, some women who used the Lact-Aid Nursing Trainer were labeled by others as dependent on the device, because totally adequate lactation was not achieved within 2 to 3 weeks of use. Likewise, infants who refused to breastfeed without the device were labeled "addicted" to or "hooked" on it.* Yet in clinical practice since 1971 and among the 606 cases surveyed in 1977,[1-4] no significant difference could be found in the amount of supplement used, or in how long it was used according to the type of container or device used for supplementation. Infants supplemented by bottle, cup, or spoon received just as much supplement and for as long as those whose mothers used the Lact-Aid Nursing Trainer.

The third issue of controversy is unsupplemented breastfeeding. Mothers ask when they can eliminate supplements. Health-care providers and lay breastfeeding advisors want to know how long it takes to be successful, to totally breastfeed, after relactation. There is no cookbook answer, no convenient timetable charted, and no clear answer for any group, situation, or individual mother. There is not even a clear definition of what unsupplemented breastfeeding means. Does it mean that the infant receives 100% of his nutrition from the mother's milk? Does it mean that liquid nutrition is breastmilk but that the infant also receives solid foods? Does it mean that the infant is breastfed but also receives solids and perhaps drinks fruit juice, water, and cow's milk by cup?

Current medical and nutritional views encourage breastfeeding of infants for at least 1 year and recognize the need for additional sources of nutrition during the latter half of the year in addition to human milk. Our clinical experience, case reports from others, and our larger survey tend to support the idea that totally unsupplemented breastfeeding may not be an appropriate objective in relactation/induced lactation situations. A pattern typical of the latter stage of normal lactation seems more appropriate. In this stage lactation is an important but decreasing factor in nutrition, whereas solid foods and other liquid foods increase as breastfeeding progresses. This more relaxed objective takes a tremendous amount of pressure off the mother to perform and leads to a more positive outcome in her evaluation of the experience. Until volumetric measurements of a significant number of cases are available, potential milk yield remains an interesting issue for speculation and debate. For susceptible infants, the benefits of some human milk from their own mother and the bonding benefits of the breastfeeding relationship should nevertheless not be discounted. In adoptive breastfeeding, lactation should be treated as a nice but lesser fringe benefit of the relationship.

EFFECT OF MENSES ON MILK YIELD

Many women attempting relactation/induced lactation have reported fluctuations in lactation related to their menstrual cycling patterns.[1-4] Typically, they reported that lactation progressed steadily but then seemed to plateau or diminish suddenly. They described their breasts as feeling full, firm, and painfully tender to the touch. Emotional

---

*Several infants thought to be "refusing" to breastfeed without the device were later identified as having neurodevelopmental oral dysfunction. Without the device present to stimulate correct suckling reflexes of tongue and jaw, infants were unable to extract milk from the breast. Their crying was thus an expression of frustration rather than breast refusal.

status was described as irritable, depressed, often on the verge of tears. When such women were counseled, they often did burst into tears while describing the situation. They felt certain that "milk is there, but it isn't coming out," and they often said they felt like abandoning the relactation effort. Early on in our clinical practice, many women did give up at this stage of their effort. While these findings come primarily from our own clinical experience, other health workers have told us about similar patterns appearing among their clients.

This phenomenon has occurred most frequently among women attempting relactation at 2 to 3 months after delivery. At first we were perplexed and could only advise the mothers to try, just a day at a time, to see if the situation might change. Some never called again, but a few persevered and reported back to us after several days. We learned that within a day or two, the women had a menstrual period, in some cases only a slight spotting on one day. Within 2 to 3 days after the onset of menses, lactation again increased at a fairly steady pace. Many women reported similar fluctuations the subsequent 2 to 3 months.

This phenonemon poses the following two questions: Is the reduction in estrogen and progesterone that occurs at the onset of menses similar in effect to the sharp drop in these hormones that occurs at birth when the placenta is expelled? Is the sudden postmenstrual increase in lactation related to an increase in prolactin secretion during the secretory phase of menstruation? Only research can provide answers to these questions. However, clinical practice often cannot wait to meet the needs of mothers seeking help for problems. Thus it is quite helpful to advise these mothers to watch for signs of menstruation, even slight spotting on 1 day. The nurse should ask them to note whether the milk supply increases after a few days, but avoid promising that it will. It is helpful to explain that the breasts and ovaries are "battling with each other to determine which will be in charge of the situation." A high attrition rate can be avoided by providing this type of anticipatory guidance to women attempting to relactate at 2 to 3 months after delivery and to others of premature infants, who often report that their infants are introduced to breastfeeding just before or during a menstrual period. Ironically this is the time that milk production is lowest.

MATERNAL EXPECTATIONS

The circumstances of prior breastfeeding experience or knowledge, cultural and educational background, and available support systems are just a few of the variables that shape a mother's expectations about relactation/induced lactation. According to these, she will develop goals that center on training her infant to suckle the breast and on stimulating and maintaining lactation in an ongoing breastfeeding relationship for some duration.

The degree to which expectations are met is a key factor in achieving a positive view of the actual outcome. If a mother's expectations are realistic, based on sound facts and not wishful thinking or individual "success" stories, her goals will be reasonably attainable and her view of the outcome will most likely be positive. However, if her expectations are based on incorrect advice and misinformation or built on false hope, she will set unreasonable goals for herself and for her infant. She will most likely view the outcome negatively, and her relationship with her infant and family may suffer. For example, women who have breastfed prior offspring are most likely to view their adoptive breastfeeding experience negatively. Many incorrectly expect to be able to dispense with supplemental feedings within a short time, particularly if they are already lactating somewhat at the time of adoption. Nulliparous women are the most pleased with their experience, since they often do not expect to achieve lactation and are not certain about being able to establish a breastfeeding relationship.

PLANNING FOR POSITIVE OUTCOMES

Whether the ultimate outcome is a decision to attempt relactation/induced lactation or to choose bottle-feeding, the key to making it a positive experience lies in realistic planning with the mother.[5,18]

Criteria for realistic planning

Identify the unique aspects of the situation. Determine the category of relactation/induced lactation. Identify special needs of the infant, the mother, and the family and help them to set realistic goals.

Review available options. Provide unbiased information about relactation/induced lactation that is relevant to the situation. Help the mother evaluate her own motives and how they relate to the information she has received.

Assess support systems. Encourage the mother to enlist her husband or other significant person for support. During the initial counseling session, this person should be present. Advise the mother to cooperate with her physician, particularly if infant illness or maternal illness is a factor. Provide information about useful equipment, educational materials, facilities, support people, and helpful organizations.

Explain the process. Give information on how to prepare for and begin. Explain potential milk production, how to train the infant to suckle, and what to look for to monitor sufficient hydration and calorie intake.

Plan for contingencies. Alert mothers to possible problems and practical alternatives. Point out the physiologic effects of relactation as they pertain to her situation. As the need arises, help the mother to reevaluate her situation and readjust objectives and methods.

Maintain a respectful attitude toward parents. Protect the parents' rights and responsibilities for making informed choices, and support their decisions. Regard them as partners in planning and management, and design advice and methods to protect and enhance the parent-infant bond.

Create a positive environment of achievement. Be honest, but present facts and advice in ways that build confidence. Tell a mother who expresses milk for her sick infant that "a whole ounce is terrific!" instead of saying, "only an ounce." If you are enthusiastic, show it. Being candid can inspire trust, even when differences of opinion arise. Regardless of the issue, always be honest. If parents ask your opinion, give it, but reveal your bias, and make it clear they are the ones who must make decisions.

Listen. Sometimes parents express desires, fears, or questions indirectly. A mother who wants to abandon relactation efforts may bring many little problems to your attention. No matter how simple the solution may be, another problem may arise as you are in midsentence offering advice. Typically, a mother may say "but" in response to each suggestion and offer a rationale as to why it may not work. It is a strong clue to listen and reassess the situation. Perhaps the mother is wanting assurance she can be a "good" mother without breastfeeding. Keep in mind that the mother who asks whether relactation is possible may be wanting to hear a "no."

TECHNIQUES FOR RELACTATION/INDUCED LACTATION

There are differences of opinion as to what specific methods should be recommended to women contemplating relactation or induced lactation, but four goals are generally recognized:

1. Stimulating the breast, particularly the nipple and areola, to increase prolactin secretion
2. Training the infant to suckle the breast and to suckle correctly
3. Providing adequate hydration and nutrition to the infant during the process
4. Ensuring that no method places the mother-infant or family relationships in danger

Women have been amazingly creative and persistent in their efforts to relactate or to induce lactation. They have applied hot or cold packs to their breasts. They have massaged their breasts, nipples, and shoulders. Some have suckled infants borrowed from other breastfeeding mothers. Husbands have been encouraged to imitate infant suckling. A variety of manually operated and electric pumps have been used in hopes of stimulating lactation.

Efforts to coax infants to accept and suckle the breast in a way that provides them with adequate nutrition have been equally ingenious. Women have applied honey (now contraindicated because of the risk of botulism), syrup, or other sweet fluid to their nipples. They have dripped milk or proprietary infant formula down their breasts toward the nipples with medicine droppers. Cups, spoons, and other assorted devices have been used to feed infants while eliminating exposure to artificial nipples.

Efforts to stimulate lactation have led women to ingest various foods, hormones, or other drugs as galactagogues. When and if lactation became evident, women engaged in a wide variety of tactics to reduce the amount of supplemental liquid, with sometimes serious results for their infants.

There is no simple recipe for managing relactation/induced lactation. However, mothers, nurses, and breastfeeding advisors all need to be aware of the availability of techniques and devices that have been tried with varying degrees of usefulness.

Breast stimulation

Suckling by the mother's own infant. Suckling 15 to 20 minutes at each breast every 2 to 3 hours is the most effective means of stimulating breasts. A longer interval between two night sucklings is acceptable so long as it is no more than 5 to 6 hours and suckling occurs at least eight to ten times within a 24-hour period. Suckling periods can be longer than 15 to 20 minutes per breast; however, continuous or "marathon" suckling is not advisable, because both mother and infant suffer fatigue, which can impair the mother's milk ejection reflex. The infant's suckling pattern in marathon suckling is frequently characterized by frantic pulling, chewing, and strong suction at the beginning, which becomes placid, ineffective suckling as fatigue progresses during each session. This erratic pattern has contributed to severe nipple soreness and maceration, in addition to further inhibition of milk let-down. Both may become extremely frustrated by the situation as well.

Suckling by a borrowed infant. The primary advantage is to demonstrate how correct suckling feels, which is important to a woman with no prior breastfeeding experience or to one whose infant is suspected of having a suckling defect. In cases in which infants have access to their mothers and are able to suckle, borrowing another infant for milk stimulation is not advised, because cross-infections can occur.[14] Neither is it advised for the adopted infant, who can become frustrated by suckling a nonlactating breast. Also, the adopting woman can become attached to the borrowed infant. A mother in my practice had such an experience, which was further complicated by the fact the borrowed infant weaned from his biologic mother first and was still suckling the adopting woman when the relationship ended. The adoptive woman felt grief similar to the loss described by mothers of infants who die.

Suckling by an adult. Many women have reported that suckling by their adult spouse/partner as part of love play had a positive role in relactation/induced lactation efforts. Although suckling probably does not accurately mimic infant suckling, such stimulation does enhance prolactin secretion just as does coitus. Many couples felt that it enhanced their feelings of closeness and of sharing, much like the experience of birthing couples who share in childbirth exercises prepartally. Explaining these facts to couples also seems helpful in their overcoming ambivalent feelings and gives them "permission" to use breasts for both nurturant and sexual functions.

Breast pumps. Both manually operated and mechanical breast pumps are useful for stimulating lactation when there is no opportunity for suckling, as in the case of the hospitalized premature infant. Techniques for their use were discussed in Chapter 12. When using pumps, women must be informed that breasts are not faucets that can be turned on at will and quickly emptied. They will need to devote as much time in pumping as it naturally takes an infant to breastfeed. In addition, women should be advised to do some gentle massage before and during pumping in motions similar to a breast self-examination. Self-stimulation of the breasts enhances prolactin secretion more than does pumping alone.[19,21]

I do not recommend using a breast pump for induced lactation to prepare for the adopted baby. In 12 years of experience, I have found that using the breast pump focuses the mother's attentions on the *milk* rather than on *bonding*.

Galactogogues. Foods, drugs, and hormones have been recommended for their reported lactogenic effects. Sound basic nutrition is the most appropriate recommendation, because a well-nourished woman will function more effectively. Use of drugs is counter to a self-care approach. It takes control from parents and places it in the hands of physicians and researchers who are more interested in expediency than in offering information, encouragement, and follow-up support. In one study,[16] for example, investigators attributed equal success for a group receiving drugs and a control group receiving placebos, to the special information and support that was provided to both groups. In another study,[15] women who used estrogens as a means of relactation/induced lactation had more difficulty initiating and enhancing lactation than those who used no drugs.

If parents' desires are given due credence, drugs should not be recommended. Mothers often express much concern about the risk to their own bodies from drugs taken before relactation and even greater concern for risks to their infants from drugs that might be excreted in the milk. Others feel it shifts their focus away from nurturing and bonding.

Among adoptive women, use of estrogens and progesterones to simulate pregnancy can mask symptoms of illness related to infertility and possibly aggravate existing conditions, such as polycystic ovary disease. A mother in my practice received high levels of such drugs for 9 months before adopting and subsequently was diagnosed as having polycystic ovary disease after an emergency hysterectomy 5 years later. Other risks are similar to those for oral contraceptives in general. Compared with other methods, drugs provide no significant advantage. Ultimately, the most effective galactogogue is the mother's own motivation and self-confidence.

Training infants to suckle at the breast while providing adequate nutrition

Lact-Aid Nursing Trainer. A device developed in 1971 has proved very effective in relactation/induced lactation.[1-4,6] Known as the Lact-Aid Nursing Trainer,* it delivers supplemental liquid food to the infant as he suckles the maternal nipple. As shown in Fig. 13-4, a presterilized disposable bag holds up to 120 ml (4 oz) of liquid, which is delivered by means of a capillary tube placed by the maternal nipple. As the infant suckles both the tube and nipple, he is rewarded for his effort and thus encouraged to continue, providing the natural suckling stimulation essential for milk secretion.

In a single feeding a healthy infant will suckle about 15 to 20 minutes on each breast to obtain 4 ounces of supplement. This approximates a typical breastfeeding for unsupplemented infants. A placid infant or one who dozes frequently will take longer to breastfeed. A high-risk infant may need to breastfeed for shorter but more frequent sessions to avoid fatigue. There is no risk of aspiration as fluid is obtained only via suckling, rather than siphoning.

Mothers using nonstandard proprietary infant formulas will need special instructions. For example, certain nonmilk formulas, such as Isomil, Cho-Free, Soyalac, and others must be slightly diluted to achieve a proper rate of flow because these are slightly thicker. Detailed instructions for this situation as well as for normal use are included with each nursing trainer kit. Meat-base formula is not suitable for use with the device, even though experimental models have been assembled with a larger orifice. The minute meat particles clump together and clog, regardless of the diameter. Women report they must repeatedly shake infant feeding bottles when using a meat formula.

Consumers and health professionals familiar with the device regard the Lact-Aid Nursing Trainer as the method of choice for managing relactation and induced lactation, as well as for other special breastfeeding problems. Most women view it as a wonderful tool of modern technology and felt very comfortable in using it. Some, however, have viewed it as a rather frightening mechanical device, particularly some mothers of high-risk infants. The manner in which it is presented to mothers may be an important factor in shaping their response. It is never a good idea to tell a mother she must use it. Always, it should simply be offered as one of a variety of available resources. Never should its use be recommended as a substitute for giving appropriate information, support, and help.

Other methods. Medicine droppers and spouted, narrow-tipped bottles have been used to drip formula or other fluid on nipples to coax infants to suckle. Mothers have been instructed to insert these devices into the corner of their infant's mouth as an encouragement to continual suckling and as a feeding method.[10,22] Mothers in general find this unsatisfactory, because suckling is erratic and does not effectively simulate breastfeeding. Many mothers also report that it is messy and confining, time consuming,

*Available from Lact-Aid Supplies Center, P.O. Box 6861, Denver, Colo. 80206.

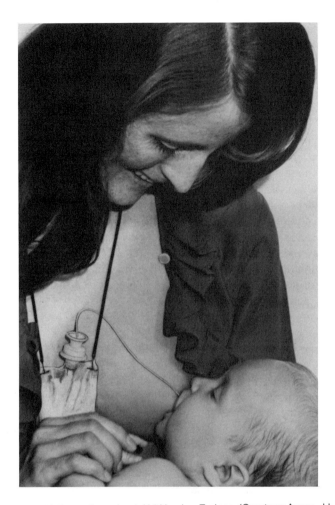

Fig. 13-4. Mother and infant using a Lact-Aid Nursing Trainer. (Courtesy Avery, J.L., Lact-Aid Supplies Center, Denver, Colo. 80206).

and that the mechanics diminish their enjoyment of their infants. Moreover, there is risk of aspiration because timing may not match infant swallowing.

Infants have been kept hungry to make them more inclined to accept and suckle the breast or to gradually decrease supplemental feedings. To do this mothers have been advised to offer minimal supplementation or to dilute supplemental food with water. Both these methods are highly dangerous, because some infants can easily starve over a brief time. Inadequate nutrition for even a day or two may have serious consequences for a high-risk infant. A variety of factors must be taken into account, and infants must be closely monitored during efforts to reduce supplemental feeding after lactation is established.

Indicators of adequate nutrition include progress in weight gain and growth, very wet diapers, clear urine, stools characteristic of breastfed infants, increase in time between individual feedings, or taking less supplement than what is offered.* In combination, these can be signs that an infant is receiving increasing amounts of breastmilk. Maternal signs are variable and are not as important but may include breast fullness and firmness, which decreases immediately after each nursing, leaking from one side while the other is suckled, and milk ejection sensations.

If supplemental bottles are necessary, a standard infant feeding bottle with a NUK orthodontic nipple has proved most effective. This nipple simulates the action of suckling a maternal nipple and reduces risk of nipple confusion for the infant. Nonorthodontic nipples do not simulate suckling a maternal nipple and may thus cause aberrant suckling such as tongue thrusting. Some mothers prefer using cups or spoons as a means of providing supplemental nutrition along with breastfeeding.

Mothers should be informed about various techniques and equipment available to assist relactation/induced lactation. They should be given information about the methods at the outset and should select one or more they wish to try first. Then, if results are unsatisfactory, they should select another to try. The offering of a potpourri of options leaves no implication that any method is less effective, simply because it might be tried second, or third, or so on. The mother should approach each with equal confidence, thereby enhancing potential effectiveness.

SUMMARY

Relactation is an old tool with modern usefulness for breastfeeding in special situations. It is truly "normal" lactation and is challenging to nurses and others who assist women in relactating. It is still uncommon in Western culture, although the practice has been increasing dramatically since the early 1970's, just as breastfeeding in general has increased from about the same time. Because most relactation situations require support, health professionals need to become more informed. The reported experiences of women can serve as a foundation for realistic planning and effective assistance for relactation.

It is very easy to launch into the how-to aspects without giving women adequate opportunity to make informed choices about whether or not to attempt relactation. Likewise, it is easy to miss cues from some women that signal that their bottle-feeding might be more appropriate than relaction for them, their infants, and families. Thus professionals and lay advisors alike must exercise caution. Assisting a woman in relactating requires genuine teamwork between the parents, the breastfeeding advisor, and all the professionals involved in their health care.

---

*Characteristically in relactation/induced lactation, morning supplements may be eliminated sooner than afternoon and early evening ones. This is a reflection of the diurnal and circadian variations in prolactin secretion. Prolactin secretion is greatest at the darkest portion of the night in humans and is also enhanced by sleep.[19,21]

REFERENCES

1. Auerbach, K.G., and Avery, J.L.: Relactation after an untimely weaning: report from a survey, No. 2, Denver, 1979, Resources in Human Nurturing International.
2. Auerbach, K.G., and Avery, J.L.: Relactation and the premature infant: report from a survey, No. 3, Denver, 1979, Resources in Human Nurturing International.
3. Auerbach, K.G., and Avery, J.L.: Relactation after a hospitalization-induced separation: report from a survey, No. 4, Denver, 1979, Resources in Human Nurturing International.
4. Auerbach, K.G., and Avery, J.L.: Nursing the adopted infant: report from a survey, No. 5, Denver, 1979, Resources in Human Nurturing International.

5. Avery, J.L.: Induced lactation: a guide for counseling and management, No. 6, Denver, 1979, Resources in Human Nurturing International.

6. Bose, C.L., et al.: Relactation by mothers of sick and premature infants, Pediatrics **67**:565, 1981.

7. Brown, R.E.: Relactation: an overview, Pediatrics **60**:116, 1977.

8. Foss, G.L., and Short, D.: Abnormal lactation, J. Obstet. Gynaec. Brit. Emp. **58**:35, 1951.

9. Greenblatt, R.B.: Inappropriate lactation in men and women, Med. Aspects Human Sexuality **6**:25, 1972.

10. Hormann, E.: Breastfeeding the adopted baby, Birth Fam. J. **4**:165, 1977.

11. Jelliffe, D.B., and Jelliffe, E.F.P.: Non-puerperal induced lactation, Pediatrics **50**:171, 1972.

12. Jelliffe, D.B., and Jelliffe, E.F.P.: Human milk in the modern world, New York, 1978, Oxford University Press.

13. Kleinman, R., et al.: Protein values of milk samples from mothers without biologic pregnancies, J. Pediatr. **97**:612, 1980.

14. Krantz, J.Z., and Kupper, W.S.: Cross-nursing: wet-nursing in a contemporary context, Pediatrics **67**:715, 1981.

15. Kulski, J.K., et al.: Changes in the milk composition of nonpuerperal women, Am. J. Obstet. Gynecol. **139**:597, 1981.

16. Lewis, P.J., and others: Controlled trial of metoclopramide in the initiation of breastfeeding, Br. J. Clin. Pharmacol. **9**:217, 1980.

17. Marieskind, H.: Abnormal lactation, J. Trop. Pediatr. **19**:123, 1973.

18. Nau, J.: Relactation: one alternative to untimely weaning, Keeping Abreast J. **2**:203, 1977.

19. Pasteels, J.L., and Robyn, C., editors: Human prolactin, New York, 1973, Elsevier North-Holland, Inc.

20. Phillips, V.: Establishment of lactation for the breastfeeding of an adopted baby, Res. Bull. Nurs. Mothers Assoc. Austr., No. 4, 1971.

21. Vorheer, H.: The breast: morphology, physiology and lactation, New York, 1974, Academic Press, Inc.

22. Waletzky, L., and Herman, E.: Relactation, Am. Fam. Physician **14**:69, 1976.

ADDITIONAL READINGS

Auerbach, K.G., and Avery, J.L.: Relactation: a study of 366 cases, Pediatrics **65**:236, 1980.

Auerbach, K.G., and Avery, J.L.: Induced lactation: a study of adoptive nursing by 240 women, Am. J. Dis. Child **135**:340, 1981.

Avery, J.L., and Fleiss, P.: Relactation: a new/old tool in managing breastfeeding in special situations. In Freir, S., and Eidelman, A.I., editors: Human milk: its biological and social value, International Congress Series No. 518, Amsterdam, 1980, Excerpta Medica.

Brown, R.E.: Some nutritional considerations in times of major catastrophe, Clin. Pediatr. **11**:334, 1972.

Brown, R.E.: Breastfeeding in modern times, Am. J. Clin. Nutr. **26**:556, 1973.

Canales, E.S., et al.: Feasibility of suppressing and reinitiating lactation in women with premature infants, Am. J. Obstet. Gynecol. **128**:695, 1977.

Choi, M.: Breast milk for infants who can't breastfeed. Am. J. Nurs. **78**:852, 1978.

Findlay, A.: The role of suckling in lactation. In Josimovich, J., et al., editors: Lactogenic hormones, fetal nutrition and lactation, New York, 1974, John Wiley & Sons, Inc.

Herman, E.: Relactation. In Waletzky, L.R., editor: Symposium on human lactation, Department of Health, Education, and Welfare Pub. No. (HSA) 79-5107, Washington, D.C., 1976.

Hormann, E.: Relactation: a guide for breastfeeding the adopted baby, Belmont, Mass., 1971, E. Hormann.

Kolodny, R.C., et al.: Mammary stimulation causes prolactin secretion in non-lactating women, Nature **238**:284, 1972.

Mobbs, G.A., and Babbage, N.F.: Breastfeeding adopted children. Med. J. Aust. **2**:436, 1971.

Newton, M.: Breastfeeding by adoptive mother, J.A.M.A. **11**:212, 1967.

Noel, G.L.: Prolactin release during nursing and breast stimulation in postpartum and non-postpartum subjects, J. Clin. Endocrinol. Metab. **38**:413, 1974.

Perlman, E.: Breastfeeding without pregnancy, Pediatrics **49**:791, 1972.

Phillips, V.: Non-puerperal lactation among Australian aboriginal women, Res. Bull. Nurs. Mothers Assoc. Austr. Nos. 1 and 2, 1969.

Weichert, C.E.: Lactational reflex recovery in breastfeeding failure, Pediatrics **63**:799, 1979.

Wieschoff, H.A.: Artificial stimulation of lactation in primitive cultures, Bull. Hist. Med. **8**:1403, 1940.

Zimmerman, M.A.: Breastfeeding the adopted newborn. Pediatr. Nurs. **7**:9, Jan.-Feb. 1981.

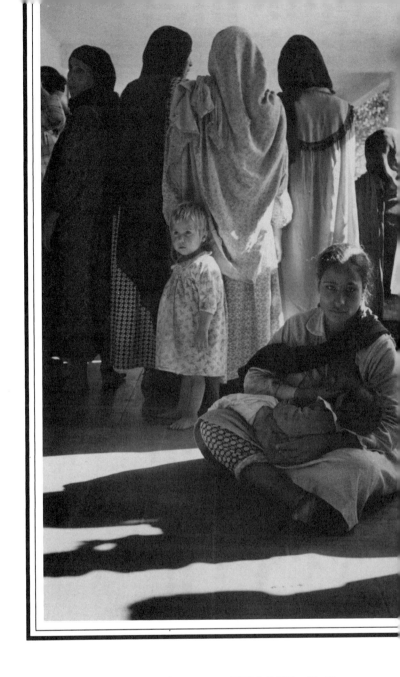

PART THREE

CROSS-CULTURAL PERSPECTIVES

As each of us grew to adulthood, we absorbed a particular cultural pattern, unaware that our corner of the world was but one small corner. For those of us who became nurses involved in maternal and child care, we first viewed our caretaking role from our own cultural perspectives. Later, as we had more contact with other cultures, our perspectives expanded to include a wider understanding of the nature of humanity. Although basic needs are met in differing ways in different cultures, we are all essentially the same: everyone eats, smiles, socializes, and makes love. Couples unite, and families are born. Everywhere there is a particular belief system for the early childbearing experience. That includes certain practices of caring for and feeding infants, especially breastfeeding, an important part of cultural belief systems and practices.

The purpose of the first chapter in Part Three is to sensitize the reader to the general impact of culture and the assessment and study of early child-rearing behaviors associated with breastfeeding. Subsequent chapters consider maternal nutrition and weaning, solid foods, and the sensuality of breastfeeding within the context of cross-cultural nursing.

The impact of culture on breastfeeding

JAN RIORDAN

In looking at breastfeeding cross-culturally, the values, customs, beliefs, and traditions of a people must be examined and understood. The broad term *culture* can be a blueprint for human behavior and can help us, as nurses, gain a clearer understanding of individual behaviors. Without understanding or knowing about the cultural health-care practices of our clients, our nursing care and interventions could possibly do more harm than good; at best, it is misguided professionalism.

Nursing education programs are beginning to emphasize cross-cultural awareness in nursing curricula. This is an important trend, especially now that an estimated 22,000 American nurses are practicing abroad.[5] A considerable number of nurses, excited by the rich diversity of cultures, are entering graduate anthropology programs. It is unusual to read through a current nursing journal without discovering an article that deals with a cross-cultural topic. Studying the universality of humankind through the blending of nursing and anthropology further broadens the dimension of nursing by providing new insights, awareness, and a holistic perspective for care.

In discussing breastfeeding from a multicultural viewpoint, I do not intend to promote the romantic illusion that children are somehow exempt from health defects in cultures in which unrestricted breastfeeding is common. Natural mothering through breastfeeding has manifold benefits, but breastfed babies can also have problems that need medical and nursing attention. An infant born with a disabling congenital heart defect is in as much danger whether he is breastfed or bottle-fed. Surgical interventions available in technologically advanced societies may actually save his life or have a rehabilitating effect. In other words, I am not suggesting the "noble savage" concept. The purpose here is to look at the process of breastfeeding as a human behavior, sensitive to cultural influence and change. The intent is to evaluate whether prevailing infant feeding practices and care are beneficial to our clients from a holistic view.

THE EFFECTS OF CULTURE ON BREASTFEEDING

American nurses increasingly have contact with people from other cultures who come here in search of a new life and opportunities. For these newcomers, adapting to our customs may include changing their attitudes about infant feeding practices. For many of them, breastfeeding becomes a choice, not a cultural norm and an economic necessity. The women may be told that it is the custom in America to bottle-feed babies (although present trends toward breastfeeding in America make this an arguable point). It is a fact, for instance, that Southeast Asian women perceive breastfeeding not as fashionable in America but as out of place and shameful.[2] In their eagerness to acclimate, many of them turn away from their cultural heritage of breastfeeding their infants.

In a local hospital, I cared for a young Vietnamese family, including an infant with severe atopic dermatitis. Since I was interested in the baby's diet, I discovered, through sign language, that the mother breastfed her firstborn child in Vietnam but was using formula for this baby. "Why not breastfeed here?" I gently ventured. She answered by shrugging her shoulders and gesturing hopelessly, "I not know." Even if an immigrant mother does breastfeed, she seems to have more problems. Another time I was referred for home visits to a mother who had breastfed another child in Vietnam but felt sure she did not have enough milk for this infant. Since she had a successful breastfeeding experience in Vietnam, her problems seemed to be related to the influences of a new culture. I considered her exposure to cultural factors, the formula discharge pack she received from the hospital in this land "where babies don't die," the stacks of formula and baby foods she saw as she did her daily shopping in the supermarket, magazine pictures of affluent American mothers bottle-feeding their babies, and so on. Perhaps these experiences caused her to doubt herself, maybe even interfering with her let-down and milk supply. I assessed her support system for breastfeeding and found she had none. Coming to this country as the wife of a serviceman, she had no female relatives or friends to support her early mothering experiences. Recognizing that English-speaking, albeit well-intentioned, American nurses could provide only limited self-care assistance, I engaged the help of a Vietnamese interpreter and was able to guide her through her breastfeeding problems. Once again she became a successful breastfeeding mother.

Well-intentioned efforts to acculturate recent immigrants can disrupt breastfeeding. For example, new Vietnamese-Americans are encouraged and sometimes even paid to attend government-sponsored English classes. Because these classes are important, new mothers should attend, but they need to be allowed to keep their babies with them in class to continue breastfeeding on demand. In cities that have adopted this policy, the rates of breastfeeding among Vietnamese women are going up.

Breastfeeding in public or in the presence of friends is also extremely sensitive to cultural norms. For instance, in Saudi Arabia it is not uncommon to see a totally veiled woman baring her breast to feed her infant in a public place, with no one taking notice—except, perhaps, the foreigners. As a contrast, in France for a woman to wear a topless swimming suit on the beaches is perfectly acceptable. However, a French woman would hesitate, or at least cover herself carefully, while breastfeeding in public—even in a restaurant across from the "topless" beach. Since breastfeeding is still not done in public very much in America, it is enlightening to read accounts of the reactions of people from other countries when they observe American women breastfeeding. "While visiting a woman from Malaya who had three small sons, I began to breastfeed my daughter, Heather," reported one woman. "My neighbor was astonished. 'I didn't know Americans did that.' "[3]

For a Spanish-speaking or an American Indian woman, breastfeeding may still be the norm in her community. Gradually her attitude may change as fewer and fewer of her peers attempt to breastfeed, and she prefers to follow what seems to be most socially acceptable—that is, bottle-feeding. Because of the Indian and Spanish cultures' respect for medical and nursing advice, a nurse who makes an attempt can make a significant difference. In these cultural groups, professional encouragement to breastfeed has an enormous impact. One example is the positive effect on breastfeeding in a small Mexican-American community when a breastfeeding support program was started at their community health clinic.[10] Another is a federally sponsored program for promoting breastfeeding among the Papago Indians in Southern Arizona. Workshops for health professionals, including hospital staff, are held on the importance of breastfeeding. Since most of the young women of the Papago tribe work at clerical jobs for the reservation, the information for health workers is directed to the type of help these women need.[12]

In working with women who speak a different language, the most effective help in communicating is having someone who can simultaneously translate for the nurse. Even better is to have the help of a translator who is an experienced breastfeeding mother. If a translator is available, it may be wise to tape-record the discussion with a mother, so that this information can be used with other women.

It is extremely helpful also to have printed materials on breastfeeding in the mother's language. La Leche League International offers information sheets on breastfeeding in 14 different languages. However, even with translations, there may be language problems, since there are a number of different dialects within some countries. Vietnam is a good example. Even if the same language is spoken, there may be different shades of word meaning from one region of the country to the next. In preparing a flip chart and audio cassette for encouraging breastfeeding among mothers in the Dominican Republic, I used the word "amamantar" to mean breastfeeding, as it does in many Spanish-speaking countries. However, much to the amusement of the Dominican mothers, it meant "milk the cow" to them. So much for the carefully planned visual aids.

Finally, it should be pointed out that significant political and social upheavals affect cultural customs, including breastfeeding and early child care patterns. For example, almost all Japanese women traditionally breastfed their infants for at least 2 years until the end of World War II. With the rapid technologic and industrial changes of postwar Japan, East met West and reflected the Western linear model of preoccupation with measurement and control. Schedules, weighing before and after each feeding, and formula-feeding became the norm. In addition, economic recovery forced many women into the workplace. Although Japanese women are returning to breastfeeding in recent years, most children are weaned by 1 year.

EVALUATING PRACTICES

One method for assessing the intrinsic value of early infant cultural practices is to evaluate them using the following four categories (beneficial, harmless, harmful, or uncertain)[13] by asking these questions:

1. *Is it beneficial?* Carrying the infant close, breastfeeding on demand, and spacing children by long-term breastfeeding would all, of course, be considered beneficial.
2. *Is it harmless?* Believing that certain foods are hot or cold and relating them to the hot-cold physical states is a harmless practice, provided that basic nutritional requirements are still being met.
3. *Is it harmful?* The value of colostrum, which has been likened to blood because

it contains so many living cells is, oddly enough, not always recognized. There are sporadic cultural customs in which colostrum is considered poisonous or bad and is discarded. The newborn is fed by a lactating relative or friend for a few days or given gruel until the "true" milk comes in, depriving the infant of the immune properties of colostrum. This is clearly a harmful practice.

4. *Is it uncertain or innocuous?* Answering this question is more difficult. Some practices fall into this "gray" area until the nurse has a more complete knowledge base for evaluation. For example, while working as a part of a nurse team in the Dominican Republic, I noted that women avoided eating fresh fruits for 2 weeks after delivery. At first glance, this practice would seem to be harmful, but there is some evidence[9] that vitamin C continues to be excreted in breastmilk for some time without oral intake. Science has yet to discover why and how. We have to ask ourselves if, through countless generations of experiential practice, this culture knows that the milk is complete even with this severe dietary restriction.

TWO TYPES OF BREASTFEEDING PRACTICE

In studying breastfeeding practices and early mothering, the nurse should consider these key questions:

- How often does breastfeeding occur in a day?
- Is the breast used as a pacifier when the baby is upset, hurt, or ill?
- How long does the breastfeeding period last before total weaning?
- What is the length of amenorrhea and spacing before the next pregnancy?
- Is the baby carried during his waking hours?
- Does the baby sleep with the mother?
- Does the woman work outside the home?

For the nurse observing maternal behavior, breastfeeding practices in different cultural settings fall generally into one of two patterns: unrestricted and restricted.

Unrestricted

Newton describes unrestricted breastfeeding as follows:

> Unrestricted breast feeding has no rules that materially restrict sucking. The infant is helped to the breast whenever he cries or fusses. He usually sleeps in the same bed, or at least in the same room as his mother, for easy access to the breast during the night. In the daytime he is carried around by his mother, or kept close enough so that his crying can be quickly quieted by suckling [Fig. 14-1].
>
> In unrestricted breastfeeding, there are typically ten or more feedings a day during the early weeks. The number gradually diminishes to about 5 or 6 feedings a day during the latter half of the first year, although more are given when the baby feels fretful or upset. No bottle feedings are given. Other foods begin to add significant amounts of calories only after the infant can swallow solids easily, and when teeth indicate the readiness to begin to chew. Breast milk continues to be a major source of nourishment beyond infancy into early childhood.[8]

During a stay in the Dominican Republic, I observed this type of breastfeeding pattern. Mothers breastfeed on street corners, in doorways, and in church. While riding on the bus one day I passed a woman galloping briskly along on a donkey while breast-

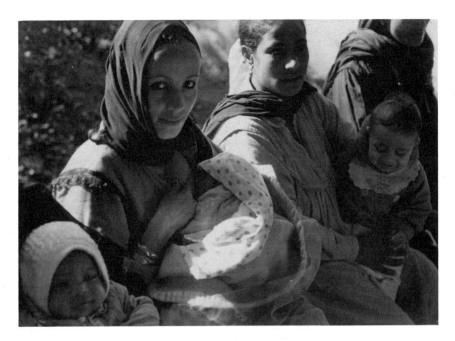

Fig. 14-1. Example of unrestricted breastfeeding. These women have brought their children to a maternal and child health center in the Nile Delta of Egypt. (Courtesy M. Jacot, WHO.)

feeding her baby. Breasts and breastfeeding are accepted in this county without a hint of embarrassment. Leininger also describes unrestricted breastfeeding in her ethnography on the Gadsup of New Guinea:

> The mother and infant establish close bonding relationships with direct skin contact (no cloth between infant and mother), for nearly two weeks. The mother holds the infant against her breast and body, and if she is doing some household task the infant lies in her lap. All Gadsup infants are breast-fed as there is no cow's milk nor infant-feeding bottles. The mothers told me they would not like to use ''such things'' as they enjoy breast-feeding their infants and occasionally feeding other infants in the village when the need arises, e.g., death or sickness of the mother, or if the mother had to leave the infant for some rare reason. The mother touches, cuddles, and talks to the infant and provides the primary care to the offspring. Much skin contact and direct facial interaction can be observed for nearly three continuous weeks.[4]

More than an act of feeding, unrestricted breastfeeding denotes a style of mothering in which care is affectionate and trust is established. The baby receives immediate nurturant response to crying and is allowed minimal restriction in movement when not being held. Unrestricted, the baby will breastfeed 3000 to 4000 times during the course of a full lactation cycle.

Swaddling the baby and carrying him close to the body typifies mothers who practice unrestricted breastfeeding. The Zambian infant is secured to his mother's body as early as 24 hours after delivery with a *dashica*, a long piece of cloth. The baby essentially rides on her hip in the dashica, and his head is not supported. As a result, the Zambian infant maintains a strong shoulder girdle to keep his head steady and develops early

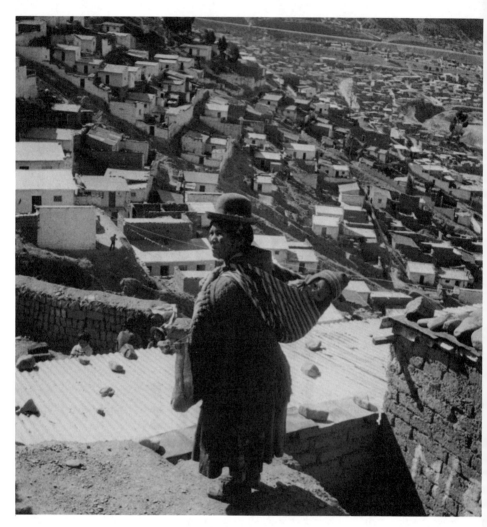

Fig. 14-2. In the high Andean plateau, a Bolivian woman carries her child in an *aguawo*. (Courtesy D. Henrioud, WHO.)

head control. A specially woven strong cotton cloth folded in a special way, the *aguawo* (Fig. 14-2), is the infant carrier of Bolivia. The *aguawo* can be turned around to several positions to facilitate breastfeeding. In Mexico, a woman uses a long, wide shawl called a *rebozo* for carrying her infant while she goes about her daily activities. The many different types of baby carriers, seen almost everywhere now in the United States, show that American women are finally catching up with their sisters in other lands in discovering this convenience.

Carrying the infant swaddled to his mother's body, in addition to developing muscle tone, seems also to encourage alertness. Being carried about during normal daily activities offers many opportunities for tactile, visual, and social stimulation. Have you ever suddenly found yourself peering into a pair of curious eyes of a baby in a back carrier?

You may find yourself irresistibly carrying on an animated "baby talk" conversation with this little mobile creature who responds to every clever thing you have to say.

Babies in the Dominican Republic are not secured to their mothers in any fashion but are carried in their arms in a horizontal position until they are old enough to sit up by themselves. I noted that their infants had very poor head control when pulled to a sitting position, probably because of this practice. Because of the indigenous belief that babies can break their necks very easily if their heads are not held, the mothers became visibly anxious when the nurses assessed head control, and I learned to be very cautious performing this maneuver. This experience points out the necessity of incorporating cultural beliefs into nursing practice.

Restricted

Newton describes restricted breastfeeding as:

characterized by severe limitation of sucking by social custom. There are rules restricting the number of feedings, their duration, the time between feedings, and the amount of mother-baby skin contact that stimulates the urge to suck. Infants and mothers are frequently housed in different rooms. Sleeping in the same bed with the mother is considered dangerous for the infant. The strength of the infant's breast sucking is limited by teaching it bottle sucking techniques and by dulling its appetite with glucose water, formula, and semisolid foods. The practice of feeding the baby at specified times may result in a baby too worn out with crying to suck well, or a baby too sleepy to persist in strong sucking. Severe sucking limitations cause excessive engorgement of the breast, which often weakens the baby's grasp on the nipple or blocks the baby's nose. When these problems prevent the mother from establishing a secure milk supply, total weaning usually occurs within weeks.[8]

The Nacirema tribe. The Nacirema people exemplify the restricted breastfeeding pattern. These people have been studied by others,[7,11] including a nurse anthropologist,[4] but this is the first attempt to report their behaviors in regard to breastfeeding. Nacirema women deliver their babies in a temple (*latipsoh*). Shortly after birth, the babies are taken to a separate room in the temple where they are looked after by members of the Gnisrun tribe (called *sesrun*). These women perform rituals on the newborn in another part of the temple (called a *yresrun*). The rituals begin immediately after birth and include removal of the gastric content by pushing a tube through his nose to his stomach. If the Nacirema baby is healthy, he will choke and gag. Then he is given sugar and water to drink, to fill his stomach before he makes a long bumpy journey on a wheeled cart to the place where his mother waits to feed him. After he feeds from his mother, he is again fed a special food made from vegetable fats and sugars. Thus the Nacirema baby learns two ways of eating, right from birth.

The breasts of the Nacirema woman are considered sexually arousing, so they are kept hidden and bound under cloth until the baby cries to eat. Then only a portion of the breast, the nipple, is exposed and only in private places. Some Nacirema women who have broken this tribal rule have been severely criticized and even arrested by tribal police.

Nacirema women are warned that sleeping with their babies, or breastfeeding them for too long a time, will bring harm, such as suffocation, or that the boy babies will act like girls when they grow up. So only a few do this, and in secret.

By now the reader probably recognizes that Nacirema spelled backwards is American. Some, indeed, think our practices backward. Much more could be said about the role of nursing (gnisrun) and the helping professions (snoisseforp gnipleh) in looking at our breastfeeding practices using an ethnographic descriptive approach, but this much gives a perspective on how others could view us. Fortunately, there are changes taking place in our society and the health professions in recent years that belie this negative viewpoint.

Working women. For the woman who works outside the home, breastfeeding too often must be unnecessarily restricted by cultural expectations. The working woman is hardly a new phenomenon of the western world; from time immemorial, women have always worked. What is new is the separation of the mother-infant pair while she is working; separation that places her many miles distant from her baby and interferes with easy, accessible contact and breastfeeding.

A few modern societies are attempting to deal with the distance between the marketplace and the home by providing facilities for babies of mothers who return to work. In the People's Republic of China, the number of children a family can have is severely controlled by the government. Fifty-six days after her infant's birth, the Chinese woman usually returns to work. Often she takes the child to work with her and leaves him in a "nursing room" at work, returning several times throughout the day to spend time with and breastfeed him. The kibbutz in Israel, a collective agricultural community, provides an Infant House for babies to which the mother comes from the fields periodically to breastfeed and cuddle her baby. On their reservation, a breastfeeding nursery is provided for Papago Indian working women. When their infants awaken for feedings, they are called from work to breastfeed and spend time with them.[12] Employers in the United States are slowly responding to the need for in-house child care facilities. Hospitals and medical centers, for example, find they can attract nurses to work and retain them if they provide quality care for their children during working hours.

RITUALS AND BELIEFS

Another question must be asked: "What are the rituals and belief systems associated with breastfeeding?" Rituals have a role in the breastfeeding process as in all life roles and are fascinating to study. Unfortunately, the word *ritual* connotes a meaningless ceremonial act, when, in fact, rituals can have a significant effect if the individual believes in them. Eating a special food or praying to a patron saint to increase the milk supply are cultural rituals that may actually work. Incidentally, a shrine of the Spanish Madonna, Nuestra Señora de La Leche y Bueno Paro,* in St. Augustine, Florida, was the inspiration for the naming of La Leche League.

In Japan, figurines and paintings depicting a woman with a bounteous milk supply are displayed with the belief that they increase the mothers' milk (Fig. 14-3). The prenatal nipple preparation discussed in Chapter 4 might be considered a ritual that prepares the mother for the breastfeeding experience by familiarizing her with handling her breasts. There is, however, conflicting evidence to its physiologic effectiveness as discussed in Chapter 4. Another cultural ritual of undetermined effectiveness is a breast massage technique popular in Japan. Called the Oketani method, named after the nurse-

---

*Freely translated, "Our Lady of Happy Delivery and Plentiful Milk."

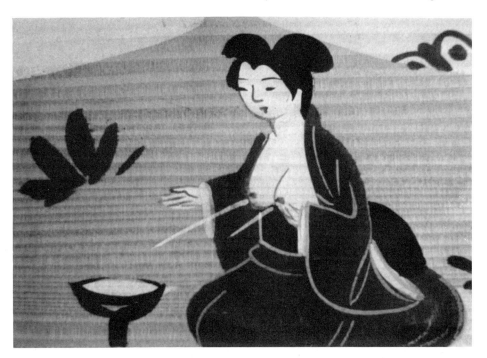

Fig. 14-3. Votive picture (*ema* in Japanese). This wooden plaque is given to the breastfeeding mother by the temple. She, in turn, prays to the plaque for sufficient milk. If her wish is fulfilled, she writes her name and age on the plaque and dedicates it to the temple. (Courtesy K. Sawada.)

midwife who developed it, the technique involves an elaborate technique of rotation and massage of the breasts. Many individuals of that country, including physicians, are convinced that it is effective for increasing the milk supply and for treatment of plugged ducts.[6]

The originality of beliefs about breastfeeding is striking and serves to explain some of the problems that occur. For example, if the baby burps during the feeding, according to one Hispanic mother, the air goes to the breast and stops the flow of milk so that her milk duct becomes plugged. To incorporate her belief it was suggested that, if this did happen, she should switch to the other breast and then back to the first breast to release the "air." This advice had the salutary effects of preventing a plugged duct and at the same time increasing her milk supply.

Another belief is the Spanish notion that the milk in the breast will go sour if a woman is upset or angry. Sour milk, of course, should never be fed to "le bebe." So if her husband is angry with her, she can avoid an argument by pleading that her milk will become sour, thereby cleverly ending the problem.[1] A number of other rituals and beliefs are discussed in the remaining chapters.

SUMMARY

In summary, culture is an individual factor that influences nursing planning and interventions for any single client. Having introduced the concept of culture, its effect on breastfeeding and early nurturing, and the assessment of practices, I turn now to weaving these ideas into other areas that interface with the breastfeeding process.

REFERENCES

1. Frantz, K.: Personal communication, Jan. 1981.
2. Gordon, V.C., et al.: Southeast Asian refugees: life in America, Am. J. Nurs. **80**:2031, 1980.
3. La Leche League International News **20**:68, July-Aug. 1978.
4. Leininger, M.: Transcultural nursing, New York, 1978, John Wiley & Sons, Inc.
5. Masson, V.: International nursing: what is it and who does it? Am. J. Nurs. **79**:1242, 1979.
6. Matsumura, T.: Personal communication, July 1981.
7. Miner, H.: Body ritual among the nacirema, American Anthropologist **58**:503, 1956.
8. Newton, N.: Key physiological issues in human lactation. In Waletzky, L.R., editor: Symposium on human lactation, Department of Health, Education, and Welfare Pub. No. (HSA) 79-5107, Washington, D.C., 1976.
9. Pajalakshm, R.: Lactation performance as a function of nutrition and social class. In Raphael, P., editor: Breastfeeding and food policy in a hungry world, New York, 1979, Academic Press, Inc.
10. Rapp, E.T.: Guadalupe, Arizona: Third World Country, U.S.A., Keeping Abreast J. **1**:288, 1976.
11. Spradley, J.: Naciremas, Boston, 1975, Little, Brown & Co.
12. Vermulapalli, C.: Cultural perspectives on child-bearing and lactation, La Leche League International, Eighth International Conference, July 1981, Chicago.
13. Wiiliams, C., and Jelliffe, D.: Mother and child health: delivering the services, Oxford, 1972, Oxford University Press.

ADDITIONAL READINGS

Ebrahim, G.J.: Cross-cultural aspects of breastfeeding. In Breast-feeding and the mother, Ciba Foundation Symposium, Series No. 45, New York, 1976, Elsevier-North Holland, Inc.

Johnson, M.: Cultural vaiations in professional and parenting patterns, J.O.G.N. Nurs. **9**:9, 1980.

Morley, D.: Pediatric priorities in the developing worlds, London, 1973, Butterworth.

Newton, N., and Newton M.: Childbirth in cross-cultural perspective. In Howells, J.C., editor: Modern perspectives in psycho-obstetrics, New York, 1973, Brunner/Mazel, Inc.

Osborne, O.H.: Anthropology and nursing: some common traditions and interests, Nurs. Res. **18**:251, 1969.

Sidel, R.: Women and child care in China, New York, 1972, Hill & Wang.

15

Maternal nutrition

JAN RIORDAN

Whether she lives on a mountaintop in remote Tibet, in a dusty Mexican village, or in an American suburb, the lactating woman produces milk that is amazingly homogeneous in composition despite the wide diversity of foods consumed. Only the woman who is poorly nourished over a long time will secrete milk that is measurably diminished in nutrient content and volume.

Obviously what a woman eats before and during her pregnancy affects her postpartum nutritional state. Chapter 4 presented a discussion of caloric intake, maternal weight, and other pertinent information on maternal nutrition during lactation. Here I concentrate on cross-cultural aspects of nutrition, since nurses need to view a mother's eating practices with an open mind while clinically eveluating her nutritional status.

A CAUTION ON ADVICE

Too often, nutritional advice to pregnant and lactating women is the simpleminded, standard fare: eat a well-balanced diet from the four basic groups and all will be well. We are all familiar with the free booklets published for new mothers by commercial formula or baby food companies. Somewhere toward the end of the booklet is advice on what she should eat if she is breastfeeding. Frequently, along with the well-worn "Basic Four" advice is a picture of a white mother about to eat from a plate holding a steak, baked potato, and two vegetables. A large glass of milk stands nearby. The Chicano or Southeast Asian mother looking at this picture can wrongly conclude that since her favorite foods are not there, she cannot breastfeed. Naturally, she has no intention of changing her food patterns. Fortunately, sensitivity to these cultural food patterns is beginning to be reflected in materials on maternal nutrition put out by governmental agencies and by universities. It is wise to carefully choose those that address themselves cross-culturally. The mother who senses criticism of practices that do not conform with our textbook or pamphlet information may summarily reject any other teaching we do. For instance, many health professionals, recognizing the concentrated nutritive value of animal milk, have been guilty of promoting its use, unmindful of the fact that more than three out of four adult people worldwide have lactose intolerance,[4] which causes belching, flatulence, cramps, and watery diarrhea from drinking milk. Instead of encouraging whole milk consumption, as promoted by the American Dairy Association, we should think of incorporating milk products or protein substitutes into their food in ways that have worked well for them over a long time. (Table 15-1 gives some examples of substitute foods.) Our effectiveness will depend on how well we can encourage optimal food practices during lactation. Our dietary recommendation must consist of food choices that are available to her. For instance, telling a mother to improve her diet does not make sense if she cannot afford the foods recommended.

CULTURAL FOODS

Part of understanding a culture is becoming acquainted with what Suitor and Hunter [10] call "foodways": those ways in which a distinct group selects, prepares, consumes, and

TABLE 15-1

Examples of cultural practices that promote adequate nutrient intake

Culture	Nutritious foods that are rarely eaten	Cultural corrections
Chinese	Milk	Cooking bones in acid solution to make soup provides an excellent source of calcium.
		Soybean products such as tofu and many Chinese greens are good sources of calcium.
Mexican	Milk	*Corn* tortillas are prepared with lime-soaked corn and therefore contribute significant amounts of calcium to the diet.*
Italian	Milk	Calcium-rich cheeses are popular.
Southern black	Milk	Buttermilk may be used occasionally.
		Calcium-rich greens are popular vegetables.
Puerto Rican	Bread	Viandas such as plantains are similar to bread in nutritive value.
		Rice is popular and is a good substitute if whole grain or enriched.

From Suitor, C.W., and Hunter, M.F.: Nutrition: principles and application in health promotion, Philadelphia, 1980, J.B. Lippincott Co.
*Lime is a calcium salt.

TABLE 15-2

Brief descriptions of an assortment of ethnic and regional foods

Grain group

Anadama: Cornmeal-molasses yeast bread (New England)

Bagels: Bread dough shaped like a donut, cooked in water, then baked; chewy (Jewish-American)

Bulgur: Granular wheat product with nutlike flavor, served like rice (Middle Eastern)

Brioche: Type of egg-rich French roll, often served at breakfast

Challah: Braided eggbread

Chapatis: Unleavened bread used by Indians

Croissants: Flaky crescent-shaped rolls (French)

Crumpets: Muffinlike product cooked on griddle; often served toasted (British)

Grits: Coarsely ground hominy (corn product) (Southern USA)

Johnnycake: Cornbread (New England)

Kasha: Coarsely ground grain toasted before cooking in liquid

Latkes: Pancakes

Limpa: Rye bread (Swedish)

Mush: Cooked cereal (often cornmeal)

Pasta: Macaroni, spaghetti, noodles in variety of forms (Italian)

Polenta: Cornmeal (Italian)

Scones: Round, flat, unleavened, sweetened bread product (British)

Sopapillas: Fried bread (rich dough) (Mexican)

Tortillas: Thin rounds of leathery dough made from lime-treated corn or from wheat flour, often fried until crisp (Mexican)

TABLE 15-2—cont'd _____

Brief descriptions of an assortment of ethnic and regional foods

Fruit and vegetable group

Bok choy: Green leafy, stalklike vegetable (Oriental)

Chayote: Green or white squashlike vegetable eaten raw, cooked, or pickled (Mexican)

Dandelion greens: Young leaves from wild dandelion plants, eaten raw or cooked

Greens in "pot liquor" ("likor"): Green leafy vegetables such as kale or turnip, mustard or collard greens, cooked with salt pork, served with cooking liquid (Southern USA)

Jalapenos: Hot peppers

Kelp: Seaweed

Papaya: Large, yellow, melonlike tropical fruit

Prickly pear: Fruit of a cactus

Viandas: Starchy tropical vegetables such as sweet potato, cassava, plantain (bananalike in appearance) (Puerto Rican)

Meat group

Adobo: Meat, soy sauce (Filipino)

Chitterlings: Pork intestine, tripe (soul food)

Chorizo: Sausage (Mexican)

Escargots: Snails (French)

Falafel: Mashed chick peas mixed with other ingredients and fried (Israeli)

Feijoada: Blackbeans, meat (Brazilian)

Finnan haddie: Smoked haddock

Frijoles refritas: Refried pinto or calico beans (Mexican)

Gefilte fish: Ground or flaked fish seasoned and shaped into balls (Jewish-American)

Hog maw: Stomach of pig (Southern USA)

Jerky: Dried meat strips

Kibee: Fresh raw lamb, ground, seasoned; eaten uncooked (Middle Eastern)

Kielbasa: Polish sausage

Miso: Soybean paste

Pepperoni: Italian hot sausage

Sauerbraten: Pot roast marinated in acidic sauce (German)

Sashimi: Raw fish (Japanese)

Teriyaki: Broiled beef marinated in sweet soy sauce (Hawaiian)

Mixed dishes

Couscous: Semolina, meat stew (North African)

Goulash: Stew usually seasoned with paprika (Hungarian)

Gumbo: Okra and meat stew, thickened with filé (pulverized sassafras leaves) (Louisiana Creole)

Hoppin John: Blackeyed peas and rice (Southern USA)

Jambalaya: Rice, ham, and seafood (Louisiana Creole)

Moussaka: Eggplant casserole (Greek)

Scrapple: Pork and cornmeal (Pennsylvania Dutch)

Tacos: Fried tortillas filled with meat or beans, vegetables, hot sauce, (Mexican)

Wonton: Stuffed dough, fried or cooked in broth (Chinese)

Others

Baklavah: A layered pastry rich in honey (Greek)

Butterhorns: Sweet pastry

Cracklins: Crispy pieces left after pork fat is rendered (Southern)

Fatback: Fat from belly of pig

Kuchen: Cake

Lard: Pork fat rendered to be used like shortening

Salt pork: Salted pork fat, sometimes with bit of meat

Sofrito: Specially seasoned tomato sauce used by Puerto Ricans

Spumoni: Fruit ice cream (Italian)

Strickle sheets: Coffee cake (Pennsylvania Dutch)

Strudel: Paper thin pastry with fruit filling or cheese (German)

Tzimmes: Carrot-prune dessert (Jewish-American)

From Suitor, C.W., and Hunter, M.F.: Nutrition: principles and application in health promotion, Philadelphia, 1980, J.B. Lippincott Co.

otherwise uses portions of the available food supply. "Food behavior" denotes and describes what foodways are carried out by an individual. I use the phrase "food pat terns" to mean the characteristic daily diet. The listing of various ethnic foods in Tabl 15-2 gives an overview of the wide variety of food patterns eaten by lactating wome around the world.

For more than half the inhabitants of this planet, including lactating women, beans rice, and grains are daily fare. Fruits and vegetables appear seasonally, and meat i found in the family cooking pot only on special occasions. When it does appear, it i poultry, goat, horse, or even dog, instead of beef. In most cultures other than our own meat plays a minor part in flavoring rice, grains, and vegetables, certainly not the majo role it serves in Western industrialized countries. In the United States we repeatedl hear warnings that we consume too much meat.

The daily food pattern of a Mexican-American woman who eats very little meat an is breastfeeding would concern us if we did not have basic knowledge of amino acid and complementary proteins. Beans, a staple item in Mexican foodways, provide a incomplete protein when served alone because they are low in methionine, an essentia amino acid. However, this deficiency is corrected when they are served with anothe food high in methionine, such as whole grain breads or cereals. Complementing protein can be achieved by numerous combinations. For example, eggs or a milk product wil balance the protein and amino acids of a meal consisting primarily of plant proteins When the same logic is used, the reverse is true; that is, two protein foods canno complement each other if they have similar amino acids in their composition. For thi reason, nuts and black-eyed peas are not complementing proteins, because both legume lack the same amino acids. Some examples for using complementary proteins are give in Table 15-3. We also need to be aware that for proteins to be complementary, the must be consumed *at the same time*. Beans at lunch and unpolished rice at dinner, fo example, would not be used by the body as a complete protein.

TABLE 15-3 _____

Complementing proteins—combining proteins so that their amino acid strengths and weaknesses balance out, resulting in a mixture of foods with good biological value

Food category	Examples		Relative amino acid content	
			Lysine	Methionine
Legumes	Peanut butter	Chili beans	+ to + +	—
Grains	Whole wheat bread	Corn bread	—	+
	Combination		Adequate	Adequate
Grains	Rye bread	Puffed rice	—	+
Milk	Cheese	Milk	+ +	+
	Combination		Good	Very good

From Suitor, C.W., and Hunter, M.F.: Nutrition: principles and application in health promotion, Philadelphia, 1980, J.B. Lippincott Co.
+ The protein contains more of the amino acid than does a high-quality protein.
+ + The protein is very high in the amino acid in comparison to a high-quality protein.
— The protein is low in the amino acid in comparison to a high quality protein.

FOOD BELIEFS
Augmentation

Almost all cultures abound with a seemingly endless array of prescriptive foods for lactating women. In the United States, beer and wheat germ are touted as promoting milk secretion. In fact, the use of beer or wine as a galactagogue is common to many cultures. As a relaxant, a small amount of alcohol may well be effective in reducing the mother's anxiety, thereby enhancing the let-down reflex. Also, the B-complex vitamins in beer potentially affect the nerve impulses controlling release of prolactin. Such an unanswered question lends itself to future nursing research. Parturient mothers in a number of countries gratefully accept the chicken soup given to them. In addition to its fluid value, chicken soup, a perennially favorite medicinal food, contains calcium.

In Mexico, the use of a wide variety of galactagogues was a common practice until recent times. The herbalist's "bible" in Mexico recommends anise and cotton seeds to increase the milk supply.[11] A low-calorie diet (rice, gruel, soup, vegetables) for mothers during the immediate postpartum period was believed to help the secretion of milk in traditional (before World War II) Japan. Lactating women in Japan were also encouraged to eat lotus roots. Since the root has many holes, it was thought a preventive for plugged milk ducts.

Sawada describes another tradition in northern Japan:

> Rice or red beans are wrapped in a cotton cloth and made to look like a small breast. Many of these models are dedicated to a statue of Buddha in a temple. A woman who wishes to have enough milk for her coming baby offers one of these breast models and prays to Buddha. After she goes home, she cooks the rice or beans wrapped as a breast model and eats it. If she has had success in breastfeeding, she visits the temple again with two of the same breast models. Thus the number of models in the temple is always increasing.[9]

Ethnographic records of North American Indians show that the Navajo woman's milk supply was believed to increase if she drank broth made from blue corn meal.[7] However, the reference fails to specify whether the corn meal was fermented. The Ojibwa Indians encouraged wild rice, lake trout, and white fish, which must have been quite tasty. In the Philippines, soups containing greens such as marungay leaves and papayas are supposed to make the milk flow; sour foods, however, are believed to decrease milk and increase lochia.[1]

Taboos

Not only augmentation but also restrictions on the postpartum diet are common in many cultures. In some cases the restrictions are so severe that they cause a nutritional deprivation that seems unnecessarily harsh and difficult to understand. In South India, for example, the custom still exists for women to subsist on coffee exclusively for 3 days or more following childbirth. For as long as 6 weeks, the new mother eats only two meals a day (instead of the usual three) and omits vegetables, milk products, meat, and fish from her diet. Note how these restrictions are similar to diets for sick people. Over a long period, such limited nutrition would seriously deplete the mother's nutritional reserves, making her more susceptible to infection, exhaustion, and other effects of malnutrition. Ultimately, her ability to breastfeed would be affected.

The custom of *pautang* in Malaya includes 6 weeks of limited food intake by the postpartum mother. Many people in the United States still believe that hot spices, beans, chili, garlic, and chocolate have a deleterious effect on the milk supply. If this were true, the Spanish and Italians would have died out long ago.

Fruit restrictions are imposed on lactating women in the Dominican Republic. This practice is common in many Spanish-speaking cultures, even for those Mexican-Americans living in the United States, as recorded by Kay:

> The postpartum diet is quite restricted. Immediately after birth, the mother may be given chamomile tea. For the first 2 days, "purely" toasted tortillas and boiled milk, or atole are served. Atole is a corn gruel, thin enough in consistency to be drunk. For the next 2-3 days, the diet is increased to include chicken in pieces or in soup. No vegetables or fruits are allowed: some midwives permit oranges, but others feel they are dangerously acid or cold. Pork, chili, and tomatoes must always be avoided for the full 40 days because these may harm the breast milk.[6]

Since eating the wrong food is thought to cause breast infection, some Mexican American women are taught to avoid cold or sour foods to prevent mastitis. Some of the food taboos described here are harmless or uncertain—others are potentially harmful to the lactating mother's nutritional state. Each should be evaluated accordingly and dietary counseling directed to improving nutrition, while respecting cultural traditions.

Food balance

For many cultural groups, foodways involve a balance that must be maintained for health or restored in illness. Balance between opposing energy forces is based on the Greek humoral system, which, after centuries of dissemination throughout the world, now appears as the "hot" (caliente)-cold (frío or fresco) system in Hispanic cultures. Other peoples such as the Chinese, Indians, and Arabs, also use the hot-cold system to some extent. Classifying "hot" or "cold" foods in a given culture has little to do with their form, color, texture, or temperature, although warm foods are believed to be more easily digested than cold foods. Instead, it is based on the food's effect on an illness or condition known to be "hot" or "cold."

During pregnancy, the unborn child is believed to be "hot," and therefore the mother is in a hot state. Once the child is born, accompanied by a loss of blood, a "cold" condition exists for both. To balance this state, "hot" foods must be eaten by the lactating mother.

The traditional Chinese consider chicken, squash, and broccoli to be hot. Cold foods are melon, fruits, soybean sprouts, and bamboo shoots. In India, milk is considered to be hot or cold according to the area where a person lives.[3] In Hispanic cultures, cold foods include most fresh vegetables, tropical fruits, dairy products, beans, squash, and some meats. Hot foods—cereal grains, chili peppers, temperate-zone fruits, goat's milk, oils, and high-prestige meats such as beef—serve to balance the cold foods. Since the potential listing of hot and cold foods in any particular culture is almost endless, we must do our own ethnographic homework in regard to the belief system of the culture with which we are working.

Another belief system concerning food balance is the yin and yang theory of the Chinese. In America, the system is practiced by macrobiotic cults and Eastern philosoohy religious groups. Like the hot-cold theory, the basis of the yin-yang belief rests on a proper balance between opposing energy forces: on one side yin represents "female," a negative force (cold, emptiness, darkness); on the other side yang represents "male," a positive force (warmth, fullness, light). Too much of either yin or yang food is considered threatening to health. Whether a food is considered yin or yang depends on what effect it is thought to have on the body and again is not associated with color, texture, or other obvious characteristics. Without an extensive orientation, it is difficult to understand the yin-ness or yang-ness of food. However, we can illustrate the usefulness of this knowledge. People who believe in the importance of maintaining a balance of opposing elements may pay close attention to nutritional information if it is put into the framework of their beliefs. For example, if an anemic lactating woman is not vegetarian and if she believes anemia is a yin condition, she will more readily accept the suggestion of consuming more meat, a yang food, to improve her anemia.[10]

Traditionally, the Chinese have used herbs in teas and in foods for their yin or yang and medicinal effects. Today, herbal teas are becoming more popular in this country, especially among younger adults. Some herbs have surprising pharmacologic effects, including irritating the mucosal lining of the intestine and aiding in the release of flatus. As a result, some breastfed infants of mothers who regularly consume these teas have increased gas and loose stools. However, unless this becomes troublesome, with an allergic response, it is more important for the mother to continue enjoying her favorite teas than to stop because of her baby's minor stool changes.

VEGETARIANISM

For reasons of health, religion, ethnic values, or economy, there is a growing trend toward vegetarianism in this country. Two general classifications are recognized: (1) lacto-ovo-vegetarians, who use eggs and dairy products in addition to plant foods, and (2) vegans, who use only plant foods. Many vegetarians do not fall into either category, since they include fish and poultry in their diets.

A lactating woman who is a vegetarian and eats a wide variety of grains, legumes, nuts, fruits, vegetables, milk, and milk products can have a nutritionally sound diet. Frequently we find that families who practice vegetarianism are quite knowledgeable about nutrition. Often their knowledge is based on thorough study to overcome many obstacles encountered in our meat-oriented society. Vegetarians are rarely obese and may have superior diet patterns because they conscientiously avoid the processed, empty-calorie foods so popular in this country.

Some nurses become very concerned if a breastfeeding mother practices vegetarianism, especially since vitamin B_{12} is not found in vegetable protein, and a deficiency in the infant can have serious consequences. However, even though it is more difficult for her, the lactating woman can consume adequate amounts of protein and vitamin B_{12}, even if she is a strict vegan, providing her diet is carefully planned and supplemented. Supplemental vitamins, fortified soy milk, and fortified yeast are all good sources of B_{12}.

Nurses should be aware that women who consume large amounts of green vegetables sometimes produce milk that has a greenish tint. "Green" milk, although not harmful to the infant, can be rather unnerving to the unwary health professional and to the mother!

The basic diet guide for balanced vegetarian meals includes[8]:

1. Grains, legumes, nuts, and seeds: Six or more servings including several slices of whole grain bread, beans, and some nuts or seeds
2. Vegetables: Three servings or more, including one or more servings of dark leafy greens
3. Fruit: One to four pieces including citrus fruits for a raw source of vitamin C
4. Milk and eggs: Two or more glasses of milk if tolerated, or other dairy products or eggs to meet the milk requirement

RELIGIOUS INFLUENCES

Religion also influences the diet of the breastfeeding woman. If she is a Seventh-Day Adventist or a member of certain Eastern religious sects, she practices vegetarianism. Orthodox Muslim and Black Muslim women are expected to breastfeed their babies according to religious teachings, and Islamic dietary regulations prohibit pork, animal shortening, and products containing gelatin. No other animal meat can be eaten unless it has been slaughtered in the prescribed manner. During the month-long Ramadan fast, Muslims are not allowed to eat or drink anything between sunrise and sunset. If enforced, this certainly would impose a severe hardship on lactating women, who require a regular intake of fluid and calories.

An Orthodox Jewish mother will closely observe dietary laws that prohibit pork products and shellfish. According to these laws, meat and milk cannot be eaten at the same meal. After meat is eaten, she must wait 6 hours before consuming milk products; therefore dietary counseling must include planning her daily meals so that she takes in adequate calcium and phosphorus from milk products or substitute foods.

The use of alcohol is prohibited by some religions. Therefore it would be highly inappropriate to suggest to a breastfeeding mother who is a Muslim, Seventh-Day Adventist, or Mormon that she put her feet up and relax with a glass of wine or beer.

MALNUTRITION

It is well recognized that malnutrition is the result of a complex interplay of multiple causes: population, education, sanitation, food production, sociocultural values, and economics are of the greatest importance. In underdeveloped areas of the world, poverty and dependence on seasonal crops are related to dietary deprivations. In Western countries, where food is more plentiful, poor diets are more often the result of consuming too many sweets and empty-calorie foods.

When malnutrition and breastfeeding are discussed, there is little question that infant feeding begins before birth. Affecting the infant's birth weight and the nutrient reserves in both the infant and mother, maternal nutrition during pregnancy sets the stage for nutrition during lactation. Moreover, long-established foodways almost invariably continue throughout lactation (Fig. 15-1).

The ability of a malnourished woman to successfully breastfeed a healthy infant, however, is well known. One reason is a pregnancy "fat bank"—a store of fat that is laid down during pregnancy and that is believed to subsidize lactation for about 3 to 4 months. Despite this remarkable ability to sustain a flow of milk, there are deleterious effects when body reserves are depleted over a long time. Repeated pregnancies, without time for nutritional recovery, speed the depletion process, and clinical evidence of

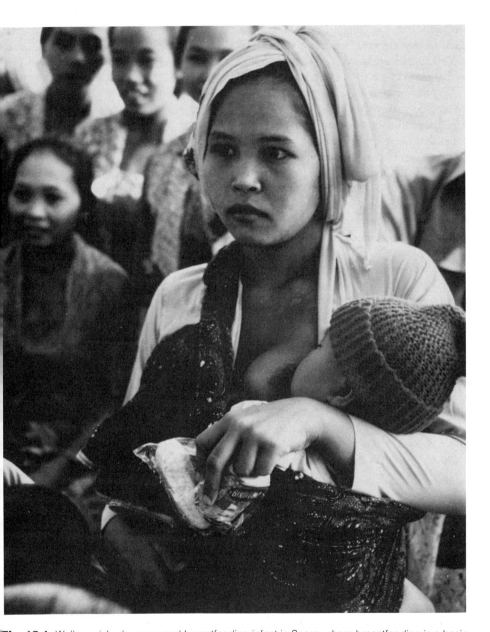

Fig. 15-1. Well-nourished woman and breastfeeding infant in Searo, where breastfeeding is a basic part of the life process. (Courtesy WHO.)

chronic malnourishment, osteomalacia (depletion of bone calcium), and nutritional edema from protein loss can result.

Milk volume and composition are also affected to a minor degree by a poor diet. The old saying "feed the mother and thereby the child" is true to the extent that milk volume increases slightly when food supplements are given to a poorly nourished woman.

In Chapter 3 it was emphasized that some nutrients in the milk, especially water-soluble vitamins, are affected by dietary intake. Total protein levels, however, are not altered by food supplementation, and if the lactating woman fails to take in adequate protein in her diet, it is taken from her body reserves for her milk.

Surprisingly, as long as the infant continues to breastfeed often, dietary food supplementation seems to have little effect on fertility. Malnourished women given food supplementation in a government program did not return to postpartum fertility any sooner than would normally be expected.[5] Apparently the level of serum prolactin is the most important factor in inhibiting ovulation and spacing children.

The quality and quantity of the mother's milk are altered in a minor way when she is malnourished. There is a greater amount of evidence that the unborn child is affected by the nutritional status of the mother during pregnancy. When this is the case, the effect of unrestricted breastfeeding in restoring infants to optimal nutritional levels after delivery can be quite dramatic. Brazelton et al.[2] carefully observed newborn infants of Zambian women who lived in urban slums and ate poorly. These babies showed strong evidence of intrauterine depletion, were dehydrated, small for gestational age, and had floppy muscle tone. After only 10 days of unrestricted breastfeeding, they filled out, their muscle tone was good, and they showed no evidence of dehydration.

SUMMARY

The additional calories (20% to 25%) needed during lactation are, when sufficient food is available, easily supplied by nutrients in a variety of foods according to the mother's cultural and personal preferences. Given that food is plentiful, the most reliable guide for the amount of food and fluids a lactating mother needs is her appetite and thirst. Nutrition education is needed when it appears that her diet is insufficient, and there are clinical signs such as anemia, excessive weight loss, or possibly a lessened supply of breastmilk. Unfortunately, maternal nutrition remains a distressing worldwide problem with overwhelming complexities. Nevertheless, nurses must be committed to its alleviation.

REFERENCES

1. Affonso, D.O.: The Filipino American. In Clark, A.L., editor: Culture, childbearing, health professionals, Philadelphia, 1978, F.A. Davis Co.
2. Brazelton, T.B., et al.: Neonatal behavior among urban Zambians and Americans, J. Am. Acad. Child Psychiatry 15:97, 1976.
3. Chen, P.E.Y.: Nondietary factors and nutrition, In Jelliffe, D.B., and Jelliffe E.F.P., editors: Nutrition and growth, New York, 1979, Plenum Press.
4. Hongladarom, G.C., and Russell, M.: An ethnic difference: lactose intolerance, Nurs. Outlook 24:764, 1976.
5. Huffman, S., et al.: Breastfeeding patterns in rural Bangladesh, A. J. Clin. Nutr. 38:144, 1980.
6. Kay, M.A.: The Mexican American. In Clark, A.L., editor: Culture, childbearing, health professionals, Philadelphia, 1978, F.A. Davis Co.
7. Moore, W.H., editor: Nutrition, growth and development of North American Indian children, Department of Health, Education, and Welfare Pub. No. 72-76, Washington, D.C., 1969, National Institutes of Health.
8. Robertson, L., Flinders, C., and Godrey, B.: Laurel's kitchen: A handbook for vegetarian cooking and nutrition, Petaluma, Calif., 1976, Nilgiri Press.
9. Sawada, K.: Breastfeeding customs in Japan. Proceedings of Eighth International Conference of La Leche League International, Chicago, Ill., 1981.
10. Suitor, C.W., and Hunter, M.F.: Nutrition: principles and application in health promotion, Philadelphia, 1980, J.B. Lippincott Co.
11. Vargas, L.A.: Traditional breastfeeding methods in Mexico. In Raphael, D., editor: Breastfeeding and food policy in a hungry world, New York, 1979, Academic Press, Inc.

ADDITIONAL READINGS

Hytten, F.E., and Thomson, A.M.: Nutrition of the lactating woman. In Kon, S.K., and Cowie, A.T., editors: Milk: the mammary gland and its secretion, New York, 1961, Academic Press, Inc.

Jelliffe, D.B., and Jelliffe, E.F.P.: Human milk in the modern world, New York, 1978, Oxford University Press.

Jelliffe, E.F.P.: Nutritional Aspects of human lactation. In Symposium of human lactation, Department of Health, Education, and Welfare Pub. No. 79-5107, Washington, D.C., 1976.

Lappé, F.M.: Diet for a small planet, New York, 1975, Ballantine Books, Inc.

California Department of Health: Nutrition during pregnancy and lactation, Sacramento, Calif., 1975, The Department.

16

Weaning

JAN RIORDAN

Weaning is a key issue in studying cross-cultural child-care practices related to breastfeeding, but before I can discuss it I must first define it. Does it mean introducing into the child's diet foods other than the mother's milk, or does it refer to the cessation of breastfeeding? For clarification, I will use the term to refer to the time beginning with the introduction of substantial sources of food other than breastmilk and ending with the last breastfeeding. Three terms will be used to describe the types of weaning: gradual, deliberate, and abrupt. Weaning gradually is over weeks or months. Deliberate refers to a conscious effort by the mother to end breastfeeding over a time. Abrupt weaning is a forced, immediate cessation of breastfeeding and is used interchangeably with "traumatic" weaning, since abrupt weaning is traumatic for a child of any culture. Other terms used in discussing weaning are nonnutritive breastfeeding, a recognition that long-term breastfeeding is more than conferring food, and closet weaning, a response to cultural criticism for breastfeeding beyond the socially acceptable time limit.

CULTURAL ISSUES

In some cultures, the issues surrounding weaning are health related, particularly in developing countries where weanling diarrhea is a prevalent health problem. In cultures in which food availability is sporadic and meager, kwashiorkor, a severe form of protein deficiency, appears as a disease occurring during the transition from breastmilk to other foods. In the Ga language of Accra, Ghana, the term *kwashiorkor* means "the disease of the deposed baby."

In technologically advanced cultures, the weaning issues are primarily psychosocial. Raised in a culture in which early weaning from both bottle and breast is the common practice, a nurse can be shocked by the sight of a walking child calmly sliding into his mother's lap for milk, deftly opening her buttons to gain access to the breast. Yet worldwide this is a common daily occurrence. In studying records from 64 primitive cultures in 1945, Ford[3] recorded 15 in which the earliest weaning age was 3 years. Another survey[1] of breastfeeding practices in non-Western cultures reveals that most children are breastfed 1 to 2 years or longer but rarely for less than a year, as with the breastfeeding women and infants in Fig. 16-1. In studying the Arapesh, Mead and Newton[7] observed in 1935 that children breastfed until ages 3 or even 4 years, providing the mother did not become pregnant again. Other field studies[7] show a reliance on prolonged breastfeeding to space children, giving the attention and nurturing to the small

318

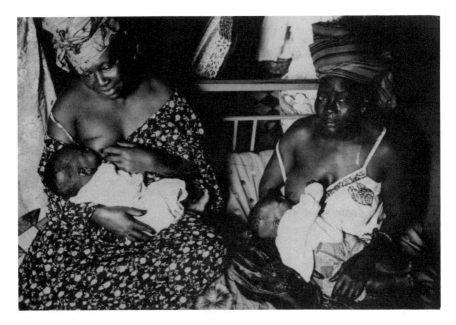

Fig. 16-1. These African children are traditionally breastfed until they are 2 years of age. (Courtesy WHO/UN.)

child before he is displaced by the next pregnancy. Considering ancient and present worldwide patterns, early weaning practices recently popular in Western countries are the exception.

Potential trauma

Examples of gradual, deliberate, or abrupt weaning may be found in any culture. Because gradual weaning has been proven to be the least traumatic approach, it is important for nurses to encourage gradual weaning from the breast over months. Weaning should proceed very slowly, dropping one feeding at a time and allowing resumption of extra feedings again if the child is ill or emotionally upset. When weaning is abrupt, the child goes through a period of grieving that can last from several days to several weeks. Rage, withdrawal, and depression are typically observable behaviors in a baby or child forcibly weaned from breastfeeding. This rejection, which perhaps is the child's first experience with betrayal of trust, is so important that it is considered the foundation of the hot-cold syndrome used in Mexico and in other Spanish-speaking cultures:

In the process of weaning, the Mexican child is subjected to a prolonged period of acute rejection. As a result of this experience, he forms strong subconscious associations between warmth and acceptance (or intimacy), on the one hand, and between cold and rejection (or withdrawal), on the other. In adult life, these associations appear in those beliefs intimately concerned with the problem of personal security; theories about nourishment and about the prevention and cure of disease and injury. On the conscious level, then, the hot-cold syndrome is a basic principle of human physiology, and it functions as a logical system for dealing with the problem of disorder and disease. On a subconscious level, however, the hot-cold syndrome is a model of social relations.[6]

Weaning customs

Often, in past civilizations, the significance of the final weaning was formally recognized as a *rite de passage*. Ancient Greek and Roman families marked the final weaning by a public ceremony much like a bar mitzvah or a christening ceremony of today. This signaled the end of one of life's passages and the beginning of another, as exemplified by Abraham, who reputedly "made a great feast the same day that Isaac was weaned."[5]

Some rather harsh techniques have been employed to bring about abrupt weaning in accordance with maternal or cultural dictates. Frequently a bitter substance was used, such as that reported in Iran,[4] where the nipple was coated with bile from a sheep's or cow's gallbladder. The public weaning rite in Grecian societies needed a little help in convincing the baby that the good old days were indeed over, and pepper or mustard was smeared over the breast. To the amusement of the onlookers, the baby recoiled in rage, although no one will ever know for sure what happened in secret once the mother and baby had returned to the privacy of their home. Another time-honored method has been called the "Spicy Burrito Method,"[2] in which a hot sauce or taco sauce is put on the nipples. The range of human innovation in such matters is endless; an exasperated mother is depicted in *A Tree Grows in Brooklyn* as dissuading her 3-year-old from breastfeeding by using stove polish to paint an ugly-teethed face on her breast.[8]

Various stages in development are sometimes used as the appropriate time to begin deliberate weaning. A common belief among African cultures is that the child should be walking before weaning is attempted. Some kind of independence is implicit in the concept of weaning, so it seems reasonable that the child be self-sufficient in locomotion before leaving the dependency of his mother's breast. In Western cultures, the eruption of teeth is a common developmental reference point when the baby is thought to be ready for weaning.

Effect of gender

Whether it is due to fear of sexual connotations or simply a buffer against harder times to come, there seems to be a tendency in many cultures to breastfeed female babies longer than males. Kendall, a nurse anthropologist in Iran, noted a significantly longer period of breastfeeding for daughters in this culture, in which sons are preferred.

> In the light of the preference for boys it seems they should be given a longer nursing period, but the mothers explained that boys receive their father's land as their inheritance, while all the girl gets is her mother's milk, hence, the reason for nursing the girl for four months longer.[4]

Baby girls in the United States also appear to be breastfed longer. Sugarman[9] in a preliminary report of a survey of mothers with breastfeeding toddlers found that boys were weaned slightly earlier.

WEANING READINESS

A subsequent pregnancy signals the time for weaning in many cultures, but not all. Usually a toddler or child will spontaneously wean with the new pregnancy. The reasons include a considerably diminished milk supply, changes in the milk composition, and a less desirable taste. One child insisted the milk tasted like apple juice.[2] Some mothers

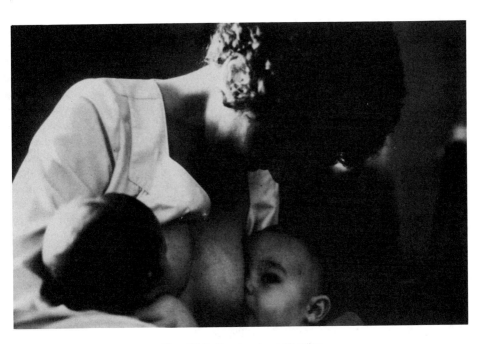

Fig. 16-2. Tandem breastfeeding.

continue to breastfeed their toddlers during pregnancy and beyond ("tandem nursing"), especially if the pregnancy is unexpectedly early. This is a common practice in India and Bangladesh and is becoming more common in the United States (Fig. 16-2); however, this double drain on the mother's body resources makes it mandatory that she take in nourishing, high-protein foods.

Ideally, the time for weaning is a collaborative effort, in which both the mother and baby reach a state of readiness to begin weaning around the same time. Unfortunately, this is not always the case. The child may be ready before his mother, but more often the mother is ready before her child. Child-led weaning should be the goal for self-care, since it is the child who expresses his needs by his behavior. But what about the mother's feelings? In cultures in which unrestricted breastfeeding is practiced with the child breastfeeding for a prolonged period, the mother feels very little guilt when she decides to wean: The Arapesh mother who tells her lusty 3-year old, "You child, have had enough milk,"[7] obviously has little ambivalence about weaning. When the cultural expectation is for early weaning, the mother often does feel ambivalent. She feels caught between her child's refusal to wean and her own mixed feelings of wanting to, yet not wanting to. Additional pressures come from her relatives, her husband, and perhaps the neighbors.

CLOSET NURSING

The term *closet nursing* refers to a practice that has evolved as a counter-cultural response to criticism of breastfeeding that extends beyond cultural expectations for weaning. With closet nursing, breastfeeding continues by mutual consent of mother and child, but only in secret, as if it were illicit. Since there is no evidence to indicate that prolonged breastfeeding is harmful, and since, in fact, it is a worldwide norm, acceptance by nurses should be matter of fact. Traditionally we have had difficulty accepting this practice and perhaps have contributed to closet breastfeeding. My personal experience described here serves as an example: During evening work in a pediatric unit I noticed that the door to Manuel's room was always closed. Whenever I pushed it open to check on him or give him medication, there was a sudden flurry of activity as Manuel moved away from his mother's lap. Finally, I realized that Manuel, who was 2 years old, was still breastfeeding and that his mother was afraid of the nurses discovering this. I decided to approach her and ask her if this was why the door was always closed. She answered "yes" rather hesitantly. Then she apologized, saying, "but there's no milk." When I told her that I had breastfed my twins until they were 2½ years old, she looked quite relieved and we talked openly about our children. She told me that they had very little money and that her children meant everything to her and her husband. She said that having children, especially this last one, made up for not having the material things they could not afford. Manuel, she confided, was closest to her because she had breastfed him longer than the rest. After that, for the remainder of the shift anyway, the door stayed open.

ACCEPTANCE BY HEALTH PROFESSIONALS

Nurses are not the only members of the health profession who find it difficult to accept late weaning. Many physicians who wholeheartedly support breastfeeding because of the superior nutritive values of breastmilk reel in horror over the nonnutritive breastfeedings of a walking child. It seems odd that professionals who would never advocate taking a security blanket away from a baby or forcing toilet training still advocate abrupt weaning. The physician's influence is so strong that negative comments to a mother about her continuing to breastfeed beyond the time when "normal" weaning occurs can be devastating. One mother, an editor, described her feelings following a dialogue with a physician whom she had consulted for a writing project:

> I suddenly stopped being a professional participating in a dialogue about breastfeeding patterns. I became a totally frightened mother, whose own mothering behaviors were being criticized. I became the hidden deviant suddenly threatened with the possibility of exposure. What would he think of me if he knew how long I nursed my babies? Would his esteem for me suddenly shatter? All those feelings and thoughts rushed through my mind. I was grateful for the telephone because if he had seen me I could not have concealed my agitation and extreme distress . . . and my anger. How dare he label me as a deviant by implication, as he talked about other mothers. How dare he, a professional grounded in applying fact and logic, make such sweeping and emotionally-laden generalizations which in fact condemned me![1]

To counteract social pressures for early weaning, mothers with breastfeeding toddlers depend on one another for moral support. La Leche League offers special group meetings, called toddler meetings, specifically to meet this need. Nonnutritive feedings are essentially a private affair in any culture and need not enter into medical or nursing judgments. When we work with a mother who is breastfeeding a walking child, our acceptance is as appropriate to the situation as the acceptance of any family tradition (Fig. 16-3).

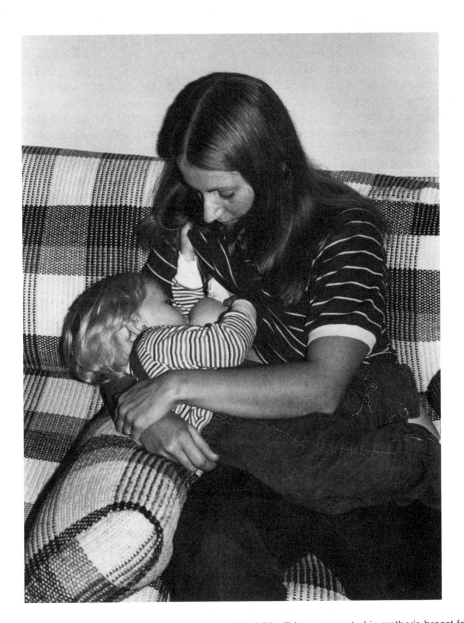

Fig. 16-3. In this American family, an 18-month-old child still has access to his mother's breast for comfort.

HOW THE NURSE CAN HELP

Nursing self-care is a positive intervention directed toward helping the mother make a self-directed choice regarding weaning, rather than one based on the culturally influenced expectations of others. It calls for active listening to her true feelings. If she feels genuine grief at the thought of weaning and enjoys meeting her baby's needs by breast-feeding but feels great pressures to wean, then pointing out cultural differences in weaning practices may be just the reinforcement she needs. On the other hand, if she expresses resentment each time the baby breastfeeds and is impatient for each feeding to end, she is undoubtedly communicating these feelings to her baby and, in this case, needs guidance for deliberate weaning techniques. It is most helpful to guide this mother by making suggestions that provide a degree of built-in flexibility:

1. Give her advice offered by La Leche League: "Don't offer, Don't refuse." This technique allows a gradual reduction in the numbers of feedings without strain or stress for either party. It may not be enough, however, and other techniques are called for. For one psychiatrist trying to wean, the "don't offer, don't refuse," technique translated as "don't wean."[10]
2. Make a contract with the child as to when breastfeeding can take place. For instance, limit breastfeeding to the privacy of the home or homes of friends.
3. Decrease the length of each feeding. After a short breastfeeding, give the child an interesting toy or suggest an activity he particularly likes.
4. Distract the child before his customary time for unimportant feedings. This takes some innovation and help: fathers can come up with wonderful and funny distractions. The most important feedings, such as the one at bedtime, will be the last to go.
5. Avoid customary favorite places of breastfeeding. Like the athlete in training, a mother diligently avoids the relaxation spots—the couch or a favorite chair, for example.
6. Reward nonbreastfeeding behavior. A favorite food, going to the park, extra cuddling, or even warmly thanking them, reinforces nonbreastfeeding and speeds the process of weaning.

SUMMARY

Whether influenced by social pressure or by potential health problems, the time and length of the weaning process varies from culture to culture and from family to family. Because of the potential psychologic trauma, the recommended style of weaning is slow, gradual, and led by the needs of the child. Examples of innovations for speeding the weaning process abound, indicating that mothers are often ready for weaning before their children are. When another pregnancy does not result in weaning the previous child, adequate maternal nutrition is a vital consideration. Weaning styles are the prerogative of the family, although when appropriate, nurses can assist by suggesting helpful techniques for slow, deliberate weaning.

REFERENCES

1. Avery, J.L.: Closet nursing: a symptom of intolerance or a forerunner of social change? Keeping Abreast J. 2:212, 1977.
2. Bumgarner, N.J.: Mothering your nursing toddler, P.O. Box 5064, Norman, Okla., 1980.
3. Ford, C.S.: A comparative study of human re-

production, Yale University Publications in Anthropology, No. 32, New Haven, 1945, Yale University Press.

4. Kendall, K.: Maternal and child nursing in an Iranian village. In Leininger, M.: Transcultural nursing, New York, 1978, John Wiley & Sons, Inc.

5. Levin, S.S.: A philosophy of infant feeding, Springfield, Ill., 1963, Charles C Thomas, Publisher.

6. Martinez, R.A.: Hispanic culture and health care: fact, fiction, folklore, St. Louis, 1978, The C.V. Mosby Co.

7. Mead, M., and Newton, N.: Cultural patterning of perinatal behavior. In Richardson, S.A., and Guttmacher, A.F., editors: Childbearing: its social and psychological aspects, Baltimore, 1967, The Williams & Wilkins Co.

8. Smith, B.: A tree grows in Brooklyn, New York, 1947, Harper & Row, Publishers, Inc.

9. Sugarman, M.: Physicians' Seminar, La Leche League International, Atlanta, 1979.

10. Walzetsky, L.: Physicians' Seminar, La Leche League International, Alanta, 1979.

ADDITIONAL READINGS

Ainsworth, M.S.: Infancy in Uganda, Baltimore, 1967, The Johns Hopkins University Press.

Amsel, P.L.: The need to wean: as much for mother as for baby? R.N. **39:**52, 1976.

La Leche League International, Inc.: The womanly art of breastfeeding, Franklin Park, Ill., 1981, The League.

Parsons, L.J.: Weaning from the breast: for a happy ending to a satisfying experience, J.O.G.N. Nurs. 7(3):12, 1978.

17

Solid foods

JAN RIORDAN

Problems encountered during the transition period from breast to solid foods, particularly weanling diarrhea, have already been discussed. In this section, different patterns of starting early solid foods with well born breastfed babies in various cultures are described, with particular attention to our western customs of early solids, or *beikost* (pronounced be-cost, a German word meaning foods other than formula). We in western nations seem to keep changing our pattern of introducing solids to our young, partly because of the influence of mass communication, advertising, and, strangely enough, competition among mothers. However, in many less industrialized countries, this is not the case, and the time of initiation of beikost given to babies stays relatively constant.

In many cultures, early solids, like other foods are often thought of in terms of the hot-cold balance described earlier, and this idea is instilled early into the belief system of the children. For example, Chen[6] reports that Malaysian toddlers are denied "cold" foods including papaya and other fruits for fear these foods will cause illness. Without fancy modern devices such as grinders and blenders for meat or foods with tough textures, earlier societies resorted to the handiest, most readily available device: their teeth. The breastfed Yuma Indian baby during the transition to adult foods ate prechewed corn, mashed peaches, and mashed juniper berries. In addition to premasticated meat, North American Indian children commonly started with gruels made of acorn flour and broth from meat or fowl.[17]

In her ethnographic account of nursing in an Iranian village, Kendall describes the local practices of initiating beikost.

> Supplementary foods are begun at four or five months. In addition to boiled water and sugar, tea and sugar are given. Bread or biscuit soaked in water is the first solid food, followed shortly by soup and rice cooked in milk. Some mothers can afford so little that they give the child neither until he can eat some of the regular adult food. Others do not feel extra food should be given until the child is almost a year old. After he has teeth he may be given small pieces of meat to chew on; the juices are considered good for him. Eggs are not given until he is weaned. They consider eggs harmful for the baby but can give no specific reason. It is the custom. In the second year of life the baby begins to eat many of the the adult foods such as rice, soup, mast (yogurt), and bread. Little meat is eaten by anyone.[13]

Sections of this chapter are taken from Guthrie, R., and Riordan, J.: Fact or fantasy: infant nutrition and solids, J. Kans. Med. Soc. **78:**388, 1977.

CUES FOR READINESS

Whatever the culture, providing the child is nourished, loved, and does not suffer from a disabling health problem, developmental milestones of childhood occur along the same pattern. Historically, nature's developmental cues for the introduction of solid food have been the fading of the extrusion reflex of the tongue, eruption of teeth, ability to sit, and development of purposeful movements of the baby's hands and fingers, all of which normally occur during the middle months of the first year of life. Also, in the full-term infant, the prenatal storage of iron acquired during the last trimester of pregnancy gradually begins to diminish by 4 to 5 months. However, some cultures wait longer. For example, the Yuma Indians generally waited until a child was ready to walk before starting solids. Since iron in breastmilk is so completely used by the infant,[16] anemia is uncommon, even if solids are delayed this long.

Going along with this approach, which suggests a developmental readiness for solids, is the notion that a baby is really an "external fetus" during the first 6 months after birth (that is, he is really as closely dependent on his mother as he was during gestation), with the breast acting as an outside placenta. Solid foods, then, have a *raison d'etre* only at the end of this extragestation.

WESTERN PRACTICES

In the Western world, "pap gruels," the forerunners of the recent early cereal feeding, were first recorded as being used in the seventeenth century, often with disastrous results. Figures compiled in Dublin during the last quarter of the eighteenth century indicate that 99.6% of hand-fed babies died. Pap was basically liquid, plus cereal, biscuits, and beer, or flour and wine. These mixtures did not contain enough calories to sustain the infant, because they had to be watered down to allow the gruel to pass through the hole in the receptacle.

Fifty years ago the milk of herd animals gradually began to successfully replace breastfeeding as the method of infant feeding in our culture. Since additional vitamins and nutrients were needed to supplement the milk of domestic animals, solids were introduced to infants earlier with each decade. A competitive spirit developed among mothers to outdo one another in initiating solid food, as if they thought that how soon an infant could eat adult food measured his maturity. And so western infants began solids increasingly early through the next several decades—a trend that finally began to reverse itself as of the late 1970's and early 1980's.

In 1935, Marriot recommended that 6 months was the optimal age for introducing beikost. Two years later the AMA Council on Foods stated that pediatricians favored the feeding of strained fruits and vegetables no earlier than age 4 to 6 months. But these recommendations went unheeded by mothers, because of a more powerful voice they were hearing at the same time. The Pied Piper baby food companies were whispering to them "convenience," and so they lined up to buy canned, strained commercial baby food, which was first introduced during the 1930's.

Warnings against this early introduction of solid food were voiced by only a few far-seeing and alert pediatricians. They argued that it was not substantiated by sound nutritional principles but was rather the result of both marketing and maternal competition. One of them, György, warned in 1957:

One of the important contributing factors in the matter of early addition of supplemental food to an infant's diet is the widespread insistence of the mother. This custom is spreading widely in modern pediatric dietetics. The argument, however, that semi-solid foods may accelerate the anatomical and physiological development of the digestive tract is not supported by the study of normal growth. The first teeth usually appear at six to seven months, a clear indication that the infant is not dependent on mastication before the end of the first half-year of life.[12]

DISADVANTAGES OF EARLY SOLIDS

Most infants will at first actively resist the advances of even the most enterprising mother in her attempts to spoon-feed him during the early months of life. Before 6 months, a baby has an extrusion tongue reflex and is unable to push food to the back of his mouth. The newspaper cartoons of a triple-bibbed infant propped in a high chair and surrounded by a wide circumference of newspaper and spit out food reflects an unpleasant reality, before the extrusion reflex begins to fade. Developmentally speaking, toleration of early solids is not evidence that early introduction of solids is advantageous. In fact, the practice may initiate a chain of disadvantages: allergies, obesity, and the disruption of natural child spacing.

For the breastfeeding mother-infant dyad, the early introduction of solids also poses the certainty of disruption of the sensitive equilibrium between supply and demand: the more solids ingested by the baby, the less he will take from the breast; the less he takes from the breast, the less milk there will be. Therefore, especially for the breastfeeding infant, beikost should be withheld until milk production is firmly established in the middle of the first year of life.

Allergies

The relationship between the time of solid food introduction and allergies has not been conclusively established; however, IgE, which is associated with allergy, rises in direct time sequence to the introduction of solid foods. IgE is also associated with skin test–positive allergy later in life. The theory to explain this phenomenon is that before the age of 6 months the infant's intestine lacks the appropriate digestive enzymes to completely digest complex proteins and starches down to amino acids and simple sugars. At the same time, the infant's intestinal mucosa is permeable to some intact proteins and starches. These incompletely digested peptides and starches can be absorbed and serve as sensitizing agents to the infantile immune system. IgE is then produced, and allergy results in some, perhaps many, infants.[18] There is some evidence that when solids, especially wheat, egg white, pork, and legumes are withheld from the potentially allergic child until the immature immunity period has passed, the symptoms are minimized or even prevented.[10-11] At age 6 months, the infant produces sufficient IgA antibody to prevent absorption of food antigens through the intestinal wall, thus reducing food allergy.

Obesity

The early introduction of baby foods is becoming crucial in the rise of obesity as a major disease of developed countries. Vigorous debate and speculation exist as to the onset of excess adipose potential that involves the nature vs. nurture controversy.[20] There is some evidence of a genetic component: children of obese parents are more likely to be overweight themselves. On the other hand, overweight mothers are likely to be more anxious about food and push their children into eating more.

According to the recommendations of the National Academy of Science, the infant from birth to 1 year requires an average of 110 to 120 Kcal/kg (50 to 55 Kcal/lb) each day for normal growth. Caloric intake above this amount results in the laying down of excess adipose tissue. Because there is a tendency for mothers to force food on the baby by encouraging them to finish the jar of baby food, without taking satiation cues from the baby, the potential for obesity increases with the giving of early solids. This force-feeding is complicated by a possibility that during the first 6 weeks of life, the appetite functions by volume, as well as by caloric intake. Foman[9] found that calorically concentrated formula results in a greater caloric intake despite a reduction in the volume of milk. Thus the use of solid foods much higher in caloric density than milk or formula greatly increases caloric intake and may lead to the tendency to lay down excess fat. In addition, this persistent food reward system establishes the conditioning of a behavior pattern that can lead to overeating for the rest of the individual's life (Fig. 17-1).

Another hypothesis is the "fat cell theory," which proposes that adipose cells are determined during the first year of life. The number of fat cells, in turn, determines the eventual amount of the adipose tissue.[4] Overfeeding, which is frequently associated with the early introduction of solids, may have the long-term, and perhaps a permanent, effect of obesity in later life. There is some scientific evidence that introducing solids is significantly correlated with obesity in the infant.[19] An obese infant, in turn, is more likely to become obese in adulthood.[5]

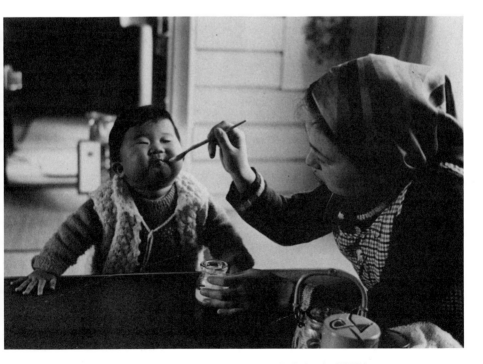

Fig. 17-1. Overfeeding. (Courtesy E. Schwab, WHO.)

How do we explain why some babies who are not given solids and perhaps are completely breastfed are yet fat? Heredity again is a factor. Just as obese parents are more likely to have obese children, slender parents who were fat as babies themselves will see this hereditary pattern repeated in their children. However, advising the mother to cut down on the number of breastfeedings to reduce an infant's weight only results in crying babies and unhappy mothers. In the final analysis, it is clear that the breast-feeding child who receives no early solids weighs less on this feeding regimen than he would on any other.

Concerned with early obesity, enlightened nurses are recommending to mothers that they delay starting solids until the middle of the first year of life.[15] The recent trend, fortunately, is away from solids, and is supported by the American Academy of Pediatrics[7] and by nutritionists. It is interesting to note that as early as 1956, La Leche League was advising delaying solids, preceding professional recommendation by 20 years. Even so, two thirds of the 1-month-old infants surveyed by Andrew et al.[2] in 1980 were given foods other than breastmilk or formula, indicating that more education is needed. Many mothers will ask about starting solids during a well baby visit—an ideal teaching opportunity for nurses. Parenting classes offer the same opportunity.

Effects on natural child spacing

Early solids have yet another disadvantage: the disruption of natural child spacing. The spacing value of lactation is most effective when, in the early months, the infant receives only human milk. The secretion of prolactin, controlled by the pituitary gland, suppresses ovulation, and higher levels of prolactin are positively correlated with the amount of sucking stimulus to the mother's nipples. When solids are delayed and breast-feeding is unrestricted, the ovulatory cycle is suppressed for many months. For the infant receiving supplementary nutrients, the sucking time and thus the child spacing effect are greatly reduced.[14]

In less technically developed countries, where contraceptive alternatives are not as available as in the United States, the impact is staggering. Taiwan scientists estimate that lactation has prevented as much as 20% of births that would have otherwise occurred. In India the same ratio would mean the prevention of approximately 5 million births per year.[3]

COMMERCIAL BABY FOODS

There are now more than 400 varieties of baby foods available on the market. In 1970, 2.7 billion jars were sold. In 1976, probably because of a drop in the birth rate and because of a burgeoning interest in home preparation of infant food, the number fell to 2 billion. Commercial baby food is generally produced by pulverizing fruit, grain, vegetable, and meat ingredients with water. Many of the baby food processors comply with the standards set up by the FDA; others do not. Of 97 baby food plants selected at random by the General Accounting Office in 1973, only 30 met FDA standards.[8] Keeping commercially prepared foods pure is impossible.

In the typical selection of strained foods purchased by the average mother, approximately 80% of the calories are in the form of carbohydrates, such as chemically modified starch and sucrose.[1] This is particularly true in combination baby foods, such as Heinz's Beef and Bacon. The caloric density of these products is about three times that of an identical home-prepared portion. In the middle 1970's, foods other than milk or formula accounted for approximately one third of the total caloric intake in 4-month-old, bottle-fed infants. This regular eating of sweetened foods by infants probably institutes an early imprinting of taste preferences that continues into adulthood.

The addition of salt to infant foods, like other ingredients such as starch and sugar, is not based on any pediatric nutritional guidance. Concern because of possible correlation with hypertension prompted the National Academy of Science Research Committee in 1970 to recommend that the level of salt be limited to 0.25%. Even that reduced amount may be excessive. As the appropriate standard, human milk contains 0.9 mEq of salt. Until 1977, 65% of the baby food from three leading manufacturers contained salt. However, in January 1977 the trend toward natural and healthy ingredients in foods had a positive effect on the baby food market. In a frenzied competition to have the most natural product, Beech-Nut announced the removal of salt from all of its 131 items and surgar from 84. Nine days later, Heinz announced the removal of salt and sugar from many of their varieties, and Gerber soon followed suit.

HOME-PREPARED BABY FOODS

As a consequence of the "less is more" naturalistic movement in our society, young families are now more frequently preparing foods for their infants at home, using baby food grinders and blenders. These foods are not only more wholesome and nutritious but also cost less than commercially prepared baby foods. Carrots and applesauce, for example, cost about one half the store price when prepared at home. Beef and chicken blended in the kitchen provide more nutrients by weight than their commercial counterparts, chiefly because they contain less water.

With the aid of an electric blender, fork, food mill, or grinder, preparing baby food is easily accomplished. The foods should be selected from high-quality fresh or frozen fruits, vegetables, or meats, with special attention to hygienic preparation and storage. For convenience, small individualized portions can be stored safely in the refrigerator or freezer for reasonable periods of time. However, if solids are introduced when the baby has teeth and is ready for them, much of the mashing and blending is not necessary.

STARTING SOLIDS

What foods should be started, when? If no solids are started until the age of 6 months, as is strongly recommended for well infants, then the sequence of solids is less critical, although even then hypoallergenic foods should be used. If solids are introduced earlier, then the following order is suggested: fruits, meats and cereals, yellow vegetables, and lastly legumes. For cereals that require mixing with a liquid, breastmilk instead of cow's milk avoids any potential allergic reaction. Egg yolk, if carefully separated from the white (which is highly allergenic), is high in protein and iron and is hypoallergenic and therefore safe. Infants need additional water when solids are started because of the added osmolar load. Juices, which are good sources of vitamin C, can be introduced when the child can drink from a cup. Using one with a tight-fitting lid or using a straw prevents excessive spilling at first.

A basic rule is to feed the infant foods in as close to a natural state as possible: pieces of raw peeled apples, banana, toasted whole wheat bread, orange sections, and a chicken leg with the skin removed can be picked up and held and are all tasty, nutritious, and satisfying to chew. Giving small amounts at first, gradually increasing the amount along with continued breastfeeding, avoids constipation. Mothers should be prepared for changes in consistency, odor, and frequency of stools when solids are begun. To test for allergy, each new food should be fed for at least 1 week before a new one is added. Generally, all foods that are eaten by his family, whatever their cultural background, can be given to the infant in a consistency he can handle. The beginning eater enjoys foods of all kinds and relishes the tactile pleasures of squeezing, smearing, and crushing his food—an activity he should be allowed with impunity, since it is also a learning experience. General guidelines for initiating solid foods are in Table 17-1.

TABLE 17-1

Introducing solid foods into a breastfed infant's diet

When to introduce	Approximate total daily intake of solids*	Description of foods and hints about giving them
6-7 mo if infant is breastfed	Dry cereal: Start with ½ tsp (dry measurement), gradually increase to 2-3 Tbsp. Vegetables: Start with 1 tsp, gradually increase to 2 Tbsp. Fruit: Start with 1 tsp, gradually increase to 2 Tbsp. Divide food among 4 feedings per day (if possible).	Cereal: Offer iron-enriched baby cereal. Begin with single grains. Mix cereal with an equal amount of breastmilk, or water. Vegetables: Try a mild-tasting vegetable first (carrots, squash, peas, green beans). Stronger-flavored vegetables (spinach, sweet potatoes) may be tried after the infant accepts some mild-tasting ones. Fruits: Mashed ripe banana and unsweetened, cooked, bland fruits (apples, peaches, pears) are usually well liked. Apple juice and grape juice (unsweetened) may be introduced. Initially, dilute juice with an equal amount of water. Introduce one new food at a time and offer it several times before trying another new food. Give a new food once a day for a day or two; Increase to twice a day as the infant begins to enjoy the food. Watch for signs of intolerance. Include some foods that are good sources of vitamin C (other than orange juice).

Modified from Suitor, C.W., and Hunter, M.F.: Nutrition: principles and applications in health promotion, Philadelphia, 1980, J.B. Lippincott Co.
*Some infants do not need or want these amounts of food; some may need a little more food.

TABLE 17·1—cont'd

Introducing solid foods into a breastfed infant's diet

When to introduce	Approximate total daily intake of solids	Description of foods and hints about giving them
6-7 mo if infant is breastfed	Dry cereal: Gradually increase up to 4 Tbsp. Fruits and vegetables: gradually increase up to 3 Tbsp of each. Meat: Start with 1 tsp and gradually increase to 2 Tbsp. Divide food among 4 feedings per day (if possible).	Meat: Offer pureed or milled poultry (chicken or turkey) followed by lean meat (veal, beef); lamb has a stronger flavor and may not be as well liked initially. Liver is a good source of iron; it may be accepted at the beginning of a meal with a familiar vegetable. Continue introducing new cereals, fruits, and vegetables as the infant indicates he is ready to accept them, but always one at a time; introduce legumes last.
7-9 mo if infant is breastfed	Dry cereal: Up to ½ c. Fruits and vegetables: Up to ¼ to ½ c of each. Meats: Up to 3 Tbsp. Divide food among 4 feedings per day (if possible).	Soft table foods may be introduced; for example, mashed potatoes and squash and small pieces of soft, peeled fruits. Toasted whole grain or enriched bread may be added when the infant begins chewing. If introduction of solids is delayed until now, it is not necessary to use strained fruits and vegetables. Continue using *iron-fortified* baby cereals.
8-12 mo	Dry cereal: Up to ½ c. Bread: About 1 slice. Fruits and vegetables: Up to ½ c of each. Meat: Up to ¼ c. Divide food among 4 feedings per day (if possible).	Table foods may be added gradually. Cut table foods into small pieces. Start with ones that do not require too much chewing (cooked, cut green beans and carrots, noodles, ground meats, tuna fish, soft cheese, plain yogurt). If fish is offered, check closely to be sure there are no bones in the serving. Mashed, cooked egg yolk and orange juice may be added at about 9 mo of age. Sometimes offer peanut butter or thoroughly cooked dried peas and beans in place of meat.

As nurses, we must take the responsibility of educating families in optimal infant feeding practices, providing rationale and support if they are needed. In teaching about solid foods, the main points to remember are the following:

1. Delay solid foods until around the middle of the first year of life when the infant indicates he is ready for them.
2. Continue frequent breastfeedings with lots of cuddling and holding. Crying may be interpreted as hunger when actually the infant needs to be held, rocked, and soothed.
3. Prepare foods for the infant in as close to a natural state as possible.
4. Introduce one new food at a time, and offer it several times before trying another new food, observing for signs of intolerance or allergy.

The following books (softcover issues available) on good nutrition and baby foods are recommended for parents:

Goldbeck, Nikki, and Goldbeck, David: Supermarket handbook: Access to whole foods, New York, Signet, 1976.

Kenda, Margaret, and Williams, Phyllis: The natural baby food cookbook, New York, 1973, Avon Books.

Lansky, Vicky: Feed me! I'm yours, Deephaven, Minn., 1974, Meadowbrook Press, Inc.

La Leche League International, Inc.: The womanly art of breastfeeding, Franklin Park, Ill., 1981, The League.

Turner, Mary, and Turner, James: Making your own baby food, rev. ed., New York, 1977, Workman Publishing Co., Inc.

REFERENCES

1. Anderson, T.A.: Commercial infant foods: content and composition, Symposium on Nutrition in Pediatrics, Pediatr. Clin. North Am. **24**:39, 1977.
2. Andrew, E.M., et al.: Infant feeding practices of families belonging to a prepaid group practice health care plan, Pediatrics **65**:978, 1980.
3. Berg, A.: Economics of breastfeeding: excerpt from the nutrition factor, Saturday Review of Science **1**:29, 1973.
4. Brook, C.G.D.: Fat cells in childhood obesity, Lancet **1**:224, 1975.
5. Charney, D., et. al.: Childhood antecedents of adult obesity, N. Engl. J. Med. **295**:6, 1976.
6. Chen, P.C.Y.: Nondietary factors and nutrition. In Jelliffe, D.B., and Jelliffe, E.F.P., editors: Nutrition and growth, New York, 1979, Plenum Press.
7. Committe on Nutrition, American Academy of Pediatrics: On the feeding of supplemental foods to infants, Pediatrics **65**:1178, 1980.
8. Echols, B., and Arena, J.M.: Food additives and pesticides in foods, Symposium on Nutrition in Pediatrics, Pediatr. Clin. North Am. **24**:185, 1977.
9. Foman, S.F.: Infant nutrition, ed. 2, Philadelphia, 1974, W.B. Saunders Co.
10. Fruthaler, G.J.: Can allergy be prevented? South. Med. J. **58**:836, 1965.
11. Glaser, J.: Prophylaxis and allergic disease in infancy and childhood: allergy and immunology in children, Springfield, Ill., 1973, Charles C Thomas, Publisher.
12. György, P.: Trends and advances in infant nutrition, W. Va. Med. J. **53**:121, 1957.
13. Kendall, K.: Maternal and child nursing in an Iranian village. In Leininger, M.: Transcultural nursing, New York, 1978, John Wiley & Sons, Inc.
14. Kippley, S.: Breastfeeding and natural child spacing, New York, 1974, Harper & Row, Publishers, Inc.
15. Markesbery, B., and Wong W.: Watching baby's diet: a professional and parental guide, M.C.N. **4**:177, 1979.
16. McMillan, J., Landon, S., and Usk, F.: Iron sufficiency in breastfed infants and the availability of iron from human milk, Pediatrics **58**:686, 1976.

17. Moore, W.H.: Nutrition, growth and development of North American Indian children, Department of Health, Education, and Welfare Pub. No. 72-76, Washington, D.C., 1979.
18. Rosenberg, T.: Breast milk and the potentially allergic child, Paper presented at Conference on Breastfeeding and Infant Nutrition, Wichita, Kansas, 1975.
19. Shukla, A., et al.: Infantile overnutrition in the first year of life, Br. Med. J. **4:**507, 1972.
20. Taitz, L.S.: Obesity in pediatric practice: Symposium on Nutrition in Pediatrics, Pediatr. Clin. North Amer. **24:**107, 1977.

ADDITIONAL READINGS

La Leche League International, Inc.: Baby's first solid food, Franklin Park, Ill., 1975, The League.
Whaley, L.F., and Wong, D.L.: Nursing care of infants and children, ed. 2, St. Louis, 1983, The C.V. Mosby Co.

The sensuousness of
breastfeeding

JAN RIORDAN

Human biology and life patterns are constantly in cyclic progression. We sleep, wake, and experience changes in body temperature, blood sugar, and blood pressure in a synchrony of predictable rhythms. These cycles and rhythms, in their certain inevitability, have use for our life functioning.

It can also be said that in feminine reproductive functioning there are five cycles: ovarian, intercourse, pregnancy, childbirth, and lactation.[10] Each of these has purpose and brings pleasure if experienced at an optimal level of function for the individual.

In this chapter I explore the notion that one of these, breastfeeding, in addition to providing nourishment, can be pleasurable for the mother. This pleasure has a purpose; in fact, the very survival of homo sapiens has been dependent upon pleasurable reinforcements of breastfeeding. As Newton[10] so aptly put it: If it were not so, man would have joined the dinosaurs in extinction long ago.

That sexual pleasure should occupy the minds of breastfeeding women may come not only as a novel but as a shocking idea. Yet in perusal of the many paintings of nursing dyads that abound in collections of great art, we may note a mood of introspection and a faint, bemused expression of pleasure on the mother's face.

As a corollary, these energies being channeled into the breastfeeding experience are shunted away from other forms of sexual expression such as coitus, and that this, coupled with the suppression of the ovarian cycle, prolongs spacing between pregnancies, thus helping to ensure nourishment and nurturing for the infant for a longer period of time.

CULTURAL PERSPECTIVES

Because cultural attitudes are intimately associated with the expression of feminine biological functions, sensual enjoyment during breastfeeding must be examined from a cross-cultural perspective. Attitudes toward breastfeeding and sensuality show considerable variation among different cultures—being developed in some, muted in others. The Navahos, for instance, have highly developed sexual innuendos. Kluckhohn[7] ob-

---

Sections of this chapter are taken ftom Riordan, J., and Rapp, E.T.: Pleasure and purpose: the sensuousness of breastfeeding, J.O.G.N. Nurs. **9:**109, 1980.

served that boy babies were observed to have erotic interchanges with their mothers with penile erection during breastfeeding.

In most cultures, however, if specific sensual feelings are ever discussed, it is usually with hesitation and embarrassment and in privacy. One mother stated, "My breast and especially my nipples are more sensitive in sex, now that I've nursed two babies than before. Somewhere along the way, I learned that sucking felt good." Our own cultural denial of sensuality during breastfeeding is revealed in the almost absence of reference to it in the growing body of sex literature. As an example, Richard Green, the male author of two major books on sexuality, limits his discussion of sexuality during the postpartum period to: "Sexual interest in women will probably be low in the immediate postpartum period. The return of sexual interest in coitus is variable."[4] Recognition of sensuality during breastfeeding is not broached in any of the major textbooks on sexuality—an astounding myopia. Indeed, most research and observations are derived from the single biological function: orgasm through intercourse or masturbation. Is this glaring omission the result of ignorance, or is it threatening that the feminine sexual cycles are so rich and varied?

MATERNAL ROLES

Evidence suggests that attitudes to maternal function are related to breastfeeding behavior. Newton[9] reports that aversion to breastfeeding is related to dissatisfaction with the woman's lot in life, longer labors, smaller size of families, and the actual amount of milk ejected during let-down. On the other hand, Newton found that women who were positive toward breastfeeding were more likely to feel that women had at least as satisfying a time in life as men, had shorter labors, and let down their milk more efficiently.

Another factor has been the emphasis which some members of the women's movement have given to liberation from maternal roles. These individuals fear that a recognition of the nonorgasmic aspects of female sexuality would be counterproductive, leading to a return of the "motherhood myth" which domesticates women and limits their potential outside the home. Instead, orgasmic liberation, rather than the fight for women's rights to give birth and breastfeed free of medical (and mainly male) interference and cultural pressures, has received the most emphasis.[5]

EROTIC STIMULATION

The close relationship between sensual feelings and sucking at the nipple is real enough. The nipple is well supplied with nerve endings, and their stimulation by the nursing baby causes uterine contractions which, in the early postpartum weeks, helps involution of the uterus to its pre-pregnancy state. This interrelationship between the breast and the lower reproductive tract has been repeatedly demonstrated. Oxytocin, the hormone released during the ejection of milk or let-down, causes the uterine muscle fibers to contract rhythmically during breastfeeding. During the early feedings following birth, these contractions are usually felt as strong and painful cramps—and are not at all pleasurable; later the contractions become painless and even pleasurable continuing for about twenty minutes after the feeding. Conversely, failure to experience uterine contractions can indicate inadequate let-down which leads to engorgement which in turn leads to inadequate milk supply. Further evidence of this relationship is the effect of lower reproductive tract stimulation on milk flow. For example, vaginal stimulation is a recognized way for dairy farmers to induce milk flow in cows, by stimulating a physiologic and endocrine response. Likewise, many human mothers describe dripping or spurting of milk during heightened sexual response and orgasm.[2]

Other similarities of physiologic responses between sexual arousal and breastfeeding are the erection of the nipples with marked vascular changes, lengthening of the nipple, rhythmic stroking of the nipple during sucking, and extensive skin-to-skin contact. Masters and Johnson found that this stimulation was reported by some women to have brought them to plateau levels of sexual response and on several occasions, to orgasm.[8] Since birth is the beginning of a long intimate relationship between a mother and her baby, is it unreasonable to expect it to be physiologically pleasurable like the sexual pleasures at the beginning of a long, intimate, and committed relationship with a mate?

Despite this tenable notion, guilt is a common response to these feelings. Six of the twenty-five breastfeeding women studied by Masters and Johnson expressed guilt feelings over their sexual arousal. Just as some religious beliefs prescribe procreation as the *raison d'etre* for the enjoyment of intercourse, nourishment is often regarded as the sole purpose of the breastfeeding act.

The exact nature of the sensual feelings during breastfeeding should be differentiated from coital arousal. Interviews with lactating women indicate that sustained erotic stimulation and/or orgasm is not the usual experience and contradict the Masters and Johnson report. Although the nipple itself is very sensitive during feedings, much stimulation falls upon the areola, which is comparatively insensitive to touch.[13] Intense anticipatory erotic sensations are unlike the tranquil and peaceful sensual feelings described by mothers following the let-down of the milk. In response to a question regarding erotic feelings during feeding, one mother stated:

> If I don't have the baby positioned right, and he starts gumming the nipple, sure, I begin to feel just like I do when my husband stimulates my breasts when we make love. But it gets in the way, this feeling, as here I am sitting and waiting to let-down my milk and I'm getting more and more tense. I just shift the baby around until he's got the entire areola and then we have a good feeding.[12]

Unfortunately, some women who experience sensual feelings during breastfeeding feel guilty to the point that they voluntarily wean their babies early and refuse to breastfeed future children.

The question now arises: Why don't some women feel sensual during breastfeeding even though they have breastfed several months? Are they intimidated by social expectations and not admitting it, or in fact, is non-sensuality just another response in the wide range of possible feelings? One such mother confided, "Although I breastfed, I never felt that it was in any way sexual for me. It brought me no particular pleasure but on the other hand, it wasn't unpleasant either." One possible explanation is that a woman whose breast and nipples are not normally erogenous zones is not likely to become erotically stimulated by breastfeeding.

SEXUAL RELATIONS

Pressures and problems of sexual relations while lactating are as ancient as woman herself. Physicians during the 17th Century recommended breastfeeding, but insisted that sexual relations during lactation would spoil the milk and endanger the life of the child. Even the alternative of coitus interruptus was not feasible; it was the sexual excitement, not intercourse itself, that was thought to ruin the milk.

A woman's early weaning to accommodate her husband's desires meant a certain health risk to her child, since the artifically-fed infant of that time was likely to become ill and even die. To alleviate the dilemma, wet nurses were employed. Husbands of that period were accused of insisting on employing wet nurses who charged high rates and dominated households with a complaint that "Many a tender mother is prevented by the misplaced authority of her husband."[14] Although in contemporary times, sexual relations are usually resumed during breastfeeding, and before return of the menses, this is not the case for all cultures. A number of societies that feel strongly about child spacing insist upon sexual abstinence from a few weeks to a year or longer. In a few instances, returning to coital activity is determined by a development milestone of the child such as cutting a tooth, crawling, or walking.[3]

Receptiveness of the breastfeeding woman to coitus and sexual expression with her mate is reported in the literature to be increased or diminished depending upon the source. Masters and Johnson found that breastfeeding women as a group reported a prompt return of sexuality and "interest in as rapid return as possible to active coition with their husbands."[8] However, these responses were not measured physiologically. In another study,[6] three-fourths of the sampled mothers reported that breastfeeding had little effect on their sexual lives. My own experience and that suggested by Newton[11] seem to indicate that sexual desire, at least on the part of the nursing mother, lessens considerably during lactation. Describing her feelings during this period, a mother reported:

> When you are home and you touch, hold, hug, and nurse all day, you're not so interested in it when your husband walks through the door. But then his day has been all talk all day and no touch, and he's ready. It creates a problem.

There are other detractors. Some couples swear that infants have radar—that when they begin to make love, their infant rouses and begins to cry.

This mother gave a different view:

> To me sex is best of all during the later breastfeeding period because I feel physically better than at any other time, and there is no need for contraceptives because for me, breastfeeding is a 100% effective contraceptive for about a year. There's something about nursing a little baby that gives you an "all's right with the world" feeling. I feel so happy and loving toward my whole family as well as the baby. Sex just seems to be a nice, natural expression of this good feeling.

This apparent wide variance of sexual responsiveness may be due to the following reasons. First, because of the importance of the Masters and Johnson research as a whole, any data derived from their studies is frequently referred to, and is accepted, as valid. However, in the Masters and Johnson study cited above, only 24 reports by lactating women were studied, hardly a population sample for any statistical significance—a point which the authors themselves clearly make in the text. Also, the halo effect of participation in one segment of much wider sex studies cannot be discounted.

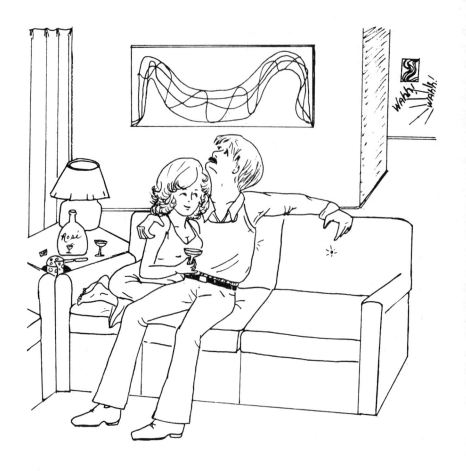

Radar. That kid has radar.[*]

On the other hand, when physiological changes were measured on the nursing breast during sexual tension from general stimulation, no consistent size increases were noted in the Masters and Johnson studies.[8]

Second, the Ford and Beach theory,[3] that the clear-cut relationship between fertility and sexual responsiveness in lower mammalian species is less well-defined in subhuman primates and is completely obliterated in the human female, may account for the heightened sexual response reported by some women. It could be that women who choose to breastfeed, as a group, possess a greater interest in coitus throughout their entire reproductive cycle than women who, because they are uncomfortable with their

---

[*]Reproduced with permission from McCartney, J.: The other side makes chocolate, Middlesex, N.J., 1981, Dään Graphics. Copyright © 1981 by Joan McCartney.

sexuality or body image, prefer to bottle feed. The woman with excessively large breasts who finds breastfeeding aversive is a case in point.

Certainly the exhaustion and anxiety of the new mother with an added work load, interrupted sleep, and concern about her ability to care for her baby would understandably cause a "drain" on her libido and sexual responsiveness. As stated by one mother:

> In the early weeks after resuming sex, the baby herself did not intrude on our relations, but my exhaustion and discomfort did. The tenderness from the episiotomy lasted a good deal longer than six weeks and this surprised me. More importantly, my total absorption in the baby and mothering drastically cut my interest and desire for sex.[2]

FEELINGS TOWARD THE INFANT

As individuals we accept the notion that love leads to sex but ignore the corollary—sex leads to love. The sensual feelings the mother experiences during breastfeeding, if they are accepted as a natural, gratifying maternal experience, strengthen the feeling of tenderness and commitment to her baby. A number of studies[11,15] have revealed that mothers who are breastfeeding tend to interact with their infants with different behaviors from bottle-feeding mothers. In one study,[1] breastfeeding mothers, observed while feeding their babies at specific intervals in the first ten days after birth, were noted to touch their infants more when feeding was not taking place, feed for longer periods of time with resultant increased holding, cuddle and rock their babies more, and sleep with their infants more often than bottle feeders.

Members of the helping professions have, in recent years, become aware of the importance of maternal-infant bonding. Through a deepened psychosocial relationship and fulfillment of physiological needs, bonding is intensified into a kind of symbiosis between the breastfeeding mother and infant. The strength of that bond is demonstrated when abrupt weaning must take place. The baby may cry for days and completely refuse the bottle. The mother, too, can grieve, and for years afterwards harbor feelings of resentment and sometimes hatred if she later realizes the weaning was not necessary after all.

In conclusion, it can be said that sexual feelings take a variety of forms. Some feelings are arbitrarily accepted as cultural norms, and others are considered as deviant. Sensual feelings during the breastfeeding cycle can and should be viewed by nurses or any member of the health-care team as a natural and important integral maternal response that can strengthen attachment to the infant. Anticipatory guidance regarding changes in sexuality after childbirth and sensual feelings during breastfeeding helps the breastfeeding mother to deal with them.

REFERENCES

1. Bernal, J., and Richards, P.: Effect of bottle and breastfeeding on infant development, J. Psychosom. Res. **14**:247, 1975.
2. Bing, E., and Colman, L.: Making love during pregnancy, New York, 1977, Bantam Books, Inc.
3. Ford, C., and Beach, F.: Patterns of sexual behavior, New York, 1950, Harper & Row, Publishers, Inc.
4. Green, R.: Human sexuality: a health practitioner's text, Baltimore, 1975, The Williams & Wilkins Co.
5. "How's your sex life?" Special issue on sexuality, MS, Nov. 1976.
6. Kenny, J.A.: Sexuality of the pregnant and breastfeeding mother, Arch. Sex. Behav. **2**:215, 1973.
7. Kluckhohn, C.: Some aspects of Navaho infancy and early childhood, Psychoanal. Soc. Sc., pp. 37-86, 1947.

8. Masters, W., and Johnson, V.: Human sexual response, Boston, 1966, Little, Brown & Co.
9. Newton, N.: Maternal emotions, New York, 1955, Paul B. Hoeber, Inc.
10. Newton, N.: Breastfeeding, Psychology Today, p. 34, June 1968.
11. Newton, N., et al.: Psychological and behavioral correlates of mother's choice of postpartum nearness to infant. In Harsh, H., editor: The family, Proceedings of the Fourth International Congress on Psychosomatic Obstetrics and Gynecology, Basel, 1974, S. Karger.
12. Rapp, E.T.: Female sexuality and lactation, Unpublished paper, Phoenix, Ariz., 1976.
13. Robinson, J., and Short, R.: Changes in breast sensitivity at puberty, during the menstrual cycle and parturition, Br. Med. J. p. 1198, 1977.

14. Stone, L.: The family, sex and marriage: in England 1500-1800, New York, 1977, Harper & Row, Publishers, Inc.
15. Thoman, E.B., et al.: Neonate-mother interaction during breastfeeding, Dev. Psychol. **6:**110, 1972.

Additional Readings

Deutsch, H.: The psychology of women, vol. 2, Motherhood, New York, 1945, Grune & Stratton, Inc.
Mead, M., and Newton, M.: Cultural patterning of perinatal behavior. In Richardson, R.A., and Guttmacher, A.F., editors: Childbearing: its social and psychological aspects, Baltimore, 1967, The Williams & Wilkins Co.
Pryor, K.: Nursing your baby, New York, 1975, Harper & Row, Publishers, Inc.

This part has attempted to provide a worldwide look at early mothering patterns that are related to breastfeeding. It is hoped that the world of tomorrow will be built on experiences learned from today and yesterday, and will be inhabited by people capable of creating life-styles that use the best of the past. In calling American nurses to come together with other nurses of the world for a renewed sense of purpose at the 1981 International Council of Nurses held in Los Angeles, Nichols, ANA President, reflected:

One of the astronauts who orbited the moon said that seen from that distance the world looked small and very dear. We share our profession, our love for people, our concern for health care and our skills with women and men of many lands. We are all part of that network of nurses caring for people in the mountains and deserts and on the seacoasts, in forests, amid farmlands, in sprawling cities and little villages of that small, dear planet.

Assessment form for breastfeeding evaluation

UNIVERSITY HOSPITAL
University of California
Medical Center, San Diego

LACTATION CLINIC
DATA BASE

SEEN BY

| Source | Date | Patient Identification |

FAMILY ADDRESS   PHONE

FAMILY INFORMATION

FAMILY MEMBERS (name)   AGE: OTHER HOUSEHOLD MEMBERS (name, age, relationship)

Mother:

Father:

Children:

PREFERRED LANGUAGE   PEDIATRICIAN, OBSTETRICIAN AND/OR FAMILY DOCTOR
☐ English   ☐ Spanish   ☐ Other:

INSTRUCTIONS: Please answer the following questions by circling either YES or NO. For any questions answered YES, please give additional information as indicated.

SUBJECTIVE INFORMATION

MATERNAL HISTORY

1. Do you have any health problems? . . . . YES NO
   If yes, what ____
   a. Have you ever had thyroid or other gland problems? . . YES NO
      If yes, what ____
      when ____
   b. Have you ever had blood pressure problems? . . . . . . YES NO
      If yes, what ____
      when ____

2. Are you presently on any of the following diets? . . . . . . YES NO
   ☐ to lose weight   ☐ to gain weight
   ☐ diabetic   ☐ low salt
   ☐ vegetarian   ☐ other ____

3. Were you on any of the following diets during your pregnancy? . . . . YES NO
   ☐ to lose weight   ☐ to gain weight
   ☐ diabetic   ☐ low salt
   ☐ vegetarian   ☐ other ____

4. Do you take any of the following nutritional supplements? . . . . YES NO
   ☐ calcium   ☐ iron
   ☐ multi-vitamins/   ☐ other ____
   minerals

5. a. Do you believe your present diet is . . . .
      ☐ excellent   ☐ good   ☐ just adequate   ☐ poor
   b. Are you able to have relaxed regular meals? . . . . YES NO

6. Would you find it helpful to talk with a nutritionist about
   ☐ weight gain   ☐ proper nutrition while you
   ☐ weight loss   are breast feeding
   ☐ other, please describe ____   ☐ your family's diet

7. Please note any medicine which you take:
   WHAT   HOW MUCH   HOW OFTEN
   aspirin
   cold/cough medicine
   laxative (please name)
   water pills
   other

8. Do you smoke? If yes, how many packs a day? ___ . . . . YES NO

9. Do you drink coffee? If yes, how many cups a day? ____ YES NO
10. Do you drink tea? If yes, how many cups a day? ____ YES NO
11. Do you drink beer, liquor and/or wine? . . . . YES NO
    ☐ occasionally   ☐ frequently   How much ____
12. Have you had any difficulty since your delivery with
    ☐ urinating,   ☐ bowel movement? . . . . YES NO
13. Has vaginal bleeding stopped? . . . . YES NO
    If yes, when ____
14. Are you using any family planning method now? . . . . . YES NO
    If yes, what method? ____
    If no, do you plan to? What method? ____ YES NO
15. Have you felt "blue" or depressed since your delivery? YES NO
16. Are you sleeping well at night? . . . . YES NO
17. Are you able to rest during the day? . . . . YES NO
18. Have your menstrual periods returned? . . . . YES NO
19. Have you ever had any breast problems or breast surgery? . . . . YES NO

INFANT HISTORY

1. Baby's name ____ Birth weight ____ ☐ boy
   Date of birth ____ Discharge weight ____ ☐ girl
2. Where was the baby born? Hospital ____
   City, State ____
3. Was the baby born ☐ on time   ☐ early   ☐ late
4. Did you have any problems during pregnancy and/or
   labor and delivery . . . . YES NO
   If yes, please describe ____
5. What type of delivery did you have?
   ☐ Cesarean   ☐ vacuum
   ☐ vaginal (normal)   ☐ forceps
   ☐ vaginal (breech)   ☐ other ____
6. Were you and your baby discharged at the same time . . . YES NO
7. Did your baby have any newborn problem? . . . . YES NO
   If yes, briefly describe ____
8. Was the baby planned . . . . YES NO
9. Is there a history of allergy on either side of your
   baby's family? . . . . YES NO
10. In general, how are the members of your family or household adjusting to having a new baby at home? (check one)
    ☐ Very well   ☐ reasonably well   ☐ poorly   ☐ very poorly

D1212(R3-81)6

<table>
<tr><td rowspan="2">SUBJECTIVE INFORMATION (Continued)</td><td>

BREAST FEEDING

1. Have you breast fed a previous baby? . . . . YES NO
   If yes, for how long? _____
   Why did you stop? _____

2. Why do you wish to breast feed your present baby?
   _____

3. Is there anyone in your household who feels you should
   not breast feed this baby? . . . . YES NO
   If yes, who? _____

4. For how long do you plan to breast feed your baby?
   (Circle the approximate number of months)
   less than 1 2 3 4 5 6 7 8 9 10 11 12 more than 12

5. Why do you think you will discontinue breast feeding at
   that time? _____

6. When did you decide to breast feed your present baby?
   Before pregnancy ☐
   During first three months of pregnancy ☐
   During second three months of pregnancy ☐
   During last three months of pregnancy ☐
   After delivery ☐

7. Have you read any books, articles or pamphlets about
   breast feeding . . . . YES NO

8. During your pregnancy did you do any kind of breast or
   nipple preparation for nursing your baby? . . . . YES NO
   If yes, during which prenatal month did you begin?
   (circle one)   1 2 3 4 5 6 7 8 9

9. Approximately how soon after your baby was born did
   you have your first opportunity to nurse him/her?
   _____

10. Do you have a quiet, comfortable place at home for
    nursing your baby? . . . . YES NO

11. Have you had any tenderness and/or redness of your
    breasts or nipples? . . . . YES NO

</td><td>

12. Have you had any other problems with breast feeding? YES NO
    If yes, what? _____

13. How many times in 24 hours do you feed your baby? ___

14. What is the longest time between feedings? . . . . ___

15. How long does your baby nurse on each breast? . . . . . ___

16. Does your baby seem to have a preference for either
    breast? If yes, which one . . . . . . YES NO

17. When your baby nurses do you feel any
    ☐ tingling   ☐ burning   ☐ filling sensations? . . . . YES NO

18. While your baby nurses at one breast does milk drip
    from the other breast? . . . . YES NO

19. Does your baby sleep well between feedings? . . . . . . YES NO

20. How many wet diapers has your baby had in the last
    24 hours? . . . . ___

21. How often does your baby have a bowel movement? . . . ___

22. Do you find your baby needs a pacifier? . . . . YES NO

23. Does your baby spit up? ☐ occasionally ☐ often. . . . YES NO

24. At home has your baby received . . . . YES NO
    ☐ water   ☐ liquids other than formula
    ☐ any solids   ☐ supplemental formula

25. In the hospital did your baby receive
    ☐ water   ☐ formula . . . . YES NO

26. Has your baby had any prolonged crying spells? . . . . . YES NO

27. Is your baby taking any medication? . . . . YES NO
    If yes, what? _____

28. Do you have any special concerns about yourself or your
    baby or your family's health which you would like to
    discuss during your appointment? . . . . YES NO
    If yes, what? _____

</td></tr>
</table>

<table>
<tr><td rowspan="8">OBJECTIVE INFORMATION</td><td rowspan="8">MOTHER</td><td colspan="2">POST-PARTUM
Weeks:
Days:</td><td>PRE-PREGNANT WEIGHT</td><td>AT TERM WEIGHT</td><td>PRESENT WEIGHT</td><td>HEIGHT</td><td>B.P.</td><td>TEMP.</td></tr>
<tr><td colspan="8">GENERAL</td></tr>
<tr><td colspan="4">BREASTS</td><td colspan="4">NIPPLES</td></tr>
<tr><td>R</td><td colspan="3"></td><td>R</td><td colspan="3"></td></tr>
<tr><td>L</td><td colspan="3"></td><td>L</td><td colspan="3"></td></tr>
<tr><td colspan="2">ABDOMEN</td><td>FUNDAL HEIGHT</td><td colspan="2">TENDERNESS</td><td colspan="3">LOCHIA</td></tr>
<tr><td colspan="4">ASSESSMENT</td><td colspan="4">PLAN</td></tr>
<tr><td colspan="2">NEXT APPOINTMENT FOR MOTHER</td><td colspan="3">WHERE</td><td colspan="3">WHEN</td></tr>
</table>

D1212(R3-81)6

From Naylor, A., and Wester, R.: Lactation Clinic, University Hospital, University of California Medical
Center, San Diego, Calif.

	AGE	TEMP	HEAD CIRC	LENGTH	BIRTH WEIGHT		DISCHARGE WEIGHT	PRESENT WEIGHT	TOTAL WEIGHT GAIN/LOSS SINCE BIRTH

OBJECTIVE INFORMATION (Continued)

INFANT

GENERAL

	Normal	PROBLEM		Normal	PROBLEM
Head			Heart		
Eyes			Pulses		
Ears			Abdomen		
Nose			Genitalia		
Mouth			Extremities		
Thorax			Neuro		
Lungs			Skin		

INFANT BEHAVIOR

Sleepy	Mellow	Active, Content	Fretful	Very Fussy

ASSESSMENT	PLAN

NEXT APPT. FOR INFANT	WHERE	WHEN

BREAST FEEDING OBSERVATION

INFANT

INTEREST							STRESS LEVEL					
Very	5	4	3	2	1	None	5+	4+	3+	2+	1+	0

MOTHER

LATCH-ON

Excellent	Drops Back	Needed Help

INFANT/MATERNAL INTERACTION

SUCKLING TECHNIQUE

Very Effective	5	4	3	2	1	Not Effective

HAND EXPRESSION TECHNIQUE

Instruction Needed: Yes ☐   No ☐

GENERAL

ASSESSMENT	PLAN

RETURN VISIT TO LACTATION CLINIC	INFANT ☐ No ☐ Yes When:	MOTHER ☐ No ☐ Yes When:

DATE	CLINICIAN

D1212(R3-81)6

Audiovisual aids

FILMS

Babe at the Breast
  8 minutes, black and white
  La Leche League International
  Marell Schmidt
  1900 Swarthmore Drive
  Aurora, Ill.0506

The Bond of Breastfeeding*
  21 minutes, color
  Perennial Education, Inc.
  477 Roger Williams
  Highland Park, Ill. 60035

Breastfeeding
  18 minutes, color
  Professional Research, Inc.
  12960 Coral Tree Place
  Los Angeles, Calif. 90066

Breastfeeding
  8 minutes, color
  Cinema Medica
  2335 Foster Ave.
  Chicago, Ill. 60625

Breastfeeding Experience
  31 minutes, color
  Parenting Pictures
  121 N.W. Crystal St.
  Crystal River, Fla. 32629

Breastfeeding, A Family Experience
  12 minutes, color
  CEA of Seattle
  1443 N.W. 54th St.
  Seattle, Wash. 98107

Breastfeeding for the Joy of It*
  31 minutes, color
  Cinema Medica
  2335 Foster Ave.
  Chicago, Ill. 60625

Breastfeeding: Nutrition, Nursing, and the Working
    Mother
  22 minutes, color
  Case Western Reserve University
  Rm. WA-6434
  University Circle
  Cleveland, Ohio 44106

Breastfeeding Prenatal and Postpartal Preparation
  26 minutes, color
  Polymorph Films
  118 South St.
  Boston, Mass. 02111

Breastfeeding: A Special Closeness*
  23 minutes, color
  Motion, Inc.
  4437 Klingle St. N.W.
  Washington, D.C. 20016

Breastfeeding Your Baby
  Wayne State University, Audio-Visual Utilization
    Center
  5448 Case Ave.
  Detroit, Mich. 48202

Comparative Biology of Lactation†
  25 minutes
  G. Maloof
  1515 Sloat Blvd.
  San Francisco, Calif. 94132

Learning to Breastfeed
  22 minutes, color
  Polymorph Films
  118 South St.
  Boston, Mass. 02111

Mother and Child*
  15 minutes, color
  Mary Jane Co.
  P.O. Box 736
  N. Hollywood, Calif. 91609

*Also available for rental from La Leche League International, 9616 Minneapolis Ave., Franklin Park, Ill. 60131.
†For professional use.

Mothering Through Breastfeeding
14 minutes, color
La Leche League International
Marell Schmidt
1900 Swarthmore Dr.
Aurora, Ill. 60506

Mother Love
20 minutes, black and white
New York University Film Library
26 Washington Pl.
New York, N.Y. 10003

The Nursing Family*
15 minutes, color
Mary Jane Co.
P.O. Box 736
North Hollywood, Calif. 91609

Preparation of the Breast for Breastfeeding*
10 minutes, black and white
Mead Johnson Laboratories
Manager, Meetings and Exhibits
2404 Pennsylvania St.
Evansville, Ind. 47721

Preparation for Breastfeeding*
11 minutes, color
Education Graphic Aids
1315 Norwood Ave.
Boulder, Colo. 80302

Talking About Breastfeeding*
17 minutes, color
Polymorph Films
118 South Street
Boston, Mass. 02111

SLIDES

The Beauty of Breastfeeding
18 minutes, 66 slides/tape
Helen Quimby
2791 Cedar Ave.
Long Beach, Calif. 90806

Best for Baby . . . Best For You
18 minutes, 56 color slides/tape
Marell Schmidt
1900 Swarthmore Dr.
Aurora, Ill. 60506

Breast Feeding
Medical Electronic Educational Series
1802 W. Grant Rd., Suite 119
Tucson, Ariz. 85705

Breastfeeding
100 slides
Lifecircle
2378 Cornell Dr.
Costa Mesa, Calif. 92626

Breastfeeding: A Family Event
18 minutes, 52 color slides/tape
Babes
Deanna Sollid, RN
59 Berens Dr.
Kentfield, Calif. 94904

Breastfeeding Series*
22 color slides/tape
Photoview Instructional Aids
27935 Roble Alto
Los Altos Hills, Calif. 94022

Breastfeeding Works for Cesareans, Too
15 color slides
Kittie Frantz
P.O. Box 7247
Burbank, Calif. 91510

Correct Positioning at the Breast
12 black and white slides
Kittie Frantz
P.O. Box 7247
Burbank, Calif. 91510

Lecture Slides on Breastfeeding: Basic Concepts, In
Hospital, Problems of Mother, Infant Feeding
Problems, Jaundice, Mastitis, Failure to
Thrive†
330 slides (only)
Edward Cerutti, M.D.
2405 Queenston Rd.
Cleveland, Ohio 44118

Fact and Fantasy: Infant Nutrition†
Department of Pediatrics
The University of Kansas-Wichita
1001 N. Minneapolis
Wichita, Kan. 67214

Preparation for Breastfeeding*
20 minutes, tape, 45 color slides
Educational Graphic Aids
1315 Norwood Ave.
Boulder, Colo. 80302

---

*Also available for rental from La Leche League International, 9616 Minneapolis Ave., Franklin Park, Ill. 60131.
†For professional use.

Preparing for Breastfeeding
90 minutes, audiotape only and booklet
Embrace International
P.O. Box 2075
Bloomington, Ind. 47402

TEACHING CHARTS AND AIDS

The breast (demonstration)
Hand washable
Chris Preble
9 Sandy Creek Rd.
Savannah, Ga. 31410

Breastfeeding teaching aids
15 charts
Vis-U-Lac
653 Bowen Street
Dayton, Ohio 45410

Demonstration Doll (for breast positioning)
Cindy Gonzales
P.O. Box 7247
Burbank, Calif. 91510

Low weight gain and postpartum breast care
Wall charts
Health Education Associates
520 School House Lane
Willow Grove, Pa. 19090

Visual aids for group meetings
15 charts
La Leche League of Ohio, South
1956 Elaina Dr.
Springfield, Ohio 45503

SPANISH

The Beauty of Breastfeeding
18 minutes, slide/tape
Helen Quimby
2791 Cedar Ave.
Long Beach, Calif. 90806

Best For Baby . . . Best For You
18 minutes, color film; 18 minutes slide/tape
La Leche League International
Marell Schmidt
1900 Swarthmore Dr.
Aurora, Ill. 60506

Breastfeeding
18 minutes, color film; ¾" videocassette
Professional Research, Inc.
12960 Coral Tree Pl.
Los Angeles, Calif. 90066

Dar Pecho (Breastfeeding)
10 minutes, color film; ¾" videocassette
Videograph
2833 25th St.
San Francisco, Calif. 94110

VIDEOTAPES

Breastfeeding
15 minutes
Video Education
46 Elgin St., Suite 45
Ottawa, Ontario KIP SK6

Breastfeeding for the Joy of It
8 minutes
Cinema Medica
2335 W. Foster Ave.
Chicago, Ill. 60625

Breastfeeding is Best Feeding
Learning Resources
1542 Tulane Ave., Rm. 703
New Orleans, La. 70112

Breastfeeding: Nutrition, Nursing, and the Working
  Mother
Case Western Reserve University
Rm WA-6434
University Circle
Cleveland, Ohio 44106

Helping the Mothers of Prematures to Breastfeed†
University of Colorado, Health Services Center,
  Department of Biomedical Communications
4200 East Ninth St.
Denver, Colo. 80262

Should I Nurse My Baby?
22 minutes
MEDIREC
3453 S. 300 West
Salt Lake City, Utah 84115

---

*Also available for rental from La Leche League International, 9616 Minneapolis Ave., Franklin Park, Ill. 60131.
†For professional use.

Milk banks

BRAZIL
Parana

Hospital Victor do Amaral
Nelio Ribas Centa, M.D.
Av. Iguacu, 1953
Curitiba-Parana-80.000-Brasil

Rio de Janeiro

Instituto da Puericultura e Pediatria Martagao
 Gesteira
Universidade Federal do Rio de Janeiro
Cidade Universitaria
IIha do Fundao
Rio de Janeiro, Brasil

Instituto Fernandes E Figueira
Maria Rita Gallotti
702 Ruy Barbosa Ave. 20,000 Rio de Janeiro,
 Brasil

São Paulo

Banco de Leite Humano do Hospital do Servidor
Publico Estadual
R. Pedro de Toledo, 1800 - C.P. 8570
São Paulo, SP, Brasil

Lactario de Santa Casa
Rua Marques de Itu 695
São Paulo, SP, Brasil

CANADA
Alberta

Calgary Mother's Milk Bank
c/o Foothills Hospital
1403 29th St. N.W.
Calgary, Alberta T2N-2T9

Holy Cross Hospital
2210 Second St. S.W.
Attention: Anne Porter
Calgary, Alberta T2S-1S6

University of Alberta Hospital
Adeline Nitska, Charge Nurse, I.C.N.
112 St. and 84 Ave.
Edmonton, Alberta T6G-2B7

Royal Alexandra Hospital
Attention: Mrs. MacMillan, Mother's Milk Bank
Kingsway Avenue and 103 St.
Edmonton, Alberta T5H-3V9

Edmonton General Hospital
1111 Jasper Avenue
Edmonton, Alberta T5K-OL4

Misericordia Hospital
16940 87th Ave.
Edmonton, Alberta T5R-4H5

British Columbia

Vancouver Children's Hospital
Aggie Radcliffe, Coordinator, Mother's Milk
 Bank
250 West 59th
Vancouver, B.C. V5X-1X2

Royal Inland Hospital
Kamloops, B.C.

Manitoba

University of Manitoba
Faculty of Medicine
Dr. Jim Hawarth, Department of Paediatrics
685 Bannatyne Ave.
Winnipeg, Manitoba R3E-0W1

Mrs. Edith Parker
Maternity Ward
St. Boniface General Hospital
409 Tache Ave.
Winnipeg, Manitoba R2H-3C1

Newfoundland

Janeway Health Centre
Pleasantville
St. John's Nfld. A1A-1R8

Northwest Territories

Marjorie McClelland, RN
Coordinator, Breast Milk Bank Program
Stanton Yellowknife Hospital, Box 10
Yellowknife, N.W.T. X1A-2N1

Nova Scotia

Izaak Walton Killam Hospital for Children
5850 University Ave., P.O. Box 3070
Halifax, N.S. B3J-3G9

Grace Maternity Hospital
5821 University Ave.
Halifax, N.S. B3H-1W3

Ontario

Mr. Jim Nasso
National Baby Formula Service of Canada, Ltd.
365 Midwest Rd.
Scarborough, Ontario MIP-4T8

Saskatchewan

Saskatoon City Hospital
701 Queen St.
Saskatoon, Sask. S7K-0M7

Regina General Hospital
1400 14th St.
Regina, Sask. S4P-0Y7

Holy Family Hospital
675 15th St. S.W.
Prince Albert, Sask. S6V-3R8

Melfort Union Hospital
317 Bemister W.
Melfort, Sask. SO3-1A0

Yorkton Union Hospital
270 Bradbrooke Dr.
Yorkton, Sask. S3N-2K6

Weyburn Union Hospital
201 First Ave., N.E.
Weyburn Sask. S4Y-1P7

St. Joseph's Hospital
1401 First St.
Estevan, Sask.

Nipawin Union Hospital
Mother's Milk Bank, c/o White Fox Kinettes
Nipawin, Sask.

DENMARK

Modermaelkcentralen
Bomehospitalet pa Fuglebakken
DK-2000 Kobenhaven F
Denmark

Modermaelkcentralen
Arhus kommunehospital
DK-8000 Arhus C
Denmark

ENGLAND

Kings College Hospital
Dr. H.R. Gamsu, Department of Child Health
Denmark Hill, S.E.
London SE5 7DG England

Queen Charlotte's Maternity Hospital
Dr. David Harvey
Goldhawk Road
London W6 0XG England

Whipps Cross Hospital
Gerald McEnery, Consultant Paediatrician
Redbridge & Waltham Forest Area Health Authority
West Roding District
London, E11 1NR, England

FRANCE
Bois-Guillaume

Lactarium
Chemin de la Breteque
Mme Pradeau
76230 Bois-Guillaume, France

Bordeaux

Lactarium hopital des Enfants malades
168, cours de l'Argonne
M. le professeur Bentegeat
Mme Boisseau
33000 Bordeau, France

Cherbourg

Centre hospitalier Louis-Pasteur
46, rue du Val-de-Saire
Mme Annick Marie
50107 Cherbourg, France

Clermont-Ferrand

Lactarium
3, rue du Maréchal-Joffre
Mme le docteur Wurm
63000 Clermont-Ferrand, France

Dijon

Lactarium Sainte-Anne
Rue Sainte-Anne
Mme Bancheri
21000 Dijon, France

Evreux

Œuvre du Lait maternel
15, rue Saint-Louis
M. le docteur Guillermou
27000 Evreux, France

Lyon

Lactarium
37, rue Bossuet
M. le docteur Roux
Mme Saignol
69006 Lyon, France

Marmande

Lactarium Raymond-Fourcade
Avenue des Martyrs de la Resistance
M. le docteur Kandel
Marmande, France

Nantes

Lactarium Jacques-Grislain
C.H.R., quai Moncousu
Mme Delvaux
44000 Nantes, France

Orleans

Lactarium du Centre hospitalier
Maison de l'Enfance
B.P. 719, 89, Faubourg Saint-Jean
45032 Cedex Orleans, France

Paris

Centre de coordination
26, boulevard Brune
M. le professeur Satge
Mme J. Bertrand
75014 Paris, France

Saint-Etienne

Lactarium départemental
24, boulevard Pasteur
M. le professeur A. La Selve
Mlle Maisonneauve
42100 Saint-Etienne, France

Strasbourg

Lactarium de l'Institut de Puériculture
23, rue de la Porte-de-l'Hopital
M. le professeur M. Levy
Mlle Lauer
67005 Cedex Strasbourg, France

Tours

Lactarium Centre hospitalier
Regional Bretonneau
Mme Coquillaud
37033 Cedex Tours, France

Versailles

Lactarium départemental
46, rue Lamartine
Mme Dautun
78000 Versailles, France

Villeneuve d'Ascq

Lactarium régional
Centre, Environnement et Santé Publique
de l'Institut Pasteur
Domaine du C.E.R.T.I.A
369, rue Jules-Guesde
59650 Villeneuve d'Ascq, France

ISRAEL
Jerusalem

Shaare Zedek Orthodox Hospital

UNITED STATES OF AMERICA
California

Mother's Milk Bank of Monterey County
Mary Madruga, RN, Coordinator
Childbirth Education League of Salinas
P.O. Box 1423
Salinas, Calif. 93901

San Diego Mother's Milk Bank, University Hospital
Brian Saunders, M.D., Coordinator
225 West Dickinson St.
San Diego, Calif. 92103

Mother's Milk Bank, Inc.
Children's Hospital, Suite 110
3700 California St.
San Francisco, Calif. 94118

Mother's Milk Unit, North California Transplant Bank
Maria Teresa Asquith, Coordinator
751 South Bascom Ave.
San Jose, Calif. 95128

District of Columbia

Carol Crichton
Georgetown University Medical Center
Department of Nursing/Milk Bank
3800 Reservoir Rd.
Washington, D.C. 20008

Georgia

Mother's Milk Bank
The Medical Center
Julie Miller, RN, Coordinator
P.O. Box 951
Columbus, Ga. 31902

Hawaii

Nursing Mothers Association, Inc. (Milk Bank)
DeEtta Cunningham, Coordinator
Hilo Hospital
1190 Waianuenue Ave.
Hilo, Hawaii 96720

Hawaii Mother's Milk, Inc.
Randi Silleck, Coordinator
226 North Kuakini St.
Honolulu, Hawaii 96817

Illinois

Milk Limited
Box 263
Kenilworth, Ill. 60043

Iowa

Variety Club Breast Milk Bank
Iowa Methodist Medical Center
1200 Pleasant St.
Des Moines, Iowa 50308

Kansas

Denise Link
Box 94
Stilwell, Kan. 66085

Kentucky

Louisville Breast Milk Program
Mrs. Patricia Stiebling
Norton Children's Hospitals, Inc.
P.O. Box 655
Louisville, Ky. 40201

Massachusetts

Central Massachusetts Regional Milk Bank
Miriam Erickson, Coordinator
Hahnemann Hospital
281 Lincoln St.
Worcester, Mass. 01605

Minnesota

St. Paul Children's Hospital Milk Bank
Sue LaRock, RN, Coordinator
311 Pleasant Ave.
St. Paul, Minn. 55102

New Hampshire

Dartmouth Medical School
Laurie Rippe, RN, Nurse Consultant
Department of Maternal and Child Health
Hanover, N.H. 03755

New York

Milk For Life
Maria Mathisen, Coordinator
R.D. No. 2, P.O. Box 278-2
Catskill, N.Y. 12414

North Shore University Hospital Milk Bank
Judith Palsgraf, RN, Coordinator
300 Community Dr.
Manhasset, N.Y. 11030

North Carolina

Piedmont Mother's Milk Bank
Mary Rose Tully, Coordinator
4025 Greenleaf St.
Raleigh, N.C. 27606

Oklahoma

Eastern Oklahoma Perinatal Center
Sue Knotts, RN
St. Francis Hospital
6161 So. Yale Ave.
Tulsa, Okla. 74136

Texas

Providence Memorial Hospital
Mother's Milk Bank
Belinda Brice, RN
2001 No. Oregon Street
El Paso, Texas 79902

Jefferson Davis Hospital
Dr. John Kenny
1801 Allen Parkway
Houston, Texas 77019

Virginia

Children's Hospital of Kings' Daughters
Frederick Wirth, M.D.
609 Colley Ave.
Norfolk, Va. 23507

Conversion tables

TABLE D-1

Conversion of pounds to kilograms for pediatric weights

Pounds→	0	1	2	3	4	5	6	7	8	9
0	0.00	0.45	0.90	1.36	1.81	2.26	2.72	3.17	3.62	4.08
10	4.53	4.98	5.44	5.89	6.35	6.80	7.25	7.71	8.16	8.61
20	9.07	9.52	9.97	10.43	10.88	11.34	11.79	12.24	12.70	13.15
30	13.60	14.06	14.51	14.96	15.42	15.87	16.32	16.78	17.23	17.69
40	18.14	18.59	19.05	19.50	19.95	20.41	20.86	21.31	21.77	22.22
50	22.68	23.13	23.58	24.04	24.49	24.94	25.40	25.85	26.30	26.76
60	27.21	27.66	28.12	28.57	29.03	29.48	29.93	30.39	30.84	31.29
70	31.75	32.20	32.65	33.11	33.56	34.02	34.47	34.92	35.38	35.83
80	36.28	36.74	37.19	37.64	38.10	38.55	39.00	39.46	39.91	40.37
90	40.82	41.27	41.73	42.18	42.63	43.09	43.54	43.99	44.45	44.90
100	45.36	45.81	46.26	46.72	47.17	47.62	48.08	48.53	48.98	49.44
110	49.89	50.34	50.80	51.25	51.71	52.16	52.61	53.07	53.52	53.97
120	54.43	54.88	55.33	55.79	56.24	56.70	57.15	57.60	58.06	58.51
130	58.96	59.42	59.87	60.32	60.78	61.23	61.68	62.14	62.59	63.05
140	63.50	63.95	64.41	64.86	65.31	65.77	66.22	66.67	67.13	67.58
150	68.04	68.49	68.94	69.40	69.85	70.30	70.76	71.21	71.66	72.12
160	72.57	73.02	73.48	73.93	74.39	74.84	75.29	75.75	76.20	76.65
170	77.11	77.56	78.01	78.47	78.92	79.38	79.83	80.28	80.74	81.19
180	81.64	82.10	82.55	83.00	83.46	83.91	84.36	84.82	85.27	85.73
190	86.18	86.68	87.09	87.54	87.99	88.45	88.90	89.35	89.81	90.26
200	90.72	91.17	91.62	92.08	92.53	92.98	93.44	93.89	94.34	94.80

TABLE D-2
Conversion of pounds and ounces to kilograms for pediatric weights

Pounds	Kilograms	Ounces	Kilograms	Pounds	Kilograms	Ounces	Kilograms
1	0.454	1	0.028	9	4.082	9	0.255
2	0.907	2	0.057	10	4.536	10	0.283
3	1.361	3	0.085	11	4.990	11	0.312
4	1.814	4	0.113	12	5.443	12	0.340
5	2.268	5	0.142	13	5.897	13	0.369
6	2.722	6	0.170			14	0.397
7	3.175	7	0.198			15	0.425
8	3.629	8	0.227				

From Whaley, L.F., and Wong, D.L.: Nursing care of infants and children, ed. 2, St. Louis, 1983, The C.V. Mosby Co.

Breast feeding policy for full-term normal newborn infants

Definition and purpose: To promote a philosophy of maternal and infant care which advocates breast feeding and supports the normal physiologic functions involved in this maternal-infant process. The goal is to assure that all families who elect to breast feed their infants will have a successful and satisfying experience.

POLICY

1. Infant will be put to breast as soon after birth as feasible for both mother and infant. This will be initiated in either the delivery room or recovery room.
2. Every mother will be instructed in proper latch-on technique and re-evaluated before discharge to assure that this technique is understood.
3. Upon admission to the post-partum unit, each mother will receive two pamphlets: "How the Breast Functions," and "Instructions for Nursing Your Baby." The Nursery day Charge Nurse will be responsible for assuring that each mother has this information.
4. All breast feeding infants will be taken to their mothers every 2½-3 hours around the clock, mother's condition permitting.
5. No supplementary water or milk will be given unless specifically ordered by the Physician or Nurse Practitioner.
6. If supplements are ordered, they are to be administered via slow syringe to avoid nipple confusion.
7. To avoid nipple confusion, pacifiers will not be used routinely unless specifically requested by the mother.
8. The suckling time at each feeding should be approximately 15 minutes per side.
9. Infants will feed from both breasts at all feedings.
10. Mothers of boarder babies will be instructed on how to maintain lactation.
11. All mothers will be given information on, and the option of attending, the Lactation Clinic. Appointments will be made by the Newborn Nursery staff as close to one week after discharge as possible.
12. Each patient will have the Lactation "hot line" number made available to her upon discharge.
13. These same policies will be in effect even if the mother and infant are not in the same unit.

From Lactation Clinic, University Hospital, University of California Medical Center, San Diego, Calif., 1980.

EQUIPMENT
Extra pillow
Pamphlets

Action	Rationale—essentials
1. Position mother comfortably.	Mother's physical comfort will promote relaxation and assist the let-down reflex.
2. Place infant in mother's arms if sitting up or next to her if lying down.	Infant's head should rest in crook of mother's arm if she is sitting up.
3. Position infant so that his/her arms do not interfere with mouth to breast contact.	
4. Have the mother hold her breast with four fingers below and nipple and thumb above.	Proper hand positioning assists in eliciting the rooting reflex and allows the infant easy access to the nipple.
5. Mother touches the infant's nearest cheek with her nipple.	In the root reflex, the infant will turn his/her head to make contact with the nipple and will then open his/her mouth widely.
6. Mother brings infant in close to her body.	Encourage proper latching on. The whole nipple and part of the areola should be in the infant's mouth.
7. Mother then removes her hand from around the breast, still supporting the infant's head to insure proper nipple contact.	
8. To remove the infant from the breast, the mother inserts one finger into the corner of the baby's mouth.	Breaking the suction helps prevent sore nipples.
9. Infant is then burped.	
10. Nursing Staff to check mother's breast each shift for nipple soreness, cracking or engorgement.	Early recognition and treatment of these problems allows for easier resolution and prevention of secondary difficulties.
11. When supplementing with a syringe place tip of syringe barely inside cheek.	To prevent infant from expecting nourishment from a firm object, rather than the mother's soft nipple.

GENERAL INSTRUCTIONS
1. Mothers are encouraged to wash their hands before beginning to nurse.
2. All mothers are encouraged to wear a bra at all times.
3. Mother may use one finger to depress her breast so that the infant's nostrils are unobstructed.
4. All staff in Delivery, Recovery, Post-Partum and Well Baby Nursery are to be well-educated in all aspects of lactation. Suggested current readings are to be found in the Newborn Nursery.

NDEX

Medela electric breast pump, 245
Medical interventions
  in jaundice in normal healthy infant, 207-208
  for mastitis, 152
Medical practice, 102-103
Medications, 138-145
  for cesarean mothers, 56
  for colic, 66
  and foods for mothers, 264
  during pregnancy and slow weight gain, 232
  and slow weight gain, 224, 231
Mellaril; see Thioridazine
Melphalan, 141
Memories after death of infant, 168-169
Meningitis, 174-175
Menses, effect of, on milk yield, 285-286
Menstruation changes in relactation/induced
    lactation, 278
Meperidine, 140
Meprobamate, 145
Mesoridazine, 145
Metabolic disease and liver disease, 203
Metabolic dysfunction, 190-194
Metabolic functioning and endocrine function-
    ing, alterations in, 130, 132-134
Metabolic problems, 204
Metabolism, inborn errors of, 190-192
Metandren; see Methyltestosterone
Methadone, 138, 140
Methdilazine, 140
Methionine, 310
Methocarbamol, 142
Methotrexate, 141
Methyldopa, 142
Methyltestosterone, 143
Metronidazole, 141
Mexican-American women, 310
  taboos among, 312
Mexico, infant carrier in, 302
Milk
  collected in breast cups, 117
  collection and storage of, 249-252
  composition of, effect of mastitis on, 149
  cow's; see Cow's milk
  expressed
    storage of, 251
    transportation of, 251
    warming, 251-252
  expression of, problems during, 252-255
  fat content of, 254-255

Milk—cont'd
  flow of, and breast and nipple shields, 121-122
  "green," 313
  human; see Human milk
  for lactating women, 307
  let-down reflex and slow weight gain, 225
  magic, 167-168
  of magnesia, 144
  manual expression of, 24-25
  mother's, sulfisoxazole in, 130
  nitrogen in, 239
  preterm and full-term, 239-240
  production of, and blood glucose level, 132
  pumping, after death of infant, 168
  stasis of, 24
  sucking, controlling amount of, 24
  supply of
    of hypothyroid mother, 133
    and stress, 163
  volume of, 260
    and composition and malnutrition, 315
    decreasing, and infant's condition, 253-254
    in relactation, 282-284
  yield of, effect of menses on, 285-286
    potential, in relactation/induced lactation,
      284-285
Milk banks, 168, 350-353
Miltown; see Meprobamate
Mineral oil, 144
Minocin; see Minocycline
Minocycline, 142
Minor tranquilizers, 145
Mismanagement of breastfeeding, 233
Model program of education, 91, 93
Modern applications of relactation, 276-277
Monilia, 127
  as cause of sore nipples, 124
  in diabetic mothers, 132
Monotropy, 58
Montgomery, tubercles of, 21
Morphine, 140
Mortality in America, 6
Mother(s); *see also* entries under Maternal
  anxious, 65
  cesarean, self-care for, 50-56
  diabetic, breastfeeding for, 132
  food-related problems of, 63
  foods and medications for, 264
  nutritional state of, and dental caries, 190

Stress(es)
  and breastfeeding, 163
  and father, 163
  and mastitis, 154
  maternal, and slow weight gain, 216
  and milk supply, 163
  parental, during hospitalization, 162-164
  and Selye, 162
  and sex, 163-164
  and slow weight gain, 225-226
Stretching, nipple, 118
'Stroking,'' 94, 95
Subclinical mastitis, 151, 152
Successful La Leche League meetings, 105-106
'Suck, reflex,'' 228
Sucking; *see also* Suckling
  ability and neurological deficits, 177
  action of, 218
    of breastfeeding compared to bottle-feeding, 26-27
  as control of amount of milk produced, 24
  of infant with congenital heart defect, 183
  of infants with Down's syndrome, 177
  time allowed, limited, 217-218
  and transition from bottle to breast, 262
Suckle, willingness of infant to, 281-282
Suckler, lazy, 233
Suckling; *see also* Sucking
  by adult in relactation/induced lactation, 289
  by borrowed infant in relactation/induced lactation, 288-289
  ineffective, and slow weight gain, 227
  negative "flutter," 219
  by own infant in relactation/induced lactation, 288
  patterns of, faulty, 47-48
  poor, and slow weight gain, 215
  and poor weight gain, 228-229
Suction device as intervention for nipple inversion, 118-119
Suction for infant with cleft lip and palate, 187
Suctioning for infant with respiratory infection, 173
Sudden infant death syndrome (SIDS), 197
Sulfa drugs, 139
  and kernicterus, 203
  for urinary infections, 130
Sulfamethoxazole, 142
Sulfamylon; *see* Mafenide

Sulfaquinadine, 6
Sulfisoxazole, 130, 142
Sulfonamides, 142
Sump tube, 185
Sunlight
  for sore nipples, 124
  for thrush, 127
Supplemental bottles, 218
  for premature infants, 262
Supplementation, food, 316
  in hypoglycemia, 194
  and slow weight gain, 227
Supply-demand response, 23
Support for hospital-based programs, 82, 83
Support groups, 65
Support system
  with high-risk infant, 243-244
  self-care, 261-262
Surgery
  for cleft lip and palate, 186
  for hydrocephalus, 181
  for infant with congenital heart defect, 183
  for myelomeningocele, 180
  for pyloric stenosis, 186
Survey, mastitis, 152-155
Survey methods in relactation/induced lactation, 281
Swaddling and unrestricted breastfeeding, 301
Swallowing and slow weight gain, 227-228
"Switch nursing," 228
Symptoms
  allergy, 194
  of mastitis and fever, 149
Symptothermal method, 136
Syndrome, magic milk, 167-168
Synthyroid; *see* Crystalline sodium levothyroxine
Syntocinon; *see* Oxytocin

T

T_3T_4, 133
Taboos, 311-312
Tacaryl; *see* Methdilazine
Tachycardia, 183
Tachypnea, 183
Tagamet; *see* Cimetidine
"Tandem nursing," 321
Taurine in breastmilk, 30
^{99m}Tc, 143
T-E fistula; *see* Tracheoesophageal fistula